MUSCLE
FOR
LIFE

Also by Michael Matthews

Bigger Leaner Stronger

Thinner Leaner Stronger

The Shredded Chef

The Little Black Book of Workout Motivation

Beyond Bigger Leaner Stronger

The Year One Challenge for Men

The Year One Challenge for Women

Fitness Science Explained

MICHAEL MATTHEWS

MUSCLE FOR LIFE

GET LEAN, STRONG, AND HEALTHY AT ANY AGE!

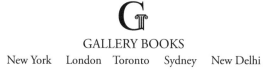

GALLERY BOOKS

New York   London   Toronto   Sydney   New Delhi

G

Gallery Books
An Imprint of Simon & Schuster, Inc.
1230 Avenue of the Americas
New York, NY 10020

First Gallery Books hardcover edition January 2022

GALLERY BOOKS and colophon are registered trademarks of Simon & Schuster, Inc.

For information about special discounts for bulk purchases,
please contact Simon & Schuster Special Sales at 1-866-506-1949
or business@simonandschuster.com.

The Simon & Schuster Speakers Bureau can bring authors to your live event.
For more information or to book an event, contact the Simon & Schuster Speakers Bureau
at 1-866-248-3049 or visit our website at www.simonspeakers.com.

Interior design by Davina Mock-Maniscalco

Manufactured in the United States of America

10 9 8 7 6 5 4 3 2 1

Library of Congress Cataloging-in-Publication Data
Names: Matthews, Michael, 1984– author.
Title: Muscle for life : get lean, strong, and healthy at any age / Michael Matthews.
   Description: New York, N.Y. : Gallery Books, [2022] | Includes bibliographical references and index. |
Identifiers: LCCN 2021018674 (print) | LCCN 2021018675 (ebook) | ISBN 9781982154691
   (hardcover) | ISBN 9781982154714 (ebook)
Subjects: LCSH: Weight training. | Physical fitness. | Nutrition.
Classification: LCC GV546 .M324 2022 (print) | LCC GV546 (ebook) | DDC 613.7/13—dc23
LC record available at https://lccn.loc.gov/2021018674
LC ebook record available at https://lccn.loc.gov/2021018675

ISBN 978-1-9821-5469-1
ISBN 978-1-9821-5471-4 (ebook)

Thank you to everyone who helped me create this book, including Karyn, who first made this project possible and then made it a joy; Rebecca, who made me sound smarter than I am; Mary and Armi, who did yeoman's work like always; and everyone else who helped get this work into your hands.

And thank you, dear reader, for your support, and thank you to all the guys and gals who have carried my banner over the years and inspired me to keep learning and teaching.

This is for you.

Contents

MUSCLE
FOR
LIFE

Foreword

Dr. Spencer Nadolsky

I've known Mike and followed his work for years, and he's one of the most authentic and effective educators in the evidence-based fitness space. His mission is to spread the gospel of healthy, successful, and sustainable eating, exercising, and supplementing, and thanks to books like this one, he's making major inroads in achieving his goal to help millions of everyday people get into the best shape of their lives.

Unlike many fitness books, *Muscle for Life* isn't an assortment of shameless pseudoscience and dubious anecdotes used to sell you on restrictive diets, unproductive exercise routines, or overhyped supplements. Instead, it's a panoramic, penetrating, and—most important—practical analysis of the art and science of gaining muscle and strength, and getting and staying lean, fit, and healthy for life. No matter your age or circumstances, the simple but powerful principles and practices taught in this book *will* transform your body—and *fast*. They work exactly as Mike describes in every person, every time. Full stop.

So, read this book, implement its teachings, and you'll never look back. With your health and fitness fully under your control, your body, and likely your life, will never be the same.

Good luck, and enjoy your journey. You're in great hands.

Dr. Spencer Nadolsky
Board-certified family, obesity, and lipidology physician

PART 1

WHAT'S IN THIS FOR YOU?

IT WORKS!
ORDINARY PEOPLE,
EXTRAORDINARY RESULTS.
WILL YOU BE NEXT?

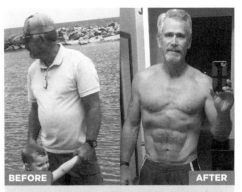

BEFORE
AFTER

"I am living proof that even at the age of sixty-two, you can have a strong, healthy body that you can be proud of."
LANNY W.

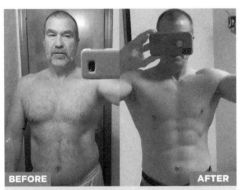

BEFORE
AFTER

"I am definitely more confident and have more energy, and having people compliment me on my body has been a morale booster."
DARREL S.

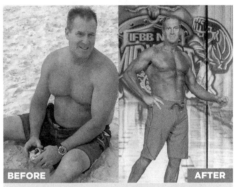

BEFORE
AFTER

"THIS PROGRAM WORKS! Just apply the principles that Mike has laid out for you— trust me, the sky is the limit."
BRANDON W.

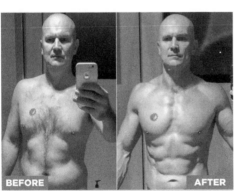

BEFORE
AFTER

"I have more energy; I wake up and practically jump out of bed (except for after leg day). I feel great, I don't get tired in the afternoons, I can't wait to knock off work and get into my workout. I'm in the best shape of my life."
DANIEL F.

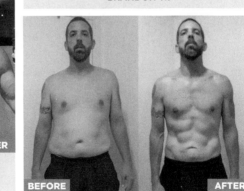

BEFORE
AFTER

"I now get asked all the time by friends and coworkers about what I am doing and how I am getting in shape, and I always point them toward Mike Matthews."
CHAD P.

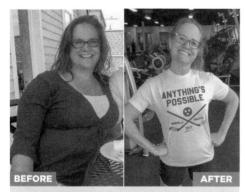

BEFORE AFTER

"I have more confidence, great clothes are easier to find, I have more energy, and my marriage is better. Food used to be my addiction; now it is finding new challenges and ways to surprise myself about what I am capable of."
STEFANIE C.

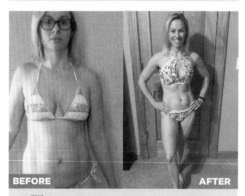

BEFORE AFTER

"This program is superior to any program out there. It wasn't just about dropping weight either—it was about taking time for myself as a mom and finding one way to put myself first. I'm most proud of my strength and that my kids ask me to flex on the daily—especially my girls."
AMBER L.

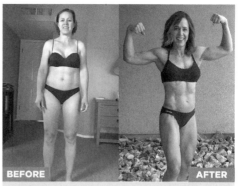

BEFORE AFTER

"I have more energy than ever. My confidence is the highest it's ever been. I have people ask me all the time what I do to stay in such good shape, and a lot of them are half my age. Shopping is more fun now, too!"
JEAN G.

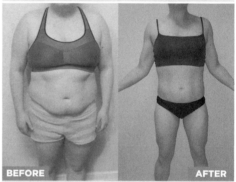

BEFORE AFTER

"I have higher confidence, energy, and I've proven that if I can do it, then anyone CAN do it, too! Seriously, this program is the easiest way to lose weight. If you stick to it, you will be able to do it, EVEN WITH YOUR FAVORITE FOODS!"
TINA H.

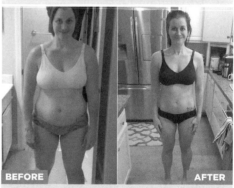

BEFORE AFTER

"I've noticed my energy levels have increased, my overall mood has changed for the better, I don't fight unhealthy cravings the way I used to— overall I just feel so much better."
JENNA H.

The men and women you just saw are like you. They're in their thirties, forties, and fifties, and they come from all walks of life and levels of fitness. Some of these people were once fit, others were always flabby; some folks had tried many diet and exercise routines before and failed, others were brand-new to it all; and some of them had plenty of time and energy for working out, others had very little.

What they all have in common, though, is that they've used my diet and exercise principles and programs to build bodies they're proud of. They've dropped pounds of unwanted fat, added pounds of lean muscle, and dramatically reduced their risk of disease and dysfunction, and they did it eating foods they love, doing workouts they dig, and taking few, if any, supplements.

I want to introduce you to a few of them whose stories have inspired and touched me, and who are definitive proof that with the right know-how and guidance, *anyone* can achieve stellar fitness. If they can do it, why not you?

AMBER'S STORY (42 YEARS OLD)

"I really never struggled with weight until after my third baby. In the two years after she was born, I ran a half marathon and did other weight-lifting programs to no avail. I was completely defeated and almost resigned to the belief that it was just my age or stage of life.

"When I couldn't drop the weight, I felt terrible about myself. I was constantly beating myself up because I had never struggled before the way I was struggling now.

"Then I started Mike's program for women, and I was shocked at how quickly the weight fell off. I dieted for eight weeks and lost fourteen pounds, and I haven't gained any weight for a year. I'm also proud of the amount of weight I can lift. I'm a little person by bone structure, but I feel SO STRONG!

"It wasn't just about dropping weight either—it was about taking time for myself as a mom and finding one way to put myself first. I love my strength and that my kids ask me to flex on the daily—especially my girls. Ninety-nine percent of the time after my workouts, I'm happy, energized, and ready to conquer my two jobs, kids, home life, and everything else on my plate.

"The thing I've repeated to myself over and over is 'trust the process.' I trust Mike Matthews and his no-nonsense, 'this is science' approach. Read the book, apply it, and you WILL see results."

BRANDON'S STORY (54 YEARS OLD)

"Before discovering Mike's work, my excuses and untrained mind (conditioned to give up easily) prevented me from attaining my goals. I used my shoulder surgery, my drinking problem, and my lack of wanting to change my lifestyle as excuses. Then I stumbled upon Mike's website and books, and my life changed.

"I'm a former Marine, Gulf War veteran, husband, and father to three beautiful children, and my best friend's name was 'beer.' Sick and tired of how I was living, I had to change my ways, my attitude, and my approach. I was worried I would end up like my father—dying at forty-six from abusing alcohol.

"I finally started using the knowledge Mike shares to overcome anything that was in my way—cravings, urges, and thoughts that had held me back in the past. I haven't looked back since September of 2016, and now I'm unstoppable. The support I have received from Mike saved my life!

"So, take it from me—MIKE'S PROGRAMS WORK! Just apply the principles that he has laid out for you (don't change, add, or subtract anything), and trust me, the sky's the limit.

"Remember, too, that this is NOT a quick fix, Hollywood diet, or fad weight loss program. This is the beginning of a lifestyle change you can maintain for the rest of your life to be happier and healthier.

"This program saved my life! A BIG and SINCERE thank you to Mike—I owe you big time!"

JENNA'S STORY (36 YEARS OLD)

"I was sick of spending hours in the gym doing CARDIO, CARDIO, CARDIO and not getting results. It worked okay for me when I was younger, but after getting older, it just wasn't working, and I felt stuck at a certain number on the scale.

"Since starting Mike's program for women, I've lost thirty-five pounds in six months! I've also noticed that my energy levels have increased, my mood is better, and I don't fight unhealthy cravings the way I used to. Overall, I just feel so much better.

"This program is also truly a lifestyle that's completely sustainable. I'm not quite at the maintenance stage yet, but I know it'll be even more flexible once I get to that point. I have so much more to learn and new goals to set, but I'm genuinely enjoying the process. I really appreciate the self-discipline this program has taught me.

"By following Mike's advice, you're building the body you want for the rest of your life, and it takes time, consistency, and patience. But it's worth it. Watching your body change is an amazing thing and very empowering."

DAN'S STORY (52 YEARS OLD)

"I turned fifty years old, and I weighed two hundred thirty-five pounds at six foot two. I had a daughter who was nineteen and two sons who were twelve and fourteen, and I realized I needed to make some serious changes if I wanted to be more actively involved in these important years in their lives.

"Then a close friend told me about Mike Matthews. I had become fairly cynical about the newest, 'best,' and most 'cutting-edge' fitness and training programs, but after seeing how Mike's program worked for him, I knew I had to give it a try. I purchased a customized meal plan the next day and began Mike's program.

"And then, just a year later, I weighed one hundred ninety pounds at nine to ten percent body fat and had gained a significant amount of strength and muscle. I was floored. And that was only the beginning.

"Now I'm in the best shape of my life since my stint as a college basketball player in the 1980s. Not only am I strong and lean (seven to eight percent body fat), the quality of my life has improved significantly too. My energy has increased, sleep quality has improved, and my joints (especially my knees and hips) ache a whole lot less! And, most important, my optimism about life as a whole is significantly better."

I'm so inspired by these outstanding men and women, and I hope you are too. What's even more amazing, though, is I hear from people with similar success stories every couple of days. Such extraordinary transformations aren't reserved only for the few. Anybody can join the club. Who knows, maybe people will be reading about *your* transformation story one day.

Anything is possible if you want it enough. And in this book, I'll show you the way.

1

Why *Muscle for Life* Is Different

If you don't risk anything, you risk even more.
—ERICA JONG

I n *Muscle for Life*, I want to prove to you that getting toned, lean, and strong isn't as complicated as you've been led to believe. It doesn't revolve around dubious "biohacks" for supercharging muscle growth, melting belly fat, or optimizing hormones. It doesn't require dietary strategies like intermittent fasting or keto, exercise techniques like muscle confusion or functional training, or esoteric pills or powders like collagen protein and exogenous ketones.

Instead, the real "secret sauce" of the fitness elite can be summed up like this:

1. They control their calorie and protein intake.
2. They mostly eat nutritious foods.
3. They work out a few hours per week, and mostly to gain muscle and strength.

In other words, the passport to the body you've always wanted is in the fundamentals, not the fringes. The devil's in the details, however, because as you'll learn in this book, there are a few correct and *many* incorrect ways of executing those strategies. It's like making music—just knowing that the process amounts to using notes to create pleasing harmonies, melodies, and rhythms isn't enough to create an earworm. You need to understand how to craft and combine those elements in very particular ways. Unfortunately, however, there's a lot more misinformation about how to get fit than about how to compose songs.

Why is that? Why are long-debunked falsehoods still trafficked by mainstream celebrities, social media "influencers," authors, and gurus?

I like to call the reason "Shiny Object Syndrome." The truth is, when millions of people are motivated to solve a problem and willing to spend large amounts of money to do it, there'll always be an abundance of things to buy and brilliant marketers to sell them. Accordingly, much of the mainstream advice featured in fitness magazines, websites, and books, which reaches millions of people every year, is informed by the need to keep you buying and subscribing.

What's the best marketing button to do this? "New." The easiest way to keep customers hooked is to give new recommendations continually—sparkly and fresh diet and training "tricks," research "breakthroughs," advanced "shortcuts," the list yammers on.

New information isn't bad per se. Health and fitness are vast subjects with myriad trails, tunnels, and caverns to explore. Most of that info won't sell subscriptions though. Your average guy or gal just wants to lose some fat and gain some muscle definition, not learn about the nuances of training periodization or nutrient partitioning, and it doesn't take a stack of books, magazines, and websites to teach someone how to build their glutes or flatten their stomach or get bigger arms or better abs.

If the fitness advice industry told the simple truth, they'd have maybe twenty-five essays to reprint, verbatim, over and over, and their teachings would be more or less identical to what you'll learn in this book. What's more, these pieces would contain "inconvenient truths," such as that you can't improve muscle tone by just working out, you can't target only belly fat for elimination, and supplements simply aren't that important.

This book, however, is different, because I have other incentives and pay-offs. I've had success as a self-published author and entrepreneur, so my work and livelihood are not beholden to publishers, advertisers, or trends. Instead, my lifeblood comes from you, based on how well I serve your interests. Thus, *Muscle for Life* can go against the grain and recommend science-based diet and exercise strategies that differ from the kind of miracle-solution promises you're used to hearing.

First and foremost, I'm going to teach you the power of building and maintaining muscle and strength—the master key to lasting and sustainable fitness and health. I'll also introduce you to a lifestyle and program that are actually doable. For example, I'll let you eat plenty of carbs while stripping fat from and adding lean muscle to your frame; I'll have you do a few hours of strength training per week and a lot less cardio (and no, ladies, this won't make you "bulky"—more on this later); and I'll recommend just a handful of simple (and optional) supplements that can enhance your physique, health, and performance.

That said, this book isn't for everyone. It's not for people who are afraid to hear hard truths and would rather swallow comfortable lies. It's not for people who are still looking for the mythical diet or exercise plan that requires no skill, struggle, or sacrifice. It's not for people who want a lot for a little. It's for people who understand that "secrets" never work unless you're willing to work for them. It's for people who are ready to screw their courage to the sticking place and step a bit outside of their comfort zone. It's for people who want to earn a healthy tomorrow by investing in it today.

Skeptical? You should be. I was when I first encountered the scientific research and practical strategies I'll share with you in this book. Take heart, though, because I'm not going to ask you to make a big leap of faith. Most of what you'll learn has been around for decades and stood the test of time, but as you're probably not an elite athlete with access to world-class trainers and dietitians, nobody has connected the dots for you the way we will here.

Moreover, *Muscle for Life* is all about getting results, and fast. That means you'll see real, tangible improvements in your body within the first thirty days of starting this program, and within three months your friends and family will want to know what the heck you're doing. Your weight will be moving in the right direction, your clothes will fit better, and you'll see muscle definition where there was little before. I promise.

And if, for whatever reason, you're not seeing these types of results, I still have good news for you: It's not because *Muscle for Life* is just another over-hyped hoax that can't deliver or won't work for you. It only means that you need some help with the implementation, and I'd be happy to give it. Simply e-mail me at mike@muscleforlife.com.

Remember, too, that tens of thousands of people (that I know of) have used the teachings in my books, articles, and podcasts to build strong and fit bodies. So, you're in good company. And soon you'll be on your way.

2

The Promise

*No matter how old you are, no matter how bad you might think
your hormones or genetics are, and no matter how lost you might feel
after trying and abandoning past diets and exercise routines . . .*

*You absolutely, positively can have the lean, defined, and healthy
body you dream about, and you're going to learn how.*

What if you could follow a science-based, doctor-approved formula for eating, exercising, and recovering that makes losing fat and adding lean muscle possible for anyone at any age—and what if you could see dramatic progress in the mirror in the first month?

What if there was a way to build your best body ever without starving or depriving yourself, putting in long hours at the gym, or doing grueling workouts that beat you up and burn you out?

What if you could also reduce your risk of just about every disease, eliminate aches and pains, and even erase the aftermath of years of physical neglect?

These may sound like outrageous claims, but this book is a realistic blueprint *anyone* can follow to realize those promises—a blueprint quite unlike what you normally find in a book like this. I won't give you dietary "hacks," quick fixes, or other unsustainable regimens that produce fast but fleeting changes, and I won't ask you to give up all the foods you like.

Instead, I'll provide you with nutritional guidelines and meal plans with enough structure to get results and enough flexibility to accommodate your eating preferences, schedule, and lifestyle. This way, you can look forward to every meal, every day, and, quite frankly, never feel like you're "on a diet" ever again.

I also won't try to force you into a one-size-fits-all training program that may or may not meet your needs or liking. Instead, I'll first show you why your primary fitness goal should be *getting strong*, and then I'll give you three workout programs to choose from—one for beginners, one for intermediates, and one for advanced trainees. This way, you can enjoy your training and never feel like you're working too hard or not hard enough.

I'll also be your guide the whole way, encouraging you to discover what you're truly capable of; helping you overcome obstacles and setbacks like emotional eating, spotty consistency, and nagging stiffness and soreness; and showing you how to avoid pitfalls like negative self-talk, stifling perfectionism, and impractical expectations, leading you to realistically achieve your goals.

"But what if it's too late?" many middle-aged people I've worked with have asked before starting their journey. You might be thinking the same. I understand. Most of these people had tried many diet and exercise programs already, and the outlook appeared grim. Everything they ate seemed to stick to their stomach, hips, and thighs. Their body didn't respond to exercise the way it once did. Their metabolism felt sluggish, their hormones screwy. And so they were reluctant to pick up a book like this. They didn't want to fail again, or worse, get hurt, and feel weak, confused, and vulnerable. They didn't want to waste their time chasing a mirage.

If you're nodding your head, you're not entirely mistaken. The body does change in undesirable ways as it gets older—ways that do conspire against your health and fitness. That doesn't mean it's too late to get fit, however; it's only too late to get fit *the way you used to*. When you were younger, you may have eaten what you wanted, lived how you wanted, and enjoyed the body you wanted. For most people, this formula consisted of eating out regularly, going for occasional runs or bike rides, and flaunting lean, defined muscles—a recipe that no longer works and never will again once you hit middle age.

Think of it this way: the springtime of your life was like the star in Super Mario that makes you temporarily invincible. Eventually, however, the aura quietly disappears, and all of a sudden, the game changes in ways you don't understand. Mysteriously, your body no longer responds to your usual tricks.

If you can learn what happened and what to do about it, though, you can reclaim youthful fitness and vitality. While I can't promise you can feel like you're twenty again, no matter how much you've snubbed your wellness in the past, you can cancel much of or even all the fitness "debt" you've accrued easier—and faster—than you think. For many people, it only takes months, not years. And if you're still in the flower of your youth but don't quite look or feel that way, this is your chance to bloom before life interferes.

This isn't just my opinion, either. More and more scientific research is showing that while "aging" isn't optional, genetics affect wellness and longevity far less than most people believe. Simply put: what appears to most influence how we age isn't time, but lifestyle. We get heavier and weaker not because of the sands of time, but because we stop exercising and overeat; our joints fall into disrepair because we weigh too much and move too little; and we develop disease and dysfunction because we allow our bodies to stagnate and sour.

So, while we can't change our chronological age, studies show that we can reverse our biological age and restore much of the vigor of our younger years.

In fact, more or less every negative aspect of aging can be mitigated by proper exercise (especially strength training), diet, sleep, and supplementation.

For example, it's often said that you lose about 1 percent of your muscle mass per year after age 30, and even more after age 50. And that's true . . . if you don't train your muscles, eat enough protein, or get enough sleep. What happens if you do, though? Research shows that you can not only prevent muscle loss in your forties and beyond, but can gain muscle and strength as effectively as when you were in your twenties.

In a study conducted by scientists at the University of Oklahoma, one group of men aged 18 to 22 and another, nearly twenty years older, 35 to 50, made nearly identical muscle and strength gains after eight weeks of following the same strength training routine. Similar results were seen in a study conducted by scientists at the University of Maryland, where women aged 65 to 73 gained just as much muscle after nine weeks of strength training as women nearly forty years their junior, aged 23 to 28.

There are many other such experiments in the scientific literature, and the message is clear: it's never too late to build a strong, toned, and functional body.

Additionally, strength training does much more than pump your muscles and harden your bones—it fundamentally changes the way nearly every organ, tissue, and cell in your body functions. There's a lot of talk these days about the relationship between aging and *telomeres*, the "end caps" that hold our chromosomes together. Every time a cell replicates, telomeres lose a bit of their length, and when they get too short, the cell dies. Since telomeres were discovered in the early eighties, scientists and anti-aging enthusiasts have been trying to increase their length and decrease shrinkage, and marketers have made a fortune promoting dubious methods of accomplishing the same.

We now know that one of the most powerful ways to increase telomere length is simple and free: exercise. In a study conducted at Brigham Young University, Dr. Larry Tucker analyzed the telomere length and activity levels of 5,823 adults of all ages. The results show why many researchers now call exercise a "wonder drug." Dr. Tucker found that the telomeres of people in the high physical activity group looked *nine years* younger than those of people in the sedentary and low physical activity groups, and, surprisingly, seven years younger than those of people in the moderate physical activity group.

That is, highly active 50-year-olds had the telomeres of sedentary or lightly active 41-year-olds and moderately active 43-year-olds. And the best part? "Highly active" in this study was equivalent to just thirty minutes of moderate exercise per day for women and forty minutes for men—about as much as the *Muscle for Life* program will entail.

Regular exercise—and strength training in particular—is also a remarkable defense against the "middle-age spread." Many people think their metabolism is programmed to crash as they get older, making it impossible to "eat the way they used to" without gaining weight.

While it's true that metabolic rate often declines as people get older, it's less than they realize, and it mostly occurs because of the loss of muscle mass. A study conducted by scientists at the University of Giessen measured the metabolic rates of a group of men and women aged 60 to 90, and then took the same measurements again eight years later. The average drop in the men's daily resting metabolic rate (the amount of energy burned at rest) was just 8 calories per year, and in the women, about 4 calories per year. In other words, after eight years, the men were burning about 70 calories less per day, on average, which is the food equivalent of a small apple; and the women were burning only 30 fewer calories per day, or about four almonds.

There's more to the story, too. The researchers also found that these people had lost about a quarter pound of muscle per year and replaced it with fat, which could account for all the metabolic slowdown. As scientists at Hiroshima University observed in another study on this topic, losing muscle mass as we age may be "wholly responsible for the age-related decreases in basal metabolic rate." This is great news for us because if you can maintain your muscle, you can maintain your metabolism, and *Muscle for Life* will show you how to do just that and much more.

You should know, though, that there are no shortcuts to optimal health. You can think of managing your fitness like managing your finances. Just as you can't count on winning the lottery, you can't stumble into an extraordinary body. Prudence, patience, and persistence are the watchwords of the hardy and healthy.

It all begins with a workable plan, and here's ours:

1. Do a lot of strength training.
2. Do some cardio.
3. Eat a high-protein, plant-centric diet.
4. Get enough sleep.

If you can follow those four steps, you can have a strong, beautiful, and dynamic body that's remarkably resistant to decay, disease, and dysfunction. For the rest of your life.

Chances are you're not surprised by these tactics because "everyone knows" that eating well and exercising are "good." What they don't know, though, is how to turn this advice into anything but a straitjacket. I, however, want to show you how to weave these threads in a new and versatile way that allows for endless variation in form and fit so you never feel smothered or squirrelly. This is *Muscle for Life*, after all, in the senses of both duration and purpose.

Let's explore my methodology one step at a time, starting at the top.

1. The King of Anti-Aging Fitness: Strength Training

You've probably heard that "exercise is medicine," but most people don't know that not all exercise is equal—especially when combating aging. And ironically, the champion of medicinal and anti-aging exercise—strength training—is something few middle-aged people do.

Strength training is exercise that involves moving your body against resistance (like machines, weights, or just your bodyweight), and it's as close to a magic bullet for optimizing health and fitness as you'll ever find. When you get strong, miraculous things happen to your body.

In a study conducted by scientists at Brigham and Women's Hospital, overweight, sedentary police officers with no history of strength training were divided into three groups: they all limited their calorie intake, and the first group did no exercise, while the second and third groups did four strength training workouts per week. After just twelve weeks, the first group lost 5.5 pounds on average, including 1 pound of muscle, whereas the second and third groups lost about 12 pounds of fat while gaining around 7 pounds of muscle.

In fitness lingo, this effect is known as *body recomposition*, and this study and others like it show that by regulating what you eat and doing strength training, as you will in the *Muscle for Life* program, you can essentially "trade" fat for lean muscle, thereby transforming how your body looks, feels, and performs.

More muscle and strength and less fat is good for more than a mere ego boost, too—it also means fewer physical limitations, accidents, and disabilities. In an extensive five-year study involving 3,069 men and 589 women aged 30 to 82, scientists at the University of South Carolina found that those who best maintained their strength as they aged were three times less likely to experience any kind of physical impairment or disability later in life than those who least maintained their strength. One of the reasons for this is that strength training is exceptional for beefing up your bones, and this greatly reduces the risk of fracture as you get older.

Strength training has still more gifts to bestow upon you: it also helps fight heart disease and diabetes. Heart health is an essential aspect of longevity (heart disease is the number one killer in the developed world), and strength training reduces cholesterol and blood pressure levels, which are vital components of cardiovascular health.

Diabetes is another disease that takes millions of lives every year, and strength training combats it by reducing blood sugar levels and improving insulin sensitivity. What's more, studies show that strength training is as effective, if not more so, than cardiovascular exercise for reducing blood sugar levels and diabetes symptoms.

Finally, strength training can help maintain healthy brain function into old age. In a study conducted at the University of British Columbia with 155 women aged 65 to 75, researchers found that women who did just one or two strength training workouts per week for a year improved cognitive function by about 12 percent. However, women who followed only a stretching-and-balancing routine experienced a 0.5 percent decrease in cognitive function.

Some women also received MRI brain scans to measure their volume of white matter, which is brain tissue that helps pass messages between different parts of the nervous system, and which declines with age. Several years later, researchers analyzed these scans and found that the women who did two strength training workouts per week kept more of their white matter than those who didn't.

So, the bottom line is that strength training is the single best way to improve nearly every aspect of your health, fitness, and well-being. With just a few hours per week, you can . . .

- Lose fat and gain muscle
- Improve strength and endurance
- Reduce the risk of physical limitations, accidents, and injuries, as well as many chronic diseases like diabetes, heart disease, and osteoporosis
- Lower LDL ("bad") cholesterol levels, and raise HDL ("good") cholesterol levels
- Enhance brain function, and protect against cognitive decline
- Enhance sleep quality
- And more

All that is why the *Muscle for Life* program revolves around strength training. If we can make you strong, we can unlock lifelong fitness and vitality.

2. The Queen of Anti-Aging Fitness: Cardio

When most people think of "exercise," they think of cardiovascular exercise or "cardio," which involves maintaining an elevated heart rate for extended periods of time. A more accurate term would be "endurance training" or "aerobic exercise," but I'll call it cardio for the sake of familiarity. Running, swimming, cycling, rowing, hiking, tennis and other team sports, and even brisk walking all qualify.

For decades, most doctors recommended cardio over strength training because they believed it produced more health benefits, stressed the body less, and was more popular among the public. We now know that strength training has multiple major advantages over cardio, and if you had to pick just one kind of exercise, it should be strength training. That said, there are good reasons to include cardio in your exercise routine as well.

First, as the term implies, cardio boosts the health and function of your cardiovascular system. For instance, while cardio and strength training are about equally effective for reducing blood pressure, research shows that doing both reduces blood pressure the most.

Additionally, cardio—but not strength training—helps keep your arteries flexible and responsive to changes in blood flow. Hence, studies show that people who do the most cardio have the supplest arteries, which is crucial for maintaining healthy blood pressure levels and minimizing stress on your heart and blood vessels.

Another circulatory downside to aging is the reduction of the capillary health and density of your muscles and other tissues, and research shows that cardio can significantly increase capillary density (the number of capillaries in an area of the body) in muscle in just a few weeks.

Cardio also burns substantially more calories per unit of time than strength training does, which can help you lose fat faster and keep it off more easily. And by combining strength training and cardio in the way I'll teach you in this book, you can maximize fat loss without hindering muscle or strength gain.

So, here's the takeaway: with moderate, sustainable, and effective doses of strength training and cardiovascular exercise, you can build a body that looks, feels, and functions like a well-oiled machine.

3. The Almost Nearly Perfect Diet: High-Protein and Plant-Centric

This is the essence of healthy eating—not fad dieting or giving up sugar, carbs, or meat, or subsisting on a short list of special "superfoods."

Protein is vital because it helps you build and preserve muscle as you get older, which is the high road to remaining almost "ageless." A study conducted by scientists at Wake Forest University examined the relationship between protein intake and lean body mass in 2,066 men and women aged 70 to 79. Over a three-year period, those who ate the most protein lost 40 percent less muscle than those who ate the least. Little wonder, then, that other research shows that older men and women who eat a high-protein diet have the lowest risk of physical disability and are notably less likely to become physically impaired.

The fact is that high-protein dieting beats low-protein dieting in every meaningful way, and in chapter 6, you'll learn more about why (and why common criticisms of eating protein, including animal protein, are unfounded).

After adequate protein, the other prime directive of wholesome eating is including plenty of plant-derived foods in your diet. In fact, out of all the variables scientists have investigated regarding the relationship between diet and health and longevity, eating plants is the standout. An extraordinary amount of evidence shows that people who eat more fruits, vegetables, whole grains, nuts, seeds, beans, and other plants are healthier, live longer, and enjoy a lower risk of high blood pressure, heart disease, stroke, cancer, osteoporosis, cognitive decline, and dementia.

Further, research shows that the consequences of eating too little fruit, vegetables, and other plant-based foods can be disastrous. A team of scientists from around the world conducted a study that looked at how fifteen different dietary factors predicted the risk of death in 195 countries. They found that poor diet (characterized primarily by a low intake of whole grains, fruits, nuts and seeds, vegetables, and seafood) accounted for around one in five deaths, killing some 11 million people in 2017 alone. Additionally, according to studies conducted by scientists at the University of Washington, the US Centers for Disease Control and Prevention (CDC), and the National Cancer Institute, only about a third of adults over the age of 65 meet the bare minimum requirements for fruit and vegetable intake.

Why are plants so good for us? First, they provide an abundance of essential vitamins, minerals, and other nutrients that are hard to get in sufficient amounts from animal foods, such as vitamin C, magnesium, and fiber. Plants also contain a wide variety of beneficial substances called *phytonutrients*, which aren't necessary for life but are still healthful.

A diet rich in fruits, vegetables, whole grains, and other plants is also fantastic for controlling calorie intake and avoiding chronic hunger or cravings. Studies have shown repeatedly that people who eat the most plants have the easiest time losing weight and keeping it off, and the principal reason for this is simple: most plant foods have a very low *energy density*, meaning they contain very few calories relative to their weight and volume. A cup of watermelon has about 50 calories, for instance, whereas a cup of shredded cheese has about 400 calories. This is important because how full we feel after a meal is affected more by volume (how much space the food fills in our stomach) than calories. Thus, by eating plenty of plant foods, we can eat more food and feel fuller on fewer calories, which can work wonders for achieving and maintaining our desired physique.

It's not accurate to tout fruits and vegetables as "weight loss foods," however, because they don't have any special inherent fat-burning properties. They're conducive to weight loss (and maintenance), though, by helping to keep you full and prevent overeating.

So, to thrive as you get older, you *must* eat a high-protein diet rich in plant-based foods, including a variety of fresh fruits, vegetables, whole grains, nuts, seeds, and legumes. Which foods should you eat, however, and which should you avoid, and why? You'll be relieved to learn that there aren't many you "should" eat beyond what you *like* to eat, and there are even fewer you "shouldn't" eat—but we'll get into that later, in chapter 7.

4. The Unsung Hero of Health: Sleep

Sleeping enough is the ultimate "health hack." It improves fat loss, muscle growth, immunity, telomere length, and cognition, and even makes you more attractive physically. In contrast, chronically undersleeping (usually defined as getting less than six hours of sleep per night) suppresses your immune system and increases your risk of just about every disease that's been studied, including obesity, diabetes, dementia, heart disease, cancer, and even the common cold.

One reason many people don't sleep enough is they've heard that sleep needs decline with age. This is true, but it doesn't mean we can get by on minimal shut-eye. Most of us start out needing about 12 to 14 hours of sleep per night as babies, 10 to 12 hours as toddlers, and 9 to 10 hours as teenagers. Then, once we reach adulthood, most of us need 7 to 9 hours of sleep per night depending on our genetics, lifestyle, and exercise habits. So yes, we need less sleep, but not *that* much less. While there is a tiny fraction of the population that can get by with 6, 5, or even 4 hours of sleep per night, statistically, you're probably not part of that group.

So, if you're sleeping fewer than 7 hours per night, you likely aren't sleeping enough, and sleeping at least 7 to 8 hours per night will immediately enhance nearly every aspect of your well-being.

5. The Cherry (Powder) on Top: Supplements

Many supplement companies claim that with enough of their natural nostrums, we can buy our way to a better body, a sharper mind, and a longer life. Many "experts," on the other hand, allege that more or less all supplements are a waste of money.

The truth is somewhere in the middle. Most supplements don't work as promised, and some are even dangerous, but there *are* natural ingredients that can safely boost your health and fitness. The trick is knowing which are worth buying and which aren't.

For example, although protein powder doesn't have any magical properties you can't get from food, it's a tasty and convenient way to meet your daily protein needs. And *creatine*, one of the most studied compounds in all of sports nutrition, has been proven to enhance muscle and strength gain, and may also improve cognition in older people and those who get very little creatine from their diet (like vegetarians and vegans). Fish oil is another superstar because it provides the body with vital molecules known as *omega-3 fatty acids*. Research shows that most people don't get enough of these nutrients, resulting in impaired cognition, cardiovascular and immune function, fat loss, and muscle gain.

There are several other safe, effective supplements you can take to boost your health, performance, and longevity, and we'll discuss them all in chapter 15.

Imagine, in as little as just twelve weeks from now, waking up every morning and feeling powerful. Imagine losing up to 15 pounds of fat, wearing the clothes you want to wear, loving how you look, and having dawn-to-dusk energy to do all the things you want to do. Imagine how confident you'll feel when you no longer fret about your weight or how your pants fit. Imagine how well you'll sleep every night, knowing you're getting a little fitter, stronger, and healthier every day.

All that and more is what awaits you on the *Muscle for Life* program, and it's neither as difficult nor as complicated as you may think. It doesn't matter whether you're 41 or 61, or whether you're in shape or not. It also doesn't matter how busy or tired you are, or how many injuries or accidents you've sustained over the years. No matter who you are, you have the power to transform your body. Ask the many people whose lives have been changed by my work. They accepted my help, and now they look and feel better than ever before. They're the proof that this book can do the same for you.

If we're to succeed, however, I'll need a few things from you.

First, I need you to approach *Muscle for Life* with an open mind. I know others like me have made promises similar to the ones I'm making and then failed to deliver, often grossly. You've likely experienced the intoxicating rush of hope that transforms into a crushing wave of disappointment, and maybe more than once. This time will be different. By dealing with diet, exercise, and supplementation in a whole new way, you *can* break the cycle of tumbling off and clambering back onto the wagon, a little worse for wear each time. This program will teach you how to escape that terrible tailspin. It's a realistic and viable plan that men and women of all ages and circumstances can win with, but you must trust the process.

Second, I need you to show up. It's easy to buy a book with an eye to execution, but your intentions must translate into actions. And so in this book, I'll ask you to push past hopes and take concrete steps toward your new reality. Do your best, then follow the *Muscle for Life* program as I'll lay it out for you, and know that I don't need you to be *perfect* (impossible anyway)—just good enough most of the time. With that, you can reach the promised land.

Third, I'd love for you to reach out to me once you've achieved your first major milestone on this program, like dropping a size or two, leaving work full of energy, or thrilling at your newfound strength. Admittedly, this is a selfish request, but hearing from people who have used my work to get fitter, healthier, and happier is the real pay for my efforts, so I'd love to listen to your story. And, as I like to lead by example and show we're in this together, I'll quickly tell you mine.

KEY TAKEAWAYS

✦ No matter how much you've neglected your wellness in the past, it's never too late to build a strong, toned, and healthy body.

✦ Most of the negative aspects of aging can be mitigated by proper exercise (especially strength training), diet, sleep, and supplementation.

✦ Strength training enhances and preserves muscle mass, mobility, and brain function, and helps fight heart disease and diabetes.

✦ Cardio improves the health of your arteries, boosts capillary density, improves the health of your muscles and other tissues, and burns more calories than strength training.

✦ High-protein dieting beats low-protein dieting in every meaningful way.

✦ People who eat more fruits, vegetables, whole grains, nuts, seeds, beans, and other plants are healthier, live longer, and enjoy a lower risk of high blood pressure, heart disease, stroke, cancer, osteoporosis, cognitive decline, and dementia.

✦ Getting enough sleep improves fat loss, muscle growth, immunity, telomere length, and cognition, and even makes you more attractive physically.

3

Who's Mike Matthews, and Why Should I Care?

Most people overestimate what they can achieve in a year
and underestimate what they can achieve in ten years.
—UNKNOWN

'**ve made some pretty bold promises about what this book will do for you, and the reason I'm so sure of the effectiveness of my methods is they're not only science-based, but they also grew out of my own trials and tribulations with fitness. I've sifted through much of the relevant scientific literature and I've tried just about every type of workout program, diet plan, and supplement you can imagine. I can confidently say that while I don't know everything, I do know what works and what doesn't.

Like most people, I had no clue what I was doing when I started out in the gym nearly twenty years ago. I turned to fitness magazines for help, which told me to work out like a professional bodybuilder a couple of hours per day and spend hundreds of dollars on supplements per month. I did just that for almost eight years, jumping from diet to diet, workout program to workout program, and supplement to supplement. For all my efforts, I had gained about 25 pounds of muscle and novice-level strength, but I had no idea how to lose fat and keep it off, and I was spending at least ten hours in the gym per week but not gaining muscle or strength, and I didn't know why.

I then hired personal trainers for guidance, but they had me do more of the same: "fancy" training techniques like supersets, circuit training, and "metabolic conditioning" that were mostly ineffective; one style of "clean eating" after another that failed to move the needle; and herbs, vitamins, and amino acids that did little more than lighten my wallet and brighten my pee. After spending many months and thousands of dollars with trainers, not much had changed in the mirror or the gym, and I still had no idea what to do to get the bigger, leaner, and stronger body I really wanted. I enjoyed working out too much to quit, but I wasn't happy with my physique and didn't know where I was going wrong.

What I did know quite well, however, was how to fail in fitness, and ironically, that proved valuable when I finally decided that something had to change because I knew where *not* to look for answers. I ditched the trainers, threw the magazines away, and got off the Internet forums, and set out to learn the true physiology of muscle growth and fat loss.

I studied the work of top strength and bodybuilding coaches, talked to veteran natural bodybuilders, and examined the scientific evidence. Months later, a clear picture was emerging: getting into incredible shape is much simpler than many fitness experts claim. It flies in the teeth of a lot of the stuff we see on TV, Instagram, and YouTube, and read in books, blogs, and magazines. The many myths and misconceptions in those parts not only make getting superfit much harder than it should be, they also undermine our self-confidence and self-esteem, strain our social lives and relationships, and discourage future attempts at self-improvement.

When I finally broke free of all of the misinformation and completely changed my approach to eating and exercising, my body responded in ways I couldn't believe. My strength skyrocketed. My muscles started growing again. My energy levels soared. And here's the kicker: I was spending *less* time working out, doing *less* cardio, and eating *more* freely.

Along the way, my friends and family noticed how my physique was improving and began asking for advice. I became their coach, and helped them shed fat they had figured was cemented to them for good, gain strength and muscle definition they hadn't seen in years or even decades, and unlock feelings of satisfaction and self-confidence they had forgotten were possible.

A year or two later, these people started urging me to write a book. I dismissed the idea at first, but then began to warm up to it. "What if I'd had a good book for bodybuilding early on?" I thought. It would've saved me who knows how much time, money, and frustration, and I would've reached my fitness goals much faster. So I wrote a book called *Bigger Leaner Stronger*, and self-published it in January 2012.

It sold maybe twenty copies in the first month, but within a couple of months, that number was growing, and every day positive e-mails and reviews were coming in from readers. I started making notes on how I could improve the book based on feedback, and I outlined ideas for other books to write, including a fitness book for women called *Thinner Leaner Stronger* and a cookbook called *The Shredded Chef*.

A few years later, I had written and published multiple books for fitness buffs—books that have now sold more than 1.5 million copies—and I was spending a couple of hours per day replying to questions, compliments, and critiques from readers and followers. I then realized I needed to write yet another book: this one. A book that offers the same science-based approach and benefits with an easier learning curve and less intimidating regimen. I also wanted to address the unique physiological, psychological, and logistical considerations of men and women in their thirties and forties and beyond, and especially those new to my evidence-based approach to fitness.

Whereas my other books cater to a more "hard-core" crowd of guys and gals who are physically, mentally, and emotionally ready to eat and train like "lifestyle bodybuilders," this book's calibrated for everyday people who want a highly accessible fitness program that produces real and long-lasting results.

Accordingly, you can use *Muscle for Life* as a smooth on-ramp to the diet and training methods of fitness champions if you want to go there—or, if you're looking to get and stay fit, healthy, and happy without having to dedicate too much time and energy to it, this may be the last fitness book you ever need to read. After you use everything in *Muscle for Life* to get into the best shape of your life, then *you* get to decide what comes next. Either way, we can't lose.

So, are you ready to begin your adventure?

4

How to Use This Book

We who cut mere stones must always be envisioning cathedrals.
—QUARRY WORKER'S CREED

There's an old Chinese proverb that goes like this: "Tell me, I'll forget; show me, I'll remember; involve me, I'll understand."

That saying summarizes the spirit of this book. It's meant for more than just reading and reflection—its essence is action—and that has informed every decision I've made about what to include in this text and how to organize and present it. Thus, I want to share with you a road map that'll help you get the most from *Muscle for Life*.

This book contains five parts:

1. In this first part, I've given you a broad overview of the *Muscle for Life* program and lifestyle, and we're about to address the "inner game" of fitness to help you clarify your goals, boost your confidence, and strengthen your resolve. I hope that, by the end of this section, I'll have inspired you to make a simple decision: "I'll give this an honest try."

2. In the second part, you'll learn everything you need to know to forever free yourself from the stresses of restrictive eating and "dieting,"

including a simple and intuitive method of meal planning that allows for maximum flexibility and sustainability.

3. In the third part, we'll address the exercise portion of *Muscle for Life*, and I'll provide you with a simple and science-based training system to gain strength and lean muscle and lose fat like clockwork.

4. In the fourth part, I'll touch on the controversial and least important aspect of this program—supplementation—and share with you the small number of supplements that are worth considering.

5. In the fifth part, I'll equip you with more insights and tactics that'll speed up your results as well as predesigned meal plan and workout templates.

There are also two ways you can approach this book:

1. Read it in its entirety and then start the program.
2. Read and implement as you go.

I prefer the second method because after working with tens of thousands of people over the years, I've found that the sooner someone can get moving, the more likely they are to keep going. When we're in motion, the roots of doubt and despair can't ensnare us. By doing things, we can't be stopped by thinking things. Therefore I've inserted calls to action throughout *Muscle for Life* that'll ask you to stop reading and start acting. These spots aren't arbitrarily chosen—they're the points where I know immediate implementation will increase your chances of long-term success. If I were coaching you, this is exactly how I'd introduce you to the program.

As you'll see, some of these steps require writing, and although space is provided for you to write directly in this book, you may want to use a notebook instead, which can become a journal where you design your meal plans, record your workouts, and track your results. By keeping everything in one place, you can easily review your progress and revise your plans as you work toward your goals. Your notebooks will also memorialize your transformation, and if you're like many of my readers and followers, you'll come to treasure your growing collection of fitness journals as a monument to your dedication to this journey.

If you want to get going even faster, you can simply skip to the *hows* and start the program, and then learn the *whys* after. To do this, begin with chapter 8, which will teach you how to create effective meal plans to lose fat and gain muscle. Once you've made your meal plan and started following it, flip to chapters 11 and 12 to find the *Muscle for Life* exercises and workouts, which you can start right away, followed by a chapter on how to track your progress and then a quickstart guide that you may also find helpful. Finally, read chapter 15 to learn about supplementation, which is optional but worthwhile if you have the budget and inclination. Then, once you're underway, return to the beginning of this book and learn everything you'll need to know to get the most from the program.

So, use this book in the way that makes it work for *you,* whether that's taking your time reading and absorbing everything in these pages before starting, or jumping around to the actionable items and plugging them into your routine immediately.

Finally, this book contains a lot of information, including many technical details and some arithmetic, but don't let that intimidate you. This isn't a textbook full of jargon and complexity for fitness geeks—it's a practical and approachable handbook for making novices into veterans. That's why, for example, I've included "Key Takeaways" sections at the ends of most of the chapters that remind you of the most important points discussed—the information that's essential for succeeding on the program. Reference these summaries regularly while you're finding your bearings, and you'll reinforce your understanding of the material and ability to use it effectively.

Regardless of how you get off the starting line, if you commit, results will follow. Whatever doubts you may have will disappear, and you'll realize that you're more than up to the challenge of upgrading your physique. And remember, if you lose your way or find yourself in a spin, I'm just an e-mail away (mike@muscleforlife.com) and happy to help.

5

How to Master the "Inner Game" of Fitness

Any idiot can face a crisis. It's the day-to-day living that wears you out.
—ANTON CHEKHOV

In his timeless bestseller *The Inner Game of Tennis*, Tim Gallwey explained that every game is composed of two parts: an outer game and an inner game. The outer game is played against an external opponent to overcome external challenges and reach external goals, and the inner game takes place in the mind and is played against obstacles like lapses in concentration, nervousness, self-doubt, self-condemnation, and other feelings that inhibit excellence in performance.

How fitting that model is to fitness. Books, magazines, trainers, and influencers usually focus on the outer game of losing fat and gaining muscle and give little attention to the inner game, which is arguably more important. Simply knowing what to do isn't enough. You then have to actually do it—and keep doing it—every day, week, month, and year.

Priority, discipline, and motivation are the biggest inner-game barriers. Every week, people launch into new fitness programs with resolve and relish, but it often doesn't take long for their enthusiasm to sputter. They struggle to fit their diet plan into their lifestyle and squeeze their workouts into their hectic schedule; they experience more physical challenges than they anticipated; and as the days and weeks pass, they see no appreciable change in their body. In short, it's a lot of pain for very little gain, so it's no surprise that many people give up on their fitness aspirations within the first couple of months.

I've seen this time and time again. Sometimes illness disturbs someone's routine, and they never return. Other times they take a week off and forget to come back. Some simply "stop caring." Maybe you've been there yourself. I know I have. Fitness is hard, and no matter how determined you may be, if you're not seeing clear and consistent results, it's only natural for your drive to dry up.

I don't want this to happen to you. I want to do everything I can to give you your best shot at success on the *Muscle for Life* program. In fact, if I'm being honest, I want this to be the fitness program that finally makes all the difference and overdelivers. That's why this chapter will help you develop a successful mindset that'll empower you to overcome the obstacles, resist the temptations, and surmount the setbacks that we all experience in our fitness journey.

To do that, we need to tackle the three ugliest inner-game ogres standing between you and the finish line:

1. The Purpose Phantom
2. The Time Troll
3. The Consistency Creature

Let's learn how to defeat each.

PREVAILING OVER THE PURPOSE PHANTOM

People with vague, unrealistic, or uninspiring fitness goals (or none at all) are always the first to quit. These men and women show up in the gym sporadically and often leave before even breaking a sweat. They fall victim to situations and circumstances that cause them to falter (pesky office potlucks!). They're on the lookout for fast fixes and miracle methods. If you're going to succeed where the masses fail, you need to inoculate yourself against these attitudes and behaviors, and this requires a little soul-searching.

Different people have different reasons for eating well and working out. Some like how it feels to push their body to the limit. Others want to impress a potential sex partner. Many want to boost their confidence and self-esteem. Most want to improve their general health and well-being.

These are all perfectly valid reasons to get fit—looking great, feeling great, having high energy levels, being more resistant to sickness and disease, and living longer—but it's important to isolate and articulate *your* reasons. Let's do this now, starting with the dimension of fitness that most people find most alluring: the visual.

What Does Your Ideal Body Look Like?

A major reason you're reading this book is you want to look a certain way. And there's nothing wrong with that. Every fit person I know—including myself—is motivated just as much by the mirror as by anything else. Don't misread that as narcissism. There are plenty of self-absorbed fitness twits out there, but I see nothing wrong with playing a bit to our vanity if looking fantastic also helps us feel great (and it does), especially if we consider how this buoyancy enhances our ability to work, love, and play. The better we look, the better we feel, and the better we feel, the better we live. It's really that simple.

So, let's talk about you. What does your ideal body look like? Let's go beyond trite words and hazy daydreams: find a picture or two (or three or four) of the type of body you want. Then save these pictures somewhere that's easily accessible, such as your phone or Google Drive or Dropbox. You could even print a couple out and paste them in your fitness journal. Why? When you're on the *Muscle for Life* program, I want you to know you're working toward a physique that's as real as the page you're reading, not merely a figment of your imagination.

Not sure what to pick because you're not sure what's possible? Start here: How would you have to look to hit the beach in a swimsuit without self-consciousness? Find a couple pictures of that, because, trust me—that we can do.

What Does Your Ideal Body Feel Like?

A fit, healthy body is far more pleasurable to inhabit than an unfit, unhealthy one. The more in shape you are, the more you get to enjoy many advantages: higher energy levels, better moods, more alertness, clearer thinking, fewer aches and pains, and better sleep, to name just a few. And then there's the deeper stuff like more dignity, pride, and self-fulfillment.

I want you to imagine what this will be like for you, and then write it out in the form of individual affirmations, which are positive statements that describe how you want to be, like "I'm full of energy all day" and "My mind is quick, clear, and focused."

This may seem a bit woo-woo, but research shows that writing and reading affirmations can benefit you in various ways. A study conducted by scientists at the University of Pennsylvania found that people who practiced affirmations exercised more than people who didn't, and another study at the

University of Sussex found that performing self-affirmations improved working memory and cognitive performance.

I like to organize health and fitness affirmations into four broad categories:

+ Physical
+ Mental
+ Emotional
+ Spiritual

Physical affirmations are all about bodily function and physical energy levels, and they can include statements like "I wake up rested every day," "My joints are pain-free," and "I don't get sick." Mental affirmations concern your ability to focus, remember, and compute. These might be assertions like "I can focus deeply on the task at hand," "My memory is sharp," and "My mind is clear." Emotional affirmations relate to your feelings of positive or negative sensations—such declarations as "I find joy everywhere I go," "I bounce back quickly from bad news," and "I give and receive love openly." Spiritual affirmations involve your sense of purpose and motivation, and they can include pronouncements like "I embody my best self" and "I know I'll succeed."

Here are a few pointers for writing more effective affirmations of any kind:

+ Keep them short so they're easier to process and remember. Even four or five carefully chosen words can be powerful.
+ Start with "I" or "My." Affirmations are all about you, so it's best to start with you.

- Write as though you're experiencing it right now, not in the future. For example, "I fall asleep quickly and wake up feeling rejuvenated" is superior to "I will fall asleep quickly and wake up feeling rejuvenated" or "Within three months, I'm falling asleep quickly and waking up feeling rejuvenated."

- Don't begin with "I want" or "I need." You don't want to affirm needing or wanting, but *being, doing,* or *having.*

- Make sure you're choosing positive statements. Realizing your affirmations may require discarding negative behaviors and thoughts, but your words shouldn't reflect this. Think, "I'm calm, confident, and contented" and not "I'm no longer anxious and insecure"; or "I enjoy my daily workouts" instead of "I don't dread exercising anymore."

- Inject emotion by including, "I'm [emotion] about . . ." or "I feel [emotion]." For example, you could say: "I'm excited to follow my meal plan." This will make your affirmations more stimulating (and thus memorable and persuasive) and can even influence how you experience events related to whatever you're affirming (actually feeling excited to follow your meal plan, for instance).

- Make your affirmations believable. If you don't think your statement is possible, it won't have much of an effect, so make sure you can fully buy into it. If you find something particularly incredible, you can start with a qualifier like "I'm open to . . ." or "I'm willing to believe I can . . ."

So, are you ready to write your affirmations? Great! Let's start with one affirmation per category (physical, mental, emotional, and spiritual), and take as long as you need to formulate statements that resonate deeply with you. You know you've hit on something meaningful when it sparks joy and positivity.

....

....

....

....

....

....

....

....

....

Now that you've formulated your first affirmations, you may be wondering what to do with them. There are many ways to use your statements, but my favorite is reading mine every morning before starting my day and whenever I feel my spirit flagging. This keeps my intentions alive and top of mind and helps adjust my mindset when I falter. Also, feel free to create new affirmations whenever inspiration strikes!

What Are Your Fitness Whys?

Whereas the affirmations above define *what* you want to achieve, the next exercise is designed to establish *why* you want to do it.

Among my favorite things about being fit are the moments where you impress yourself; where you just stop for a second and think, "Wow, it's awesome I did that with my body." These are moments that put a smile on your face and a spring in your step, and sometimes even make your day. I'm not just talking about stuff like "turning heads in the coffee shop," but "eating desserts guilt-free," "keeping up with my kids without getting tired," and "enjoying clothing shopping more." You know, the often small but substantial things that confirm you're on the right track.

I've worked with thousands of people over the years, and here are a few examples of the fitness wins they've shared with me:

- Getting asked for advice in the gym
- Feeling more confident and competent
- Looking sexier naked
- Being more productive at work
- Savoring delicious food
- Pleasantly surprising their doctor
- Rocking their favorite clothes
- Setting a good example for their kids
- Enjoying outdoor activities again
- Feeling physically and mentally strong
- Eliminating aches and pains
- Tackling a new sport

I love these. They're great examples of personal reasons to get into killer shape—simple, specific, and sincere. How about you? Why do you want to achieve everything you just laid out in your affirmations? Brainstorm your reasons for getting fit and write them below until you feel pumped up and ready to take action, because with the *Muscle for Life* program, we'll make them all a reality.

....

....

....

....

TRUMPING THE TIME TROLL

I don't know anybody who can *find* time to exercise. I've never had anyone tell me, "Mike, I have too much free time. I think I'll spend a few hours in the gym every day to get in shape. What should I do while I'm there?" It's always the opposite. Most of us lead busy lives brimming with urgency and obligations and feel we don't have time for anything new, let alone something as "selfish" as working out. But almost always, that just isn't true. As much as some people would like to think they're too swamped to work out, when they analyze how they spend their every waking minute every day, they discover otherwise (especially when they realize how little time it really takes to get fit).

The reality is that people who have transformed their bodies have the same twenty-four hours in a day as you and me, as well as their share of daily duties to discharge. They still have to go to work, attend to loved ones, attempt a social life, and remember to exfoliate, moisturize, and have some fun now and then. The only difference is that they've decided exercise is important enough to be in the plan.

For some, that requires watching less TV or giving it up altogether. For others, it means going to bed and waking up earlier. For others still, it involves asking the spouse to handle the kids in the morning or evening, or some other solution. My point is: if you really want to carve out a couple of hours per week to train, I'm positive you can.

That's not to say that finding the will and time for fitness is easy. It's often a challenge, and the solution may not be convenient or comfortable (at first, at least), but who said it should be? No matter how difficult or daunting our circumstances may be, there's always something we can do about it. If we can accept that our well-being is worthwhile, it suddenly becomes possible. Whether we act is up to us. And let's face it—whenever someone says, "I would do X, but I can't because Y," it's almost always hogwash unless Y is "I don't really want to." There's very little we're incapable of; there's only how badly we want it. When we lie to ourselves and say otherwise, what we're saying is that we find alibis more attractive than achievements, excuses more seductive than excellence, and comfort more desirable than challenge.

Writer Steven Pressfield coined a term for this psychological friction: Resistance. Here's how he explained it in his best-selling book *The War of Art*:

> Resistance will tell you anything to keep you from doing your work. It will perjure, fabricate, falsify; seduce, bully, cajole. Resistance is protean. It will assume any form, if that's what it takes to deceive you. It will reason with you like a lawyer or jam a nine-millimeter in your face like a stickup man. Resistance has no conscience. It will pledge anything to get a deal, then double-cross you as soon as your back is turned. If you take Resistance at its word, you deserve everything you get. Resistance is always lying and always full of shit.

How do you defeat Resistance and turn an "I won't" into an "I will"? You meet it in pitched battle, and you refuse to surrender. You refuse to take the easy road out. You refuse to look for reasons to be weak. You refuse to blame anyone or anything for your condition. When you can do those things, you can tap into a primal and powerful force that sets extraordinary people apart from everyone else. That's the big secret.

What's more, the "I don't have time" excuse can't pass the straight-face test when scrutinized. Imagine that your doctor says you have a fatal disease, and the only way to cure it is to whirl around in circles for two hours per day. After accepting that you do indeed have the strangest disease in the history of the human race, what would you do? Would you slink off and resign yourself to your fate? Or *somehow* free up the time to spin widdershins?

You know without a doubt that you'd find a way, regardless of how busy you are. Maybe you'd work a bit less, banish streaming apps, or disappear from social media, but somehow you'd make the time. Now, think about that. You just admitted you have a couple of hours per day waiting in the wings, available for immediate use toward any goal of your choosing, such as transforming your body. What's going on here?

Many people understand that "I don't have time to exercise" is just another way of saying "It's not important enough to me," but they struggle with prioritizing working out when the demands of their work, marriage, children, and errands pound like jungle drums from sunrise to sunset. Some of us work more instead of working out, for instance, and others put the needs of everyone close to them ahead of their own. Also, many women don't just work full-time jobs but also carry much of the domestic load, including shopping, supervising kids, cooking, chaperoning, and cleaning.

When these people are told they don't lack the time to train, only the will, they bristle. And understandably so. On a good day, they have maybe thirty minutes to themselves, before bed, after all the important tasks on the to-do list have been checked off. Such situations can seem hopeless, but remember—every problem has a solution, even this one.

Many of these people have had to get creative. I've helped them assemble simple but effective home gyms for less than they'd pay for a year of gym dues. I've helped them create thirty-minute bodyweight and band workouts they can do at work during lunch in the privacy of their office or even broken up into several ten-minute workouts throughout the day. I've suggested finding a workout buddy with children, which allows for shared babysitting, and early-morning weekend jaunts to the gym.

The first step in all of these cases, however, was shifting how these guys and gals viewed health and fitness in relation to their lives. The time given to eating well and exercising regularly is often considered a luxury, or worse, a self-indulgence, but here's the rub: you can make your health and wellness a priority now, or it'll make itself a priority later. There is no third choice.

Unless we take effective measures to counter the decline, after about age 35, every day, in every way, our body wanes. We usually don't notice it because the changes are subtle, but just as the seasons slowly shift from warm to cold, so does our health and vitality gradually decay. Furthermore, neglecting nutrition, exercise, sleep hygiene, and muscle definition and strength speeds up the downward spiral as the years pass. Add in regular alcohol and tobacco use, and one can reach terminal velocity. Bob Dylan got it right when he said if we're not busy being born, we're busy dying.

"But wait," someone somewhere is thinking, "my friend's cousin's doctor's mom's sister is ninety-three years old and eats like a raccoon, smokes like a chimney, and drinks like a fish, and she's still as fit as a bull moose. I'll probably be fine." This is silly. Every rule has exceptions, and every group has outliers, but that doesn't negate the principles or patterns. A century of medical literature has proven that as we get older, snubbing the cornerstones of healthy living greatly increases the risk of debilitating and deadly disorders, so much so that as time goes on, if we don't get our act together, our chances of remaining healthy and well become vanishingly small. If we do nurture our body with wholesome habits like proper diet, exercise, sleep, and supplementation, however, it'll repay us with a wellspring of vigor and vivacity for living our best life.

Another important element of this discussion is quality versus quantity because our goal isn't merely to survive as long as possible but to *thrive*. Just because your heart is still beating doesn't mean you still feel *alive*. So, even if we can disregard our health and wellness long into our golden years and somehow keep death from darkening our door, how much will we enjoy the later part of life with a body that suffers and a mind that stumbles? Why choose that path when we can follow the advice in this book instead and enjoy the fruits of beauty, strength, stamina, mobility, and spirit as we get older?

So, to Mr. and Ms. "I-*really*-don't-have-time-to-eat-well-and-exercise," I say: you can choose the rigors of healthy living now or the penalties of unhealthy living later. There is no third option.

CONQUERING THE CONSISTENCY CREATURE

Raise your hand if you know the answer to this question: What's the enemy of great? Chances are a montage of social media posts, motivational speeches, and self-help books just flashed through your mind, all proclaiming that "good" is the droid you're looking for. Good, they cry, is what's holding you back from dreaming your quest and manifesting your visions into reality. Good, you must understand, is never good enough. To achieve greatness, good must die. You must strive, suffer, and surpass. You must go big or go home.

On and on this philosophy goes, winning wide approval among people from all walks of life. It rings true because it's not wholly misguided. By definition, you can't achieve the extraordinary through ordinary ideas and efforts— but there's a problem. It's impossible to be great *all the time*. Usually, good enough is all we can muster. And that's okay because, ironically, a whole bunch of "good enough" can make you great, and that's true both inside and outside the gym. In fact, it's the only way to get to great without losing your nerve or sanity.

Think about it for a minute. When was the last time you were *outstanding* in an activity? When your faucet was fully open and you were in full flow? Now consider how much effort, energy, and presence that demanded, and how drained you felt afterward. Does it make sense to expect that from yourself continually? Of course not. That's a surefire way to destroy motivation and mood and burn out, because as sexy as greatness is, it's equally elusive. Like the muse, it can't be commanded, cajoled, or contracted with. It comes and goes as it pleases.

Thus, appreciate the fleeting moments of greatness, but don't hang your hat on them. Instead, demand something else from yourself—something rather mundane but also readily achievable and sustainable: consistency. Excellence is achieved by becoming great at being consistent—not by being consistently great—and this mostly comes down to being good enough again and again. In fitness, this means following your meal plan, workout program, and supplementation routine more often than not. If you can do that, you can make steady progress that compounds over time by relieving pressure and anxiety, reducing the risk of injury and exhaustion, and providing useful feedback.

By the same token, "Did I show up and put in the work?" is a much more productive question to ask yourself at the end of every day than "Was I great?" Or even worse, "Was I perfect?" That isn't to say that standards don't matter and that going through the motions, avoiding hardship, and swallowing mediocrity is acceptable. "Good enough" is about embracing what you've got and where you are, not what you wish you had or where you wish you were. It means acknowledging the fact that you can't micro-wave real results. They take time—no matter how "optimized" your approach.

Take dieting, for example. Many people want to know the "best" diet for losing weight, and these days many of those conversations revolve around carbohydrate intake. Guess what? According to research conducted by scientists at Stanford University, how much or little carbohydrate you eat doesn't matter. What does matter is adherence to a well-designed dietary protocol, like one that controls calories and protein intake. That is, the people who lose the most weight are the most consistent with their diets, not the best at avoiding carbs or any other foods.

The same goes for training. Simplistic workout programming and rock-solid consistency beats even the most scientifically sound routines and shaky compliance every time. Thus, a few low-intensity workouts every week will always beat out a few higher-quality training sessions per month. Similarly, an obsession with colossal effort in the gym is a vice, not a virtue—one that inevitably leads to disappointment and flameout.

So, stop trying to have perfect workouts. Stop trying to be invincible. Stop trying to rush the process. Strive for consistency instead. Stay patient, and in time, once you've given enough "good enough," you'll gain entry to the hallowed halls of greatness.

Oh, and here's a spoiler: You'll make mistakes along the way. You'll eat too much sometimes, sleepwalk through or skip workouts now and then, and forget to take your supplements when you're in a hurry. Don't sweat any of that or get down on yourself when you mess up. The "damage" is never as bad as you may think, and an abusive tirade of self-criticism will only make things worse.

For example, many people worry they've "blown" their diets after a single instance of overeating, not realizing that the amount of fat they can gain from a meal is negligible (a few ounces). And even in the case of an entire day of reckless eating, you *might* be able to gain up to ½ to 1 pound of fat if you really tried.

Therefore, when you stumble (and you will), show yourself the same compassion and forgiveness you'd show a friend. Research suggests that this type of response in times of frustration and failure is associated with better willpower and self-control because it helps us accept responsibility for our actions and steam ahead, unfazed.

To help you make this mental adjustment, I'm officially giving you a stack of hall passes to use whenever they're needed, because as I'm wont to say, in fitness, you only need to get the most important things mostly right most of the time.

This attitude is especially important as we get older. The human body is rugged and resilient, but as it racks up mileage, it can't endure as much abuse as it once could. Therefore, you can't subject yourself to the punishing workouts of your twenties and expect the same results. You can train hard, gain plenty of muscle and strength, and lose plenty of fat, but it'll likely be a slower process than when you were in college. So don't view your time with *Muscle for Life* as a competition with your former self. That's a race you can't win. Instead, appreciate what you're capable of now and where you can go from here.

You also can't compare yourself to the photoshopped influencers you see on social media. Let's see them on #HumpDay when they're working sixty hours per week and considering selling a kidney to keep their kids in private school. It's also okay if you feel you've "let yourself go"—it probably wasn't merely for lack of trying. You probably didn't know what to expect as you got older or what to do to maintain your health and fitness (and probably because of all the moronic and misleading information you were fed). You probably did your best with the hand you were dealt.

The good news is that none of that matters now. Somehow you found your way to this book, and together we'll make up for lost time by putting you on the fast track to the body you've always wanted. As you can imagine, your ability to establish good habits will heavily affect your progress, so I want to share with you two powerful evidence-based strategies for making the new fitness habits I'll be teaching you stick.

Hacking Your Habits

The first technique is deceptively simple: filling out a sentence. Not just any sentence, though—a sentence that works subconsciously to reduce your need for motivation, willpower, and self-control. You can use it for many goals, including exercise, diet, health, and everything else. This sentence exists thanks to a decade of work by a team of psychologists, and it has three parts: *what*, *when*, and *where*.

A study conducted by researchers at the University of Bath demonstrates the remarkable effectiveness of this formula. In this experiment, 91 percent of participants who were asked to create an exact exercise plan ("During the next week, I will partake in at least twenty minutes of vigorous exercise on [DAY] at [TIME OF DAY] at/in [PLACE]") exercised at least once per week, compared to just 38 percent of participants who were asked to read a few paragraphs from a random novel before working out, and 35 percent of participants who were asked to read a pamphlet on the heart benefits of exercise and told that most young adults who stick to an exercise program reduce their risk of heart disease.

No, that's not a typo—by simply writing when and where exercise would occur, follow-through skyrocketed (and, curiously, education on the benefits of exercise was no better than pleasure reading as a motivator).

Similar results have been seen in other exercise studies, as well as those analyzing other positive behaviors ranging from breast self-examination to dietary adherence to condom usage and more. As it happens, there are over one hundred published studies on this phenomenon, and the conclusion is crystal clear: if you explicitly state what you'll do, when you'll do it, and where you'll do it, you're much more likely to actually do it. For example:

+ "Every Monday, Wednesday, and Friday, I'll wake up at 7 a.m., drink an espresso, and go to the gym" will be far more effective than "I'll work out a few times per week."
+ "Every evening after dinner, I'll sit on the balcony and read twenty-five pages before watching TV," in place of "I'll read every day."
+ "Every weekday, I'll eat a salad and an apple for lunch" is preferable to "I'll eat better."
+ "Every Friday after I deposit my paycheck, I'll go home and transfer 10 percent of it into my investment account" will help you grow your net worth a lot faster than "I'll invest more than I did last year."
+ "Every weekday, I'll drink from a bottle of water at my desk and refill it whenever it's empty" will outdo "I'll drink more water."

What–when–where statements are far more effective for regulating behavior than relying on inspiration or willpower to strike at the right moment because they speak the brain's natural language, creating a trigger-and-response mechanism that doesn't require conscious monitoring or analysis.

I like to take this technique even further and put my important personal and interpersonal commitments on my calendar so they stay top of mind. At the beginning of every day, I check that calendar, and every time I review my pledges, I improve my chances of following through. You can also use your phone's assistant to remind you of daily obligations so you don't accidentally forget. For instance, if your intention is to eat a nutritious breakfast every day, you can set a reminder in your phone to prepare the food the night before and grab it in the morning before you go. Don't discount the value of such spadework—it can often be the factor that leads to follow-through, even when it's as mundane as getting into your workout clothes first thing on Saturday morning so you're dressed for your lunchtime workout.

One of the hidden benefits of preparatory actions like these is they reduce the amount of *activation energy* required to follow through on our aims. This is a concept in chemistry that refers to the minimum amount of energy needed to activate a chemical reaction, and it can be more broadly understood as the minimum amount of effort it takes to start or change something. The more mental or physical energy it takes for us to get up to speed, the more susceptible we'll be to the ebb and flow of willpower and motivation, which can surge and slump for reasons best known to themselves. When resolve is high, follow-through flows like breathing; but when it's low, implementation feels like wading into a pool of glue. By taking simple steps to lessen our reliance on these fickle feelings—like those I've just shared with you—we can greatly boost our consistency, strengthen our *whys*, and affirm our priorities.

To help you further reduce the activation energy of eating and exercising according to the plan, you can use another type of statement that's scientifically proven to increase self-control: the if–then statement. An if–then statement looks like this: "If X happens, then I'll do Y." This works for the same reason what–where–when statements work (specificity of stimulus and response), and it allows you to provide for contingencies and curveballs and reduce the need for moxie when things go sideways.

Let's take a scenario given earlier: you've decided that every Monday, Wednesday, and Friday, you'll wake up at 7 a.m., drink an espresso, and go to the gym. To generate complementary if–then statements, think about what may impede your intentions, and what you'll do in each instance. Here's a good start:

+ "If I'm a little short on sleep, then I'll still get up at 7 a.m. and do my workout."
+ "If I miss a morning workout, then I'll do it after work."
+ "If I can't go to the gym after work, then I'll do the workout on Saturday or Sunday at 9 a.m."

Or what about if–then statements for the what–when–where statement "Every weekday, I'll eat a salad and an apple for lunch"?

+ "If I don't have time to make my normal lunch, then I'll go to the salad place near my office."
+ "If I have to eat out instead of following my meal plan, then I'll eat just one piece of bread and skip dessert."
+ "If a coworker offers me a pastry at lunch, then I'll politely decline."

Every what–when–where statement can be strengthened in this way, especially after you've gotten into action and unforeseen difficulties and complications require that you adjust and augment your systems. This process is akin to running mental simulations to stress-test your desired outcomes. Psychologists call it *mental contrasting*, and research shows that it can increase your motivation to overcome obstacles and achieve your goals.

———————

Remember (or even review) this chapter whenever you need a shot in the arm, and it'll help you find the power to persevere. Recall it when you're choosing meals at your favorite restaurants, staring down sugary treats at the grocery store, and rolling out of bed for your morning workout like a log off a truck. Regularly look at the pictures you've saved, read the affirmations you've written, and revisit the whys and implementation intentions you've created. Then when you encounter difficulties or setbacks, you may stagger, but you'll also be able to steady yourself, breathe wind back into your sails, and speed toward your goals.

Make no mistake, however—this transformation business takes time. We live in the Age of Impatience. These days, too many people wear themselves out chasing easy—"four-hour workweeks," "six-minute abs," and "thirty-second meals." They don't want processes and paradigms; they want shortcuts and stratagems. They don't want to plant in the spring and tend in the summer to earn a harvest in the fall; they want to shirk and slack and reap a bounty they didn't sow.

Well, I hate to be the bearer of bad news, but you can't lose 20 pounds of fat in twenty days or reshape your butt or flatten your belly in a couple of weeks. Upgrading your body is a rewarding undertaking, but you have to give a lot to get a lot. Plus, you'll learn a valuable life lesson along the way: fitness is one of those special things you can't buy, steal, or fake. There aren't any prizes for lying, complaining, or failing, nor any privileges for status, opinions, or feelings. It's called "working out" for good reason. You either put in the work or get put in your place. Fitness is nothing if not a tribute to the primacy of effort.

In this way, the gym is a lot more than a place to move, grunt, and sweat. It's a microcosm where we can make contact with the deeper parts of ourselves—our convictions, fears, habits, and anxieties. It's an arena where we can confront these opponents head-on and prove we have what it takes to vanquish them. It's a setting where we can test the stories we tell ourselves. It calls on us to demonstrate how we respond to the greater struggles of life—adversity, pain, insecurity, stress, and weakness—and, in some ways, who we really are. Hence, the gym is a training and testing ground of sorts for the body, mind, and soul.

The gym is also a source of learning, because it calls on us to constantly attempt new things. It's a forum where questions are at least as important as answers, and it cultivates what scientists call a *growth mindset* by teaching us that our abilities can be developed through dedication and hard work—a worldview that's essential for great accomplishment. The gym is practical, too, not idealistic. It's a laboratory open to all ideas and methodologies, and it gives clear, unqualified feedback: either they work or they don't.

In short, the gym can be so much more than merely a place to work out. It can be a refuge from the chaos around us, a world of our own that we create to satisfy dreams and desires. So, if you feel anxious or intimidated about getting started, brace up, because soon you'll know more about fitness than most everyone at your gym, and once you're a regular, don't be surprised if they start coming to *you* for advice.

In the next chapter, we'll get you a little closer to that milestone by exploring the science of everyone's least-favorite four-letter word: *diet*.

KEY TAKEAWAYS

+ People with vague, unrealistic, or uninspiring fitness goals (or none) are always the first to quit.

+ Different people have different reasons for eating well and working out—but it's important to isolate and articulate *your* reasons.

+ Find a picture or two (or three or four) of the type of body you want and save them somewhere that's easily accessible, like your phone or Google Drive or Dropbox.

+ Imagine what your ideal body feels like for you, and then write it out in the form of individual affirmations, which are positive statements that describe how you want to be, such as "I'm full of energy all day" and "My mind is quick, clear, and focused."

+ One of the best ways to use the statements you've formulated is to read them every morning before you start your day or whenever your spirit is flagging.

+ Use what–when–where statements to reduce your need for motivation, willpower, and self-control. Write a sentence that explicitly states what you'll do, when you'll do it, and where you'll do it. For example, "Every Monday, Wednesday, and Friday, I'll wake up at 7 a.m., drink an espresso, and go to the gym."

+ Use if–then statements to further reduce the activation energy of eating and exercising according to the plan, like, "If I'm a little short on sleep, then I'll still get up at 7 a.m. and do my workout."

PART 2

THE LAST DIET ADVICE YOU'LL EVER NEED

6

It's All in Your Body Composition: The Four-Step Formula for Less Fat and More Lean Muscle

In this age, which believes that there is a shortcut to everything,
the greatest lesson to be learned is that the most difficult way is,
in the long run, the easiest.
—HENRY MILLER

For thousands of years, a lean, toned, athletic body has been the gold standard of physical status and attractiveness. It was a hallmark of the ancient heroes, gods, and goddesses, and it's still idolized today. With obesity rates over 35 percent here in America (and rising), however, it would appear that reaching that brass ring must require youth, top-shelf genetics, or a level of understanding, discipline, and sacrifice far beyond the capabilities of most people.

This isn't true. The knowledge of how to achieve peak fitness is easy enough to gain—you'll learn everything you need to know in this book—and it doesn't require as much gumption or self-denial as you may think.

Before you can do it, though, you must disabuse yourself of some of the biggest myths and lies people are told about fat loss and gain and learn the real science of getting and staying lean for life. Addressing these fictions head-on is crucial because only a fraction of everything you could learn about fitness produces most of your bottom-line results. So long as you understand and apply *those* principles and techniques correctly, you can afford to be ignorant of most else and stay in fantastic shape for the rest of your life. Run afoul of them, however, and you'll struggle with your fitness until the end of your days.

The first mess you mustn't make is complexifying getting in shape. This tendency is exemplified by an article the *Wall Street Journal* published on January 30, 2020, titled "Weight Loss Is Harder Than Rocket Science." The gist of the piece was how the math behind the *body mass index* (BMI) is harder to apply to weight loss than the math of rocket science is to rocketry.

Many people would agree, having tried and failed to lose weight many times themselves and witnessed countless abortive attempts by others. Well, I have good news for you: while the human metabolism is complicated and weight loss isn't *easy*, the science is straightforward. It's just different from what many doctors, trainers, and coaches believe.

The emphasis on BMI is a perfect example of how many experts miss the mark. The idea behind it is this: in order to know if someone is over- or underweight, their height must be taken into account, since taller people are naturally heavier than shorter ones. To calculate BMI, you divide weight (in kilograms) by height (in meters squared), producing a number that represents the relationship between these dimensions.

Doctors often use BMI to monitor how a patient's weight is likely to affect their health, categorizing them according to simple criteria:

+ Underweight = BMI of less than 18.5
+ Normal weight = BMI of 18.5 to 24.9

- ✦ Overweight = BMI of 25 to 29.9
- ✦ Obese = BMI of 30 or greater

If your number is too high, you may be told to lose weight, and if it's too low, to gain weight. There's a kicker, however: BMI was never meant to serve as a proxy for the health of specific individuals, only to reveal trends in a population. In other words, a lone person with a high or low BMI may or may not be over- or underweight, but a large group of people with a high or low average BMI will likely include many over- and underweight individuals.

For instance, I weigh 197 pounds and have a six-pack, but my BMI is 25.29, suggesting I'm overweight and should slim down. Likewise, there are many people who have a "normal weight" BMI with the health problems of an obese person (elevated cholesterol, blood sugar, etc.). How can that be?

BMI doesn't take into account your *body composition*—how much muscle and fat you have. This is crucial because it's not excess body *weight* per se that negatively affects our health, but excess body *fat*. "Excess body weight" in the form of muscle actually has the opposite effect on the body, enhancing our health.

For this reason, one of the first major mental shifts I like to see in my readers and followers is for them to pay less attention to their weight and more to their body composition. So long as muscle and body fat levels are going in the right direction, we don't much care about your body weight. Similarly, while we may say we want to "lose weight," what we really want is to lose fat, not muscle; and if we say we want to "gain weight," we really want to gain muscle, not fat.

This is especially important to understand for people new to strength training, who can expect to gain a considerable amount of muscle in their first six to twelve months—muscle that'll mask some or even much of the fat weight lost along the way.

So, the first key to controlling your body composition is knowing how to use food to drive both fat loss and muscle growth. And how do you do that? It all starts with understanding the scientific principle of *energy balance*, which is the relationship between energy intake (calories eaten) and output (calories burned).

Most mainstream diets vilify one kind of food and claim that by removing it from your life, you can lose weight and rejuvenate your body without fussing over calories or portions. The formula used to flack one of these diets usually exploits powerful psychological pressure points and goes like this:

1. "It's not your fault you're overweight and unhealthy. You're a victim of bad advice and worse food."
2. "New research shows this heinous habit/food/nutrient/molecule is to blame."
3. "Avoid this clunker at all costs, and you'll automagically transform your body and health."

These emotion-based tactics are how marketers sold us on low-fat dieting a couple of decades ago, and how they peddle low-carb and low-sugar dieting today. Cut the vicious carbs and sugars out of your life, many pundits currently claim, and the pounds will melt away and you'll enter a new era of health and vitality. It can all sound so believable until someone comes along and points out the glitches in the matrix—like Mark Haub, a 41-year-old Kansas State University professor, who lost 27 pounds in ten weeks eating Hostess cupcakes, Doritos, Oreos, and whey protein shakes. Or 55-year-old science teacher John Cisna, who lost 56 pounds in six months eating nothing but McDonald's. Or 34-year-old fitness enthusiast Kai Sedgwick, who got into the best shape of his life while following a rigorous workout routine and eating fast food every day for a month. Or the dozens of studies that have found no difference in weight or fat loss between low- and high-carb and low- and high-sugar diets.

I don't recommend that you follow in the footsteps of Haub, Cisna, or Sedgwick (the nutritional value of your diet does matter for enhancing body composition, improving longevity, and protecting against disease), but you don't have to choose between carbs and sugars and health and wellness—between abstinence and abs. By striking the right balance between inhibition and indulgence, you can enjoy the fruits without upsetting the applecart.

Here's the first principle in play: if you consistently consume fewer calories than you burn, you'll lose fat, regardless of how much carbohydrate or sugar—or anything else, for that matter—you eat. There's a corollary here, too: if you consistently consume more calories than you burn, you'll gain fat, even if those calories come from the "healthiest" food on earth. Thus, no individual food can make you thinner or fatter. Only undereating and overeating can.

You don't have to look far for obvious evidence of this. How many people do you know who are overweight despite their commitment to "clean eating"? Have you experienced the same? And what about people who stay svelte eating many "forbidden" foods? Ever wonder how such a paradox is possible? Now you know.

Many people in the diet industry look down their noses at this model, though. Eat the right foods, many of them state, and you'll "unclog and supercharge" your hormones and metabolism, and your body will take care of the rest—music to the ears of those who want to believe they can get lean and fit without paying attention to *how much* they eat, only *what*.

Malarkey. In fact, it's worse than that. It's a blatant lie. You can't focus only on the what or the how much—you need both. As far as your body weight is concerned, how much you eat is far more important than what you eat. As far as your health and wellness are concerned, what you eat is more important than how much you eat (so long as you don't overeat to the point of obesity, which is quite unhealthy).

You can think of this relationship like the classic Chinese yin and yang symbol that represents a set of opposing and complementing principles. In this case, if you only pay attention to how much you eat, your body weight can remain balanced, but your well-being can decline; and if you only control your nutrition, your health can remain stable, but your body weight can be unpredictable. The goal, then, is to harmonize these two elements of our diet so we can optimize our body weight (read body composition) and health. And this brings us back to energy balance (calories in and out), which forms the foundation of science-based eating.

Technically, a *calorie* is the energy needed to raise the temperature of one kilogram of water by one degree Celsius. Various foods contain varying amounts of calories. For example, nuts are very energy-dense, containing about 6.5 calories per gram on average, whereas celery contains very little stored energy, with just 0.15 calories per gram. If you add up the calories you eat and drink during a period (a day, week, or month, for instance) and then compare that number to how many you burn in the same period, you'll notice one of three things:

1. You ate more calories than you burned. (You'll gain weight.)
2. You ate fewer calories than you burned. (You'll lose weight.)
3. You ate more or less the same number of calories as you burned. (You'll maintain your weight.)

This alone explains why every single controlled weight-loss study conducted in the last hundred years has concluded that meaningful weight loss requires energy expenditure to exceed energy intake. This is also why bodybuilders dating back just as far—from the "father of modern bodybuilding" Eugen Sandow, to the sword-and-sandals superstar Steve Reeves, to the iconic Arnold Schwarzenegger—have been using this knowledge to reduce and increase body fat levels as desired.

That doesn't mean you always have to count calories to lose weight, however. It just means you have to *understand* how the calories you eat and burn influence your body weight, and regulate your eating according to your goals.

Thus, it's no surprise that diets that eliminate foods or even entire food groups often work for some people but not others. By forbidding delicious, high-calorie foods people love—foods that make it easier to overeat—and forcing the consumption of less-palatable, lower-calorie fare, you may reduce calorie intake enough to produce weight loss. Hence the success stories. You can also fail to create a large enough difference between calories in and out, or any at all, by simply eating too much of the "diet-approved" food, resulting in little or no weight loss. Hence the failures. But let's not mistake correlation for causation. People who have lost weight with such diets didn't succeed because they stopped eating sugar, gluten, or carbs, per se—they lost weight because doing away with sugar, gluten, or carbs helped them consistently eat fewer calories than they burned for long enough to produce weight loss.

This has been shown in countless studies. The people who ate the least lost the most weight, and those who ate the most lost the least weight (or gained weight)—and these outcomes have been demonstrated with many diets, including Mediterranean, vegan, vegetarian, paleo, Weight Watchers, Slimming World, South Beach, Best Life, Atkins, DASH, and others.

No matter the protocol, people lose weight only if they eat fewer calories than they burn, and people who fail to lose weight fizzle because they eat too many calories too consistently, not because they fail to follow arbitrary rules strictly enough or because there's something mysteriously awry with their bodies.

You might still be skeptical, however. Maybe you've heard that energy balance is contradicted or even debunked by the latest scientific research, or maybe you know of individual stories that seem to defy its principles. For example, take people who apparently can't lose weight on very-low-calorie diets: "Jim eats nine hundred calories per day, works out several hours per week, and is *gaining* weight. How does energy balance explain this?" Mysterious indeed, until you realize the culprit virtually every time is human error, not metabolic voodoo. Aside from total ignorance of energy balance, the three most common weight loss mistakes are:

1. Underestimating calorie intake. Most people are bad at accurately evaluating how many calories they're eating, which makes it easy to overeat. Studies show that while someone may think they're eating 800 calories per day (starving themselves), it could easily be 1,200, 1,500, or more. This isn't surprising when you consider how many calories are in the more savory foods many of us like to eat. A single slice of pizza, for instance, contains 300 to 400 calories, or about as many as are burned in a thirty-minute run or sixty-minute resistance training workout.

2. Overestimating calorie expenditure. Exercise and physical activity don't burn as many calories as many people think, which makes it harder to keep calories out over calories in. In a study conducted by scientists at York University, overweight participants not at-

tempting to lose weight overestimated energy expenditure during vigorous exercise by 72 percent on average.

3. Extreme overeating. Too many "cheat meals"—or worse, "cheat days"—can set you back more than most people realize. Let's say you stick to your diet faithfully throughout the week, eating about 300 fewer calories than you burn every day, ending Friday with a cumulative deficit of 1,500 calories. Right on! That's almost half a pound of fat loss! Then comes the weekend, when you're less active and more lax with what you eat. Saturday is your cheat day, and you put down about 1,000 more calories than you burn. On Sunday, you pump the brakes, but still end up a couple of hundred calories over your expenditure for the day. What have you done here? Do the math, and you learn you've more or less erased your entire week's fat loss in two days, putting you back to square one.

These three factors account for the majority of weight loss failures everywhere and explain why so many people flounder with diets that deal in rules and restrictions instead of hard numbers.

Yet another popular refrain against energy balance is that the human body isn't a machine, so you can't treat it like one and expect predictable results. Our physiology is far more complicated than the simple heat engine that powers a refrigerator or car, we're told, so it's silly to assume they work in the same ways. This is all smoke and mirrors. While it's true the human body is more complex than a combustion engine, there's a reason that a century of metabolic research has conclusively proven that energy balance works the same in the lean and the obese, the healthy and the diseased, the old and the young.

That doesn't mean energy balance is a silver bullet, however. Just as watching your body weight tells you only about quantity and not quality (muscle versus fat), watching your calorie intake tells you only how much energy you're eating—not where it's coming from. As many critics of energy balance will correctly point out, your body doesn't process all calories the same way. Some are more beneficial to your body composition and health than others, which is why you must pay attention to not only your calories but your *macronutrients* as well.

Macro-what? The nutrients we need in relatively large amounts are called *macronutrients*, also referred to as *macros*. Technically the term includes minerals, but for our purposes here, we'll focus on the three aspects that are most relevant to body composition: protein, carbohydrate, and fat.

As you've learned, foods don't have special properties that make them "fattening" or "slimming." Instead, they have varying amounts of calories, which makes some foods more or less conducive to fat loss and gain, as well as different amounts of protein, carbs, and fat, which makes some foods better for losing fat and gaining muscle. Therefore, if your goal is to optimize your body composition (and your health), a calorie is not just a calorie, and a carefully controlled diet of junk food won't cut it. Instead, you need to follow my formula for a system that scientists refer to as *flexible dieting*.

THE LAST "DIET" YOU'LL EVER NEED

Many people eat in a haphazard manner, driven by impulse and whim rather than design and intent, and their health and fitness levels are a reflection of this. If you're one of those people, you won't be for much longer, because with *Muscle for Life*, you'll learn how to use delicious food to nourish your body, enhance your physique, and satisfy your stomach.

In the evidence-based fitness space, this routine is known as *flexible dieting*, and it has four steps:

1. Regulate your calories according to your body composition goal.
2. Eat a high-protein diet.
3. Get most of your calories from whole, nutritious, relatively unprocessed foods.
4. Find a balance of carbohydrate and fat intake that works for you.

If you can follow that simple formula, you can forever free yourself from the frustrations of fad and yo-yo dieting and develop a healthy, enjoyable, and lasting relationship with food. Let's take a closer look at each of these points.

1. Regulate your calories according to your body composition goal.

The first question to answer when creating a diet plan is what you're trying to achieve. Are you looking to lose fat? Maximize muscle growth? Maintain your body composition? Each requires a different dietary strategy, starting with calorie intake, and flexible dieting offers three different approaches depending on your goal.

To lose fat, you must consistently eat fewer calories than you burn. This produces the *calorie deficit*, as it's called, required for diminishing your body's fat stores. Without this caloric shortfall, no fat loss will occur no matter what else you do in the kitchen or gym.

To maximize muscle growth, you must consistently eat more calories than you burn. When you eat fewer calories than you burn, you lose fat, but you also impair your body's ability to build muscle. Thus, you need to ensure you're not in a calorie deficit when you want to gain muscle as quickly as possible, and the easiest way to do this is to consistently eat more calories than you burn.

"Won't that result in fat storage?" you might wonder. Yes, my astute reader, it will, but when you know how to do it correctly (as you will on the *Muscle for Life* program), you can minimize the amount of fat you gain.

If you want to neither lose nor gain fat and make slow muscle and strength gains, you want your calories in to match your calories out. Practically, you can never sync them perfectly because your total daily energy expenditure is a moving target that you can't estimate with 100 percent accuracy. You don't need to hit that bull's-eye, however. You only need to get close enough, watch how your body responds, and adjust accordingly.

2. Eat a high-protein diet.

This is the second rule for optimizing your health and body composition, and one of the simplest ways to use food to boost your fitness.

A *protein* is a compound that contains one or more long chains of *amino acids,* which are used to create body tissues such as muscle, hair, and skin, as well as various chemicals vital to life. Protein affects your body composition far more than carbohydrate or fat, and research shows that people who eat more protein . . .

- ✦ Lose fat faster
- ✦ Gain more muscle
- ✦ Burn more calories
- ✦ Experience less hunger
- ✦ Have stronger bones
- ✦ Enjoy better moods

Protein intake is even more important when you exercise regularly because working out increases your body's need for amino acids. Similarly, high-protein eating is also essential when you restrict your calories to lose fat because it helps preserve lean mass while dieting.

You may be hesitant to eat more protein, however, because you've heard it'll speed up aging by increasing the production of hormones and chemicals in the body that amplify tissue growth, oxidative stress, and cellular damage. By restricting protein intake, the story goes, we can decrease these unwanted side effects, reduce wear and tear in the body, and lower our risk of disability. It's a nice theory, but research indicates it's probably wrong.

For one thing, all of the studies suggesting that low-protein dieting can increase lifespan are in animals, mostly mice. While humans and mice share many of the same biological mechanisms, there are also key differences. We humans aren't merely big rodents. For example, mice burn about seven times more calories per pound of body weight than humans, which is important to know because the faster the metabolism, the more cellular damage that accumulates from metabolic activities. Thus, mice stand to benefit from protein restriction—which lowers metabolic activity—much more than humans do.

Additionally, while there are no long-term studies on how restricting protein intake affects lifespan in humans, statistical models developed by scientists at Texas A&M University have predicted that if you reduced your protein intake to the absolute minimum required to maintain your metabolism (about 12 percent of daily calories) at age 18, and kept it there for the rest of your life, you could *maybe* increase your lifespan by about three years.

Then again, maybe not—because the researchers didn't take into account the fact that low-protein dieting is associated with a higher incidence of muscle loss, bone fractures, and frailty, which pose a considerable threat to longevity.

Therefore, one could reasonably argue that restricting protein in hopes of living longer is stepping over dollars to pick up dimes, and that, given the current scientific evidence, the well-established advantages of high-protein eating far outweigh the theoretical disadvantages.

3. Get most of your calories from whole, nutritious, relatively unprocessed foods.

This is the third tried-and-true rule for mastering your health and body composition and unlocking lifelong vigor and vim.

By "unprocessed," I mean foods that may have undergone mechanical processing (cleaning, cutting, portioning, heating, and freezing, for example), but little or no compositional processing (added sugar, salt, preservatives, hydrogenated oils, and flavor enhancers, to name a few). Unprocessed choices are generally whole, natural foods that come from animals or the earth, and processed foods are packaged or "fast" foods.

Hitting the drive-thru or pizza joint or having some sugar or "empty calories" here and there won't hurt you in the long run, but allotting a majority of your daily calories to nutritionally bankrupt fodder absolutely will. Over time, eating too much nutrient-poor food too often can lead to nutritional deficiencies that contribute to health problems, impair mental and physical performance, and even blunt fat loss and muscle gain by slowing your metabolism and interfering with your body's ability to recover from your training.

One of many examples I could give you of the power of nutrition concerns the mineral zinc, which is abundant in foods like beef, seeds, and legumes, and required for optimal thyroid function. Thyroid hormones influence metabolic rate, so if you don't consume enough zinc, those hormone levels can drop, followed by your metabolism and rate of weight loss. In a case study conducted by scientists at the University of Massachusetts, two zinc-deficient college women received 26 milligrams of zinc per day for four months. By the end of the experiment, one woman was burning 194 more calories every day than before, and the other was burning 527 more calories per day. This is the energy equivalent of about thirty and sixty minutes of moderately intense cardio, respectively, and it would speed up fat loss by about ½ and 1 pound per week. From just correcting a zinc deficiency.

Granted, this was just a case study and so it can't support sweeping claims about nutrition and metabolism, but it's evidence nonetheless of how important it is to consider food as a source of not just energy or pleasure but crucial nutrients as well.

Think of it like this: When baking, what happens if you forget the leavener? Or if you use too much sugar? Or not enough fat? You're in a bad way because you need all of the right components in the right quantities to create a righteous batch of confections. Likewise, your body's recipe for robust health and performance calls for a lot more than mere calories and macros.

Another reason that eating mostly whole, minimally processed food benefits your body composition is because it has a higher *thermic effect of food* (TEF), which is the number of calories required to process what we eat. Whole-grain bread with less-processed (cheddar) cheese has a TEF of around 20 percent, for example, meaning that about 20 percent of the calories are burned during digestion. On the other hand, a slice of white bread with highly processed (American) cheese has a TEF of only 11 percent.

While small differences like this in a single meal are insignificant, they can add up if you're getting many of your calories from highly processed, low-TEF foods. In this case, you might burn several hundred more calories per day by swapping most of your food for less-processed fare. Instead of a sweetened breakfast cereal, you could eat oatmeal with a drizzle of honey; or instead of downing a bag of chips, you could create crispy potato wedges; and instead of snacking on a granola bar, you could munch on some homemade muesli. Bit by bit, these changes add up.

Eating plenty of unprocessed food (and plant-derived food in particular) also provides your body with enough fiber, which is an indigestible carbohydrate found in many types of plant foods. Eating enough fiber reduces the risk of many types of disease and is linked to living a longer, healthier life. Accordingly, the Academy of Nutrition and Dietetics recommends that children and adults consume 14 grams of fiber for every 1,000 calories of food eaten.

Now, you'll notice this third rule is to get *most* but not *all* of your calories from whole, nutritious, relatively unprocessed foods. The reason for this is that so long as you provide your body with an abundance of nutritive food, you can safely slip in some less-nourishing grub. The rule of thumb, then, is to get at least 80 percent of your calories from such food by mostly eating stuff you clean, cut, and cook yourself, like lean protein, fruits, vegetables, whole grains, legumes, nuts, seeds, and oils.

And what about the remaining calories? Here's your reward: you can use them for your favorite treats, if you desire. And that makes for a pretty flexible diet, wouldn't you say?

4. Find a balance of carbohydrate and fat intake that works for you.

This is the final principle of flexible dieting, and, contrary to many of the dietary dogmas du jour, the least important one for enhancing your body composition. High-carb, low-carb, high-fat, low-fat—it doesn't much matter for losing fat and gaining muscle. It *does* matter for maximizing your enjoyment of how you eat, though, because you probably like carbs. And with *Muscle for Life*, you won't just get fitter, leaner, and stronger; you'll do it while eating carbs. Lots of carbs, if you prefer, including the ones you like to eat. You'll eat dietary fat, too, because it's needed for optimal health, it helps you feel fuller, and it makes food tastier, but you won't have to eat nearly as much fat as people following the ketogenic or paleo diet if you don't want to.

To better understand why carbs aren't your enemy (and in fact are your friend when you're physically active), let's briefly discuss what a carbohydrate is and what happens in your body when you eat it.

Whether we're talking about the natural sugars found in fruit or vegetables, or the processed ones found in a candy bar, they're all digested into glucose and shipped off in the blood for use. The key difference between these forms of carbohydrate is the rate at which this conversion happens. The candy bar turns into glucose quickly, whereas the green beans take longer because they contain slower-burning sugars.

Some people say that digestive processing time makes all the difference in determining whether a carbohydrate is "healthy." The idea is "fast" carbs are "bad" and "slow" ones are "good." This is mostly wrong. A baked potato is a "fast" carb but packed with vital nutrients. Watermelon is up there in speed, too, and even oatmeal—arguably the greatest grain for human health—is digested more quickly than a Snickers bar.

The primary reason we can't replace foods like potato, watermelon, and oatmeal with candy isn't because of how quickly or slowly they're assimilated, but because our body needs vitamins, minerals, fiber, and other substances that aren't in junk food and beverages. This helps explain why there's an association between high *added sugar* intake—sugars like *sucrose* and *fructose* added to make food sweeter—and metabolic abnormalities and health conditions, including obesity, as well as varying degrees of nutritional deficiency.

There's no denying that eating too much added sugar can harm our health and that limiting it is a good idea. That doesn't mean we need to completely avoid such foods or restrict our consumption of all forms of carbohydrate, however, especially those associated with health benefits, like whole grains, fruit, vegetables, and legumes. In actuality, if you're healthy and physically active, you'll likely do better with *more* nutritious carbs in your diet, not less (especially if you're into strength training).

One substance your body creates from carbohydrate is *glycogen*, which is stored in the muscles and liver and used for fuel during intense exercise. When you restrict your carb intake, your body's glycogen stores drop, and studies show that this inhibits workout performance and genetic signaling related to muscle repair and growth. When you're exercising regularly, restricting your carbs also raises your cortisol and lowers your testosterone levels, which further hampers your body's ability to recover from your training. We shouldn't be surprised, then, that research shows that athletes who eat low-carb diets recover more slowly and gain less muscle and strength than those who eat more carbs.

"But what about insulin?" people often ask me. "Don't carbs stimulate insulin production, and doesn't that make you fat?" Not quite. Eating carbs triggers insulin production, and insulin triggers fat storage, but none of that makes you chubbier. Only overeating does.

Insulin is a hormone that causes muscles, organs, and fat tissue to absorb and use or store nutrients like glucose and amino acids. When you eat a meal containing protein or carbohydrate, insulin levels rise, and the body uses some of the energy provided by the meal to power the many physiological processes that keep us alive, and it uses some to increase its fat stores. Some people call this the body's "fat-storing mode." Once your body has finished digesting, absorbing, burning, and storing the food eaten, insulin levels fall, and you must now rely on fat stores for energy. This is sometimes called the body's "fat-burning mode."

You flip between these states every day, storing small amounts of fat after meals, and then burning small amounts after food energy runs out. Here's a simple graph of this in operation:

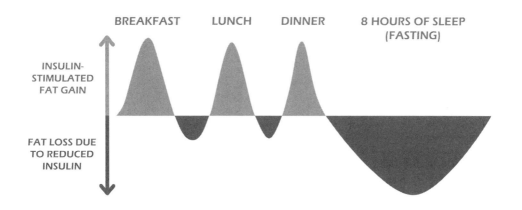

The lighter portions are the periods where you've eaten, providing your body with energy to use and store as fat. The darker parts are where food energy is absent, and fat must be burned to stay alive.

Insulin's role in this natural and inevitable metabolic process makes it an easy scapegoat for unwanted weight gain. But without excess calories, no amount of insulin or insulin-producing foods can significantly increase body fat levels. The chemical energy needed to physically produce additional body fat has to come from somewhere, and if you're burning as much energy as you're eating (or more), there's nothing left for increasing fat stores.

So, in the final analysis, you have nothing to fear from insulin, and that means you can achieve peak health and fitness while eating many of your favorite foods. If you're still skeptical, maybe because of how many experts claim otherwise, that's okay, because before long you'll have firsthand proof in the way of rapid muscle gain and fat loss as well as improvements in just about every biomarker of health you care to monitor.

Let's now talk about dietary fat, the overhyped darling of the diet industry. You should eat enough dietary fat to stay healthy, but you have no reason to follow a high-fat diet unless you enjoy it—and even then, you need to do so mindfully. To understand why, let's talk about the two different fats found in food: *triglycerides* and *cholesterol*.

Triglycerides

Triglycerides make up the bulk of our fat intake and are found in many foods, including dairy, nuts, seeds, meat, and more. There are two types of triglycerides: those that are liquid at room temperature (*unsaturated*) and those that are solid (*saturated*). Both support our health in numerous ways—absorbing vitamins, creating hormones, supporting skin and hair health, and more—but they shouldn't be eaten in equal proportions.

Saturated Fat

Since the 1950s, people have been told that saturated fat increased the risk of heart disease, but more recent research has challenged this assertion. The diet industry has exploited this shift marvelously with glittering low-carb and high-fat diets that allow (or even encourage) much higher amounts of saturated fat than previously believed to be healthy.

The problem, however, is that much of the scientific literature used to promote high-fat diets has also been criticized by prominent nutrition and cardiology researchers for various flaws and omissions, and some studies still show a weak albeit consistent correlation between high saturated fat intake and heart disease. Thus, many scientists maintain that we should follow the generally accepted dietary guidelines for saturated fat intake (less than 10 percent of daily calories) until we know more.

I agree—nobody can credibly claim that we can eat as much saturated fat as we want with no chance of negative consequences—and so I, too, recommend limiting saturated fat intake.

Unsaturated Fat

Unsaturated fat comes in two forms: *monounsaturated* and *polyunsaturated*. Monounsaturated fat is liquid at room temperature and solidifies when cooled. Foods high in monounsaturated fat include nuts, olive and peanut oil, and avocado. This is one of the best forms of fat you can eat. Research shows that it can reduce the risk of heart disease, and it's also believed to be responsible for some of the health benefits associated with the Mediterranean diet, which involves eating a lot of olive oil. Polyunsaturated fat is liquid at room temperature and remains so when cooled. Foods high in polyunsaturated fat include safflower, sesame, and sunflower seeds; corn; and many nuts and their oils.

The two primary polyunsaturated fats are *omega-3* and *omega-6 fatty acids*—designations referring to their molecular structures. These substances produce many effects in the body and are the only fats we must get from our diet, which is why they're referred to as *essential fatty acids*.

The chemistry is complex, but here's what you need to know: omega-6 fatty acids generally cause "bad" (but sometimes needed) effects in the body, including increased levels of inflammation; and the effects of omega-3 fatty acids are generally "good" (but sometimes untimely), including reduced inflammation levels.

Scientists suspect that the absolute amount of omega-3 fatty acids in the diet may be more important than the ratio between omega-3 and omega-6 intakes, and since many people don't have enough omega-3 fatty acids in their diets, a considerable amount of work has been done to boost the omega-3 content of various foods, like eggs and meat.

The takeaway? If you're like most people, you're getting enough omega-6 fatty acids from commonly consumed foods like vegetable oil, nuts, seeds, and meat, but probably not enough omega-3s. An easy fix is with an omega-3 supplement, which we'll discuss later in this book.

Cholesterol

Cholesterol is the other form of fat found in food, and a waxy substance present in all cells in the body that's used to make hormones, vitamin D, and chemicals that help you digest your food.

You've probably heard that you should reduce your cholesterol levels to lower your risk of heart disease, and that one of the best ways to do this is by eating less cholesterol and saturated fat. While this is more right than wrong, it's not entirely accurate.

One reason the relationship between cholesterol and heart health is tricky has to do with how cholesterol travels throughout your body. It's delivered to cells by molecules known as *lipoproteins*, which are made of fat and proteins. There are two kinds of lipoproteins:

1. *Low-density lipoprotein* (LDL)
2. *High-density lipoprotein* (HDL)

When people talk of the "bad" type of cholesterol, they're referring to LDL, because studies show that high levels of LDL in your blood can lead to an accumulation of fat in your arteries and increase the risk of heart disease. By the same token, food that can raise LDL levels, such as fried and heavily processed foods, is considered bad for your heart. HDL, on the other hand, is often thought of as the "good" cholesterol because it protects LDL from being chemically altered by oxygen and carries cholesterol to your liver, which flushes it from your body.

Scientists are still learning about the structure and function of lipoproteins, but the evidence is clear that you want to ensure that your LDL levels aren't too high and your HDL levels aren't too low. And what's the best way to go about this? The common practices of eating low-cholesterol foods and avoiding saturated fat won't cut it. Here's what will:

+ Exercising regularly (especially intense exercise, including strength training)
+ Maintaining healthy body fat levels
+ Getting enough sleep
+ Not smoking

And of the four, the first (regular intense exercise) is the most beneficial to cholesterol levels. What's more, you may be surprised to learn that research suggests that exercise alone can neutralize at least some of the downsides of poor lifestyle choices, like unhealthy eating. Exercise isn't a natural panacea, but it touches on that magical territory.

So, now that we've separated some key carbohydrate and dietary fat facts from falsehoods, the relaxed approach of finding a balance of each that works for you likely makes more sense. Not only does this follow the latest scientific discoveries about how these macronutrients affect health and body composition, it also allows you to enjoy your diet. This works wonders for adherence and consistency, which are critical ingredients of long-term success.

—————

With the principles of flexible dieting—using energy balance to control your calories, eating plenty of protein and carbs, and sticking mostly to nutritious foods while still making room for treats—you'll enter a new era of personal nutrition. No more crash diets, cleanses, or other rigorous regimens that deliver fast but fleeting results. With these axioms I've shared, we can create healthy and satisfying meal plans that'll enable you to switch between losing fat, gaining muscle, and maintaining your physique at will.

To do that, you need to know three things:

1. How many calories you should eat every day.
2. How to go from calories to grams of protein, carbohydrate, and fat per day.
3. How to translate those numbers into delicious and nutritious meals.

When you can do that—and soon you'll have it down—you'll enjoy higher energy levels, less hunger and fewer cravings, and better post-workout recovery. You'll sleep better. You'll look better. You'll live better—slashing your risk of illness and building a strong, resilient body that never gets in the way of the life you want to live.

KEY TAKEAWAYS

+ Controlling your body composition starts with understanding the scientific principle of *energy balance*, which is the relationship between energy intake (calories eaten) and output (calories burned).
+ The three most common weight loss mistakes are: underestimating calorie intake, overestimating calorie expenditure, and overeating during "cheat meals" or "cheat days."

+ To lose fat, you must consistently eat fewer calories than you burn. This produces the calorie deficit required for diminishing your body's fat stores.

+ To maximize muscle growth, you must consistently eat more calories than you burn. This produces the calorie surplus required for optimizing your body's "muscle-building machinery."

+ If you want to neither lose nor gain fat and make slow muscle and strength gains, you want your calories in to match your calories out.

+ Protein affects your body composition far more than carbohydrate or fat does, and research shows that a high-protein diet is superior to a low-protein one in many ways.

+ At least 80 percent of your daily calories should come from nutritious, relatively unprocessed foods that you clean, cut, and cook yourself, like lean protein, fruits, vegetables, whole grains, legumes, nuts, seeds, and oils. You can then use the remaining calories for your favorite treats, if you desire.

+ It doesn't much matter whether you eat high-carb, low-carb, high-fat, low-fat when it comes to losing fat and gaining muscle. Find a balance of carbohydrate and fat intake that works for you.

+ Much of the scientific literature shows a weak albeit consistent correlation between high saturated fat intake and heart disease. I recommend limiting saturated fat to no more than 10 percent of daily calories.

+ If you're like most people, you're getting enough omega-6 fatty acids in your diet from commonly consumed foods like vegetable oil, nuts, seeds, and meat, but probably not enough omega-3s. An easy fix is with an omega-3 supplement.

7

Welcome to the Easiest Diet in the World

A small daily task, if it be really daily,
will beat the labours of a spasmodic Hercules.
—ANTHONY TROLLOPE

I f you dread "dieting," I understand. It often feels more like self-sacrifice than self-improvement. If you want to lose fat and build lean muscle, most diets say, you can kiss just about everything you like to eat good-bye. Grains, gluten, sugar, refined carbs . . . blow 'em all out of the airlock. "Maybe I'm not up to this," you've probably thought as you contemplated starting such a program—and which you may be feeling again now.

I'm here to tell you that, yes, you are up to it. With the four pillars of flexible dieting you learned in the last chapter, you can transform your body eating foods you want to eat, every day, and turn healthy eating habits into an enduring lifestyle. And in this chapter, you'll learn how—how to turn my prescription for flexible dieting into exact numbers and inclusive food menus.

There's a catch, however: it'll require some math. Nothing more than basic arithmetic, mind you, and every step will be carefully explained and illustrated, but if your brain fogs at the sight of figures, take your time with the rest of this section of the book. I've worked with enough people to know you're more than capable of mastering the numbers (I've yet to have anyone flunk this class), and you can also breathe easy knowing that we have a fail-safe fallback: premade meal plans in the back of the book for losing fat and building muscle. You won't want to follow my ready-made plans forever, but they're great guides for finding your feet.

To give you a foretaste of the *Muscle for Life* method of flexible dieting, let's walk through what a typical day may look like. As you'll see, no utensils or gadgets will be required—your hand is all you'll need for portioning your meals. You wake up and mix a scoop of protein powder with some water, milk, or a milk substitute, and you eat a banana. That holds you over until the middle of the morning, when you enjoy a fist-sized portion of low-fat Greek yogurt and a couple of thumb-sized portions of nuts. Next is lunch, when you have a palm-sized portion of chicken or fish on a homemade salad topped with tomato, carrot, and your favorite dressing. A couple of hours later, it's midafternoon snack time, and you eat a fist-sized portion of low-fat cottage cheese on a buttered English muffin. Then, at dinner, you cook up a palm-sized portion of chicken or fish and fist-sized portions of rice and a vegetable medley. Finally, to end on a (sugar) high note, you snack on your favorite dark chocolate. Your actual mileage will vary, of course, but this example gives you a flavor of the streamlined and stress-free nature of the regimen.

So, let's begin with nailing down the first element of flexible dieting: calories.

HOW MANY CALORIES
SHOULD YOU EAT EVERY DAY?

Imagine that someone told you they want to drive across the country without paying attention to the gas tank. Their plan is to stop whenever they feel like stopping and pump as much (or as little) gas as they feel like pumping. How would you respond? You'd think they're nuttier than a five-pound fruitcake, wouldn't you?

What if they picked up on that and snapped back with something like, "I hate feeling like a slave to the oppressive fuel meter. I should be able to drive as far as I want before refueling!" What would you do then? Gather up your toys and go play with someone else, right?

The point is, when someone says they want to lose (or gain) weight without paying attention to their calories, or says that energy balance has little to do with body weight, they're being just as gonzo. If you're going to upgrade your body composition, you *must* know how many calories to eat every day, and fortunately, you don't need a degree in Excel to figure that out—just the calculator in your phone.

The first step in working out your calories is deciding what you want to do with your physique. Here are your basic options:

- *Cutting*—Whenever you want to get leaner, you want to enter a *cutting phase* and consistently eat fewer calories than you're burning.
- *Lean gaining*—If you're relatively lean and you want to maximize muscle and strength gain (and minimize fat gain), you want to start a *lean gaining phase* and consistently eat slightly more calories than you're burning.
- *Maintaining*—When you're happy with your body composition,

and you want to prevent fat gain while slowly adding muscle and strength, you should begin a *maintenance phase* and consistently eat more or less how many calories you're burning.

Essentially, the path to a toned, athletic body alternates between lean gaining and cutting phases, between focusing on gaining muscle (with some fat) and then losing fat (while retaining muscle), until you love what you see in the mirror—a powerful "I've made it" moment that'll make every calorie counted and workout wrapped worth it. Think of it like farming, where you first grow and harvest crops (lean gaining) and then separate the grain from the chaff (cutting), retaining the former (muscle) and discarding the latter (fat), and then do it all over again.

The value of this cyclical approach to improving body composition is vitally important but understood by few. When you start out with strength training, your body is hyper-responsive to it, and you can easily gain muscle and lose fat at the same time when cutting—the bodybuilding equivalent of alchemy. This honeymoon period only lasts six to eight months for most people, however, and then the only reliable way to continue gaining muscle and strength is lean gaining (and fat loss still requires cutting).

Many people don't know that and try to keep cutting for far too long or settle into eating maintenance calories and err on the side of undereating and not overeating (to prevent fat gain), and they eventually stall in the gym no matter how hard they train. Stick to the strategies and techniques I'm sharing with you, and you'll avoid those shoals of stagnation.

Your efforts will pay much larger dividends over time, too, because the fitter you get, the more you can focus on enjoying the rewards of your labor rather than the work of producing them. It takes a lot more time and effort to build your best body than to maintain it, so once you have your "body for life," you'll have even more leeway in how you eat and exercise. You'll be able to pay less attention to calories and macronutrients and eat more "intuitively" (according to your body's natural cues), and mix up your training with other activities that interest you, like yoga, calisthenics, boot camps, cross-training, high-intensity interval training, or something else.

Keep that in mind as you progress on the *Muscle for Life* program because if you stick with it, you *will* get there. It's only a matter of when.

How Many Calories You Should Eat When Cutting

We've established that you must be in a calorie deficit to lose fat, but how large should that deficit be? Ten percent? Twenty percent? Larger?

Some authorities advocate *slow cutting*, which involves mild calorie restriction and moderate (at most) exercise to whittle down fat stores over many months. The advantages of this are supposedly less muscle loss, more enjoyable workouts, and fewer issues related to hunger and cravings. There's some truth here. Slow cutting can feel easier than a more ambitious approach, but the upsides aren't significant in most people and come at a steep price: duration.

Slow cutting is, well, *slow*, and for many dieters, this causes more trouble than eating less food every day. For instance, by reducing your calorie deficit from 20 to 10 percent, you're halving the amount of fat you'll lose each week and doubling the time it'll take to reach your goal. This is a problem for most people because the longer they remain in a calorie deficit of any size, the more likely they are to backslide through life commotion, dietary slipups, scheduling snafus, and so on.

Furthermore, when you know what you're doing, you can maintain a calorie deficit large enough to produce rapid fat loss without losing muscle, suffering in the gym, or facing metabolic challenges. This means faster results and less time spent restricting calories, and thus more time doing the fun stuff (maintaining and lean gaining).

Therefore, my recommendation is an aggressive but not reckless calorie deficit of 20 to 25 percent when cutting (eating 75 to 80 percent of the calories you're burning every day).

Why this number? Research show that it works well for both losing fat and preserving muscle when combined with resistance training and a high-protein diet. A study conducted by scientists at Finland's University of Jyväskylä split athletes with low levels of body fat (at or below 10 percent) into two groups:

1. Group one maintained a 300-calorie deficit (about 12 percent below their total daily energy expenditure).
2. Group two maintained a 750-calorie deficit (about 25 percent below daily expenditure).

After four weeks, the first group lost very little fat and muscle, and the second group lost, on average, about 4 pounds of fat and very little muscle, and neither group experienced any negative side effects to speak of. This is an outstanding result—and particularly in lean athletes, because the less body fat you have, the more susceptible you are to losing muscle when cutting. Other studies on calorie restriction have echoed this finding and so has my own experience working with thousands of people. When combined with a high-protein diet and reasonable workout schedule, a calorie deficit of 20 to 25 percent allows for speedy fat loss with no significant side effects. How many calories is that for you, though? This is normally where an evidence-based fitness guy like me would begin talking about formulas for calculating how much energy your body burns at rest and during different types of physical activity. This approach has advantages, especially with experienced weightlifters, but we can take a shortcut: in most people, eating between 8 and 12 calories per pound of body weight per day creates a 20 to 25 percent calorie deficit. So, if a woman weighs 160 pounds and wants to lose fat rapidly, she should eat between 1,300 (160 x 8) and 1,900 (160 x 12) calories per day; and if a man weighs 220 pounds and wants to see his abs, he should eat between 1,800 (220 x 8) and 2,600 (220 x 12) calories per day.

Physical activity level mostly determines whether you should choose the low or high end of the range. If you're sedentary (little or no exercise or vigorous physical activity), you'd have to choose the lowest number (8) to maintain an effective calorie deficit. This can work, but it isn't optimal because it'll mean subsisting on a meager meal plan ("poverty calories," as bodybuilders like to say). If you remained sedentary and just ate slightly more every day, this becomes the slow-cutting approach we just discussed—doable but suboptimal. This is one of the many reasons I recommend that underactive folk who want to cut fat figure out a way to exercise regularly—it makes the process more sustainable and rewarding.

In *Muscle for Life*, I'll ask you to do at least a couple of workouts per week when cutting so you can eat at least 9 or 10 calories per pound of body weight per day, which is appropriate for one to three hours of exercise or vigorous physical activity per week. And if you're moderately active (five or more hours of exercise or vigorous physical activity per week), you should choose the highest number (12).

How can so simple a method work? Most of the energy you burn is driven by your basic metabolic needs for survival, not physical activity. For instance, in an average adult at rest, the brain alone consumes about 20 percent of the body's energy, and the other major organs, excluding muscle, account for another 60 percent. Thus, scientists realized long ago that with the right data, they could produce formulas for estimating how many calories people burned every day if they didn't move around much.

That was an interesting start, but as the additional energy expenditure from physical activity wasn't reflected in these new metabolic calculations, there was more work to do. So researchers set out to discover how to compute and include these extra calories in their reckonings. As they learned about the energy costs of various types of activities, their models became more accurate and useful, and eventually all that was needed to roughly predict total daily energy expenditure in most people was their gender, body weight, and total hours of light, moderate, and heavy activity per week.

This line of work caught on among bodybuilders, who were keen to use it to hone their dietary protocols for losing fat and gaining muscle. Then astute practitioners developed shorthands based on patterns they observed, like the one I've shared with you (8 to 12 calories per pound of body weight per day for cutting).

So, don't mistake this simple method as simplistic. Also, remember that all you're looking to achieve with any system of determining how many calories to eat is a reasonable starting place. You can easily adjust your numbers up or down based on how your body responds (something we'll discuss later in this book), so there's no reason to make the process more complicated than it needs to be.

How Many Calories You Should Eat When Lean Gaining

Since a calorie surplus boosts muscle growth, the easiest way to maximize muscle building is to purposely eat more calories than you're burning every day. You don't want too large of a calorie surplus, however, because after a point, eating more no longer increases muscle growth but just fat gain instead.

Research suggests that this point of diminishing returns is somewhere around 110 percent of your total daily energy expenditure. By eating 10 percent more calories than you burn every day, you'll gain just as much muscle as you would eating 20 or 30 percent more, but a lot less fat. And so that's my recommendation for lean gaining: eat about 10 percent more calories than you burn every day. For most people, this comes out to 16 to 18 calories per pound of body weight.

As with cutting, physical activity level mostly determines whether you should choose the low or high end of the range. If you're sedentary (no exercise or vigorous activity), you shouldn't be lean gaining—lean gaining only makes sense if you're doing at least two strength training workouts per week, which are what drive the muscle growth, not the extra calories. If you're lightly active (one to three hours of exercise or vigorous activity per week), choose the lowest number (and work out more if possible). If you're moderately active (five or more hours of exercise or vigorous activity per week), start with the middle number, and then if you aren't gaining weight and strength steadily, move up to the highest number.

How Many Calories You Should Eat When Maintaining

Remember that this usually comes into play after you've completed several cycles of cutting and lean gaining and more or less have the body you want. When you're maintaining, not much changes in your body composition—you don't lose any fat to speak of or gain much muscle. It's like putting your physique on cruise control.

As for how many calories you should eat when maintaining, 12 to 16 calories per pound of body weight per day is the range for most people. If you're sedentary (little or no exercise or vigorous physical activity), choose the lowest number; if you're lightly active (one to three hours of exercise or vigorous physical activity per week), a middle number; and if you're moderately active (five or more hours of exercise or vigorous physical activity per week), the highest number.

And that's it for calories. Easy enough, right? Next, you need to understand how to translate your daily calorie target into grams of protein, carbohydrate, and fat (macros), because just as calories are the simplest way of measuring your energy intake, grams per day is the easiest way to track macros. It's also a useful meal planning shortcut because, as you'll see, if you set up your macros correctly, your calories will also be correct.

HOW MUCH PROTEIN YOU SHOULD EAT

You've probably heard a lot of conflicting advice on protein intake. Some people, bodybuilders in particular, recommend sky-high amounts, up to 2 grams per pound of body weight per day. Others advocate a much lower amount, claiming that anything above 0.8 grams per pound of body weight per day is unnecessary.

A significant amount of research has been done on the protein needs of people who are physically active, and a fantastic summary of the literature was coauthored by my friend Dr. Eric Helms. In his paper, he explains that 0.55 to 1 gram of protein per pound of body weight per day—or 25 to 40 percent of daily calories—is adequate when calories aren't restricted for fat loss, and when they are, about 1 gram per pound of body weight per day works well for most people.

I prefer the top of this range when cutting, lean gaining, and maintaining because the drawbacks of not eating enough protein (less muscle growth, less satiety, and less bone density, among others) are far greater than the downsides of eating a little more protein than you need (fewer calories for carbs and fat, mostly). Thus, I recommend getting 30 percent of your daily calories from protein when lean gaining or maintaining and 40 percent when cutting. For most people, this is around 0.8 to 1.2 grams of protein per pound of body weight per day, and for people who are very overweight, it may be closer to 0.6 grams of protein per pound per day.

To put ideal protein intake into perspective, here's the protein content of popular high-protein foods:

+ A palm-sized piece of chicken, pork, fish, or beef: ~20 grams of protein
+ A fist-sized portion of low-fat Greek or Icelandic (my favorite) yogurt: ~15 grams of protein
+ A thumb-sized portion of Parmesan cheese: 11 grams of protein
+ An egg: 6 grams of protein
+ A fist-sized portion of pinto, mung, or fava beans: ~14 grams of protein
+ A fist-sized portion of green peas: 8 grams of protein
+ A fist-sized portion of cooked rice or quinoa: ~7 grams of protein
+ A scoop of whey protein powder: ~20 grams of protein
+ A protein bar: ~15 to 20 grams of protein, depending on the brand

As you can see, high-protein eating is easy enough—for most people, it entails a serving or two of meat per day supplemented with some dairy, legumes, or whole grains, and a scoop or two of protein powder in between sit-down meals. That said, this is probably more protein than you're used to eating, and if you're not big on meat and dairy (the richest whole-food sources of protein), protein powder and bars will be especially helpful because of how convenient they are.

Let's now learn how to turn "percent of daily calories" into "grams of protein per day." Say you're a 160-pound woman starting a cutting phase, and you've just determined your daily calorie target is 1,600 calories. As you're cutting, 40 percent of those calories should come from protein, so you multiply 1,600 by 0.4 to get 640. Then, since each gram of protein contains about 4 calories, you only need to divide the daily calories in protein by 4 to determine how many grams of protein to eat every day. So, you divide 640 by 4, which comes to 160 grams of protein per day.

And that's it for figuring out how much protein to eat.

HOW MUCH CARBOHYDRATE YOU SHOULD EAT

While a high-carbohydrate diet works best for most physically active people, some prefer fewer carbs, and that's perfectly fine. If you're not sure what's best for you, start here: get 30 to 40 percent of your daily calories from carbohydrate regardless of whether you're cutting, lean gaining, or maintaining. This works out to about 0.75 to 2 grams of carbs per pound of body weight per day for most people.

One gram of carbohydrate also contains about 4 calories, so to calculate your carbohydrate intake, multiply your total daily calories by 0.3 to 0.4 and then divide the result by 4. Continuing with our example above, if you're planning to eat 1,600 calories per day, multiplying by 0.3 produces 480 and dividing by 4 gives 120 (grams of carbohydrate per day). And if you wanted to increase your carbs to 40 percent of your daily calories, you'd wind up with 160 grams per day (1,600 x 0.4 divided by 4).

If you know you prefer a lower-carb diet, you can adjust that number downward. For many people I've worked with over the years who enjoyed lower-carb living, 15 to 20 percent of daily calories from carbs worked well because it allowed them to eat a healthy amount of fruits and vegetables.

Keep in mind, however, that if you reduce your carbohydrate intake from 30 percent of daily calories to less, you'll need to increase either your protein or your fat intake to hit 100 percent of your daily calorie target and ensure you don't eat too little every day. While an argument could be made for the benefits of increasing just your protein intake, you'll likely want to "trade" your carbs for more fat, not protein, and that's okay so long as you keep your saturated fat intake in a healthy range. At any rate, to successfully make the low-carb adjustment, you only need to allot the calories you're "missing" to reach the assignment of 100 percent of daily calories by reducing your carbohydrate intake to protein or fat using the methods you're learning here.

On the other hand, if you know you prefer a very-high-carb diet, especially when lean gaining (many people do), you can adjust your carb intake up to 50 or even 60 percent of daily calories. Remember, though, that you need to ensure that most of those carbs are nutritious, and you must also eat enough protein (30 percent of daily calories) and ensure your fat intake doesn't drop below 20 percent of daily calories (too low for optimal health).

HOW MUCH FAT YOU SHOULD EAT

If you're not following a low-carb diet, 20 to 30 percent of daily calories from fat works well for most people. This is usually between 0.2 and 0.4 grams of fat per pound of body weight per day. If you're following a low-carb diet, however, fat intake can rise as high as 55 percent of daily calories depending on your preferences.

One gram of fat contains about 9 calories, which means you can determine how many grams of fat to eat every day by multiplying your total daily calories by 0.2 to 0.55 and then dividing the result by 9. Thus, if your daily calories are set at 1,600, the math looks like this for 30 percent of calories from fat: 1,600 x 0.3 = 480, and then 480 / 9 = 53 (grams of fat per day, which you could round down to 50 or up to 55 for simplicity).

And just like that, we've figured out the macros for someone on a cutting phase aiming to eat 1,600 calories per day:

+ 160 grams of protein (~40 percent of daily calories)
+ 120 grams of carbs (~30 percent of daily calories)
+ 50 grams of fat (~30 percent of daily calories)

Note how the percentages add up to 100—a simple test for verifying that we didn't make an obvious mistake. Now, if our volunteer would rather eat low-carb and fill in the missing calories with dietary fat:

+ 160 grams of protein (~40 percent of daily calories)
+ 60 grams of carbohydrate (~15 percent of daily calories)
+ 80 grams of fat (~45 percent of daily calories)

To help you further understand all of this in action, I want to show you some examples of calorie and macronutrient targets (with varying ratios of carbs and fat) for different weights, goals, and activity levels. Also, if you run the numbers yourself, you'll notice I'm rounding up and down—62 grams of fat becomes 60, for instance, 278 grams of carbs becomes 280, and so forth.

Weight	Goal	Activity Level	Calories	Protein	Carbs	Fat
120 lbs	Cutting	3 hours/week	1,200	120 g	90 g	40 g
140 lbs	Cutting	6 hours/week	1,700	170 g	130 g	55 g
160 lbs	Cutting	2 hours/week	1,600	160 g	105 g	60 g
200 lbs	Cutting	5 hours/week	2,400	240 g	190 g	75 g
220 lbs	Cutting	8 hours/week	2,600	260 g	280 g	50 g
120 lbs	Lean gaining	5 hours/week	2,000	150 g	170 g	80 g
150 lbs	Lean gaining	3 hours/week	2,400	180 g	180 g	110 g
180 lbs	Lean gaining	8 hours/week	3,100	230 g	410 g	60 g

So much for the arithmetic of dieting. Now let's discuss food choices.

WHAT KINDS OF FOODS YOU SHOULD EAT

It's nice to imagine that eating a few special foods every day could super-charge your body composition, metabolism, and physical performance. But there are no individual foods that can single-handedly transform your health and fitness. Only an overall lifestyle can do that—one that revolves around eating nutritious food, exercising regularly, maintaining good sleep hygiene, and balancing stress and relaxation.

Marketers won't let a pesky fact like that thwart their designs on our paychecks, though, so we have the "superfood" phenomenon, and spinach, quinoa, kale, berries, and tea are in their heyday.

This development has encouraged many people to eat better, but it has also confused many about how their body functions and how to make it look and work better. Here's the heart of the matter: to get adequate nutrition, including vitamins, minerals, and fiber, you'll need to eat several portions of fruit and vegetables every day. Just as energy balance is a nonnegotiable aspect of weight management and high-protein dieting is vital to gaining muscle and strength, eating an abundance of fruits and vegetables is essential to staying healthy. It's also smart to eat a variety of fruits and veggies—especially colorful ones—because some are richer in certain nutrients than others. Here's a list of much of the good stuff:

- ✦ Apple
- ✦ Arugula
- ✦ Asparagus
- ✦ Avocado
- ✦ Banana
- ✦ Blackberry
- ✦ Blueberry
- ✦ Bok choy and other Asian greens
- ✦ Broccoli
- ✦ Brussels sprout
- ✦ Cabbage
- ✦ Carrot
- ✦ Cauliflower
- ✦ Celery
- ✦ Cherry
- ✦ Cranberry
- ✦ Cucumber
- ✦ Eggplant
- ✦ Garlic
- ✦ Grape
- ✦ Grapefruit
- ✦ Green bean
- ✦ Kale
- ✦ Leek
- ✦ Lemon
- ✦ Lettuce
- ✦ Mango
- ✦ Mushroom
- ✦ Onion
- ✦ Orange
- ✦ Pineapple
- ✦ Radish
- ✦ Spinach
- ✦ Strawberry
- ✦ Swiss chard
- ✦ Zucchini

It would be disingenuous to call any of these options "superfoods" in the way the term is normally used, but collectively, they're a superb category of chow.

As for your protein, if you're not going to eat a high-fat diet, most of it should come from lean sources like meat, fish, eggs, high-protein dairy products, soy, whey, casein, and plant-based protein powders; and most of your remaining calories should come from wholesome sources of carbohydrate and fat, like whole grains (brown rice, corn, oats, quinoa, barley, etc.), legumes (beans and peas), tubers (potatoes and other root vegetables), oils, nuts, seeds, and avocados.

You may have noticed I haven't endorsed caloric beverages. While they can have some nutritional value (fruit juice, milk, and sports drinks, for instance), they're usually less wholesome than and don't trigger satiety as effectively as food, making them an inferior source of calories. You can drink 500 calories of a sugar-sweetened beverage and be hungry an hour later, for instance, whereas eating 500 calories of protein-and-fiber-rich food will keep you full for hours. Hence, it's not surprising that studies show that people who drink calories are much more likely to overeat than those who don't. There's also a clear association between a greater intake of sugar-sweetened beverages and weight gain in both adults and children.

That said, you don't have to completely abstain from all caloric beverages. Except in the case of whole milk (for which we'll make an exception and label it a source of healthy fat, because it is), you just have to regard them as treats—the next and final element of *Muscle for Life* meal planning we'll discuss.

What should you mostly drink, then? You guessed it—water. In fact, drinking enough water is one of the simplest ways to immediately enhance many aspects of your health and performance. Research shows that dehydration impairs cognition and endurance, depresses mood, causes constipation, and may even increase the risk of heart disease.

Thus, the National Academy of Medicine (formerly the Institute of Medicine) recommends a baseline intake of about ¾ of a gallon (about 12 cups or 3 liters) of water per day for adult men and women, with additional drinking to replace fluids lost through significant amounts of sweating. Down an additional 1 to 1.5 liters of water per hour of sweaty physical activity, and you'll stay well hydrated.

While we're on the topic, let's also address the common myth that caffeinated beverages like coffee and tea are dehydrating. While it's true that caffeine has a slight diuretic effect, studies show that it's minimal even at high doses (up to 500 milligrams per day) and doesn't meaningfully reduce hydration status. So, good news: you can count your jitter juice toward your water intake.

WHAT ABOUT TREATS?

One of the many perks of flexible dieting is that no foods are off-limits, regardless of how "unhealthy" they supposedly are (because no individual food can harm your health, only your diet on the whole can). That's why, with flexible dieting, you can allot up to 20 percent of your daily calories to your favorite indulgences when cutting, lean gaining, or maintaining, and use them on whatever combination of protein, carbs, and fat you'd like. For instance, my favorite choices are often dark chocolate, ice cream, and restaurant meals, and at other times pancakes, pastries, and pasta.

Let's see how this might work with our 1,600-calorie cutting plan. In this case, we'd have 320 calories to give over to goodies, which provides plenty of options: nearly a pint of some brands of low-calorie ice cream, half of a bar of chocolate, three Reese's cups, a small bag of chips, or a few Oreos, for example. And yes, when you're eating more calories (lean gaining or maintaining), that means more room for delicious additions!

So, what will you reward yourself with every day? Start making your mental list now, because soon one or more will be in your meal plan!

Every so often, another headline pops up and proclaims that "diets don't work." According to one expert or another, no matter what people do, if it qualifies as "dieting," it won't result in significant and long-term weight loss. You may have concluded this yourself based on your own experiences.

The real problem isn't that "dieting" doesn't work, but that most diets suck. They restrict calories too heavily, leaving you feeling miserable; feed you too little protein, boosting hunger and muscle loss; prohibit too many foods, making them impractical and irritating; and provide no exit ramp to help you return to normal eating, increasing the likelihood of regaining some, much, or even all of the fat lost. That's why a new approach to dieting is needed—one that sets you up for a physical, psychological, and emotional victory.

The solution is flexible dieting. It truly is the easiest diet in the world because it's effective and enjoyable, no matter your goals, circumstances, and inclinations. You're about to see for yourself, too, because in the next chapter you'll turn your calories, macros, and food choices into a *Muscle for Life* eating plan that you can implement right away.

KEY TAKEAWAYS

+ Whenever you want to get leaner, you want to enter a cutting phase and consistently eat fewer calories than you're burning.

+ If you're relatively lean and you want to maximize muscle and strength gain (and minimize fat gain), you want to start a lean gaining phase and consistently eat slightly more calories than you're burning.

+ When you're happy with your body composition, and you want to prevent fat gain while slowly adding muscle and strength, you should begin a maintenance phase and consistently eat more or less how many calories you're burning.

+ To achieve a toned, athletic body, alternate between lean gaining and cutting phases, where you focus on gaining muscle (with some fat gain) and then losing fat (while retaining your muscle) until you love what you see in the mirror.

+ Use an aggressive but not reckless calorie deficit of 20 to 25 percent when cutting (eat 75 to 80 percent of the calories you're burning every day when cutting).

+ In most people, eating between 8 and 12 calories per pound of body weight per day creates a 20 to 25 percent calorie deficit.

+ For lean gaining, eat about 10 percent more calories than you burn every day. For most people, this is 16 to 18 calories per pound of body weight per day.

+ As for how many calories you should eat when maintaining, 12 to 16 calories per pound of body weight per day works well for most people.

- Get 30 percent of your daily calories from protein when lean gaining or maintaining and 40 percent when cutting. This is usually around 0.8 to 1.2 grams of protein per pound of body weight per day, and for people who are very overweight, it may be closer to 0.6 grams of protein per pound per day.

- Get 30 to 40 percent of your daily calories from carbohydrate regardless of whether you're cutting, lean gaining, or maintaining. This works out to about 0.75 to 2 grams of carbs per pound of body weight per day for most people.

- If you're not following a low-carb diet, 20 to 30 percent of daily calories from fat works well. This is typically between 0.2 and 0.4 gram of fat per pound of body weight per day.

- To get adequate nutrition, including vitamins, minerals, and fiber, you'll need to eat several portions of fruit and vegetables every day.

- Unless you're eating a high-fat diet, most of your protein should come from lean sources like meat, fish, eggs, high-protein dairy products, soy, whey, casein, and plant-based protein powders.

- With flexible dieting, you can allot up to 20 percent of your daily calories to your favorite indulgences when cutting, lean gaining, or maintaining, and use them on whatever combination of protein, carbs, and fat you'd like.

8

The *Muscle for Life* Meal Plan

There's more to life than training,
but training is what puts more in your life.
—BROOKS KUBIK

How important is your diet to achieving your health and fitness goals? Some people say it's everything. Others say it's not as important as exercise, genetics, or some other factor. Still others say it's 70, 80, or even 90 percent of the game. I say it's 100 percent. And training properly? That's another 100 percent. Having the right attitude is 100 percent too. And let's not forget getting adequate rest and sleep, because that's also 100 percent. (I know, we're at 400 percent so far. . . .)

We need a different paradigm because the building blocks of a great body are more like pillars than puzzle pieces. If you weaken one enough, the whole structure collapses. Your body composition won't progress if you don't regulate your calories and macros. You won't recover from your training if you don't support it with proper nutrition. You won't gain much muscle or strength if you don't train correctly. Your compliance won't hold up if you have the wrong attitude. Your workout performance won't improve if you don't generally get enough sleep.

That's why I want you to go all-in on achieving your fitness goals. I want you to give 100 percent in each part of the *Muscle for Life* program and achieve 100 percent of the potential results. Let other people train at just 60 percent, diet at just 30 percent, and give just 20 percent of their spirit. They'll make you look that much better.

All that aside, here's the practical answer to how important diet is in your fitness journey: your diet either works for you or it works against you, multiplying or dividing the bottom-line results you get from your training. You can think of diet as a series of tollbooths along the highway of fat loss and muscle gain. Training moves you forward, but if you don't stop and pay your dues, you don't get to go any farther.

No matter how much you get right in the gym, you'll never be fully satisfied with the results unless you also get things right in the kitchen. This is why so many people spend so much time exercising yet look like they've never even seen a barbell or bicycle, let alone touched one.

Here's another helpful perspective on the relationship between diet, training, and body composition: diet is primarily how you lose fat, maintain a desirable body fat level, and boost muscle growth, while training is primarily how you gain and maintain strength, muscle mass, and endurance.

Many people get this mixed up. They think that working out is mostly for calorie and fat burning and fall into a frustrating and ultimately fruitless cycle of grueling exercise just to keep pace with all their eating. This is mentally and physically exhausting, and when taken to the extreme endangers one's long-term health and well-being. Fortunately, that won't happen to you on my program—with *Muscle for Life*, you'll be permanently protected from this trap.

In the last chapter, you learned about three phases of dieting depending on your goals, as well as rough guidelines for when to use each:

1. Cutting—for getting leaner
2. Lean gaining—for gaining muscle as quickly as possible
3. Maintaining—for slowly gaining muscle or maintaining muscle gained while staying lean

Now you'll decide where to start your *Muscle for Life* journey (cutting, lean gaining, or maintaining) and then create a meal plan with the right numbers of calories and macronutrients.

SHOULD YOU CUT, LEAN GAIN, OR MAINTAIN?

If you're unhappy with your body fat percentage and want to get lean, you want to cut first. There's no reason to get fatter (which will happen when you lean gain because even a slight calorie surplus produces some fat gain) just to gain muscle a little faster if that's not your primary concern right now. Similarly, if you're very **overweight**, you also want to cut first. This is the healthiest and smartest choice, even if your long-range goal involves gaining a fair amount of muscle mass.

If you're thin or lean and want to focus on gaining muscle and strength, you want to lean gain. And if you follow my advice, it'll truly be a *lean* gain, as research shows that for the first couple of months, people new to strength training gain very little fat while in a calorie surplus.

Finally, if you're in the middle—if your body fat is in a normal range and you also want more muscle definition—whether you should cut, lean gain, or maintain first is dictated by your body fat percentage. If you're a man at 15 percent body fat or higher or a woman at 25 percent or higher, I recommend you start by cutting down to around 10 percent body fat (men)/20 percent (women), for two reasons:

1. You'll be happier with how you look. We don't have to be ripped year-round, but at least half of the reason we stick to a meal plan and bust our butt in the gym is to look good. Once you get above 15 percent body fat (men)/25 percent (women), you can start feeling overweight, and this can make it harder to stay the course. At some point, you'll question why you're working so hard to look and feel like *that*. By never letting your body fat percentage go too high, however, you'll find it easier to stay motivated.

2. You'll have an easier time cutting. The longer you remain in a calorie deficit, the more likely you are to struggle with hunger, cravings, and the other unwanted side effects of dieting. Thus, when you gain too much fat, you set yourself up for a longer, more difficult cut. If you always keep your body fat at a reasonable level, however, your cuts will be shorter and more manageable, both physically and psychologically.

Lastly, if your body fat percentage is somewhere between 10 and 15 percent (men) or 20 and 25 percent (women), you can choose to cut, lean gain, or maintain, based on what's most appealing to you. What gets you most excited and ready to begin? Pick that.

To help you determine your current body fat percentage, consult the following images.

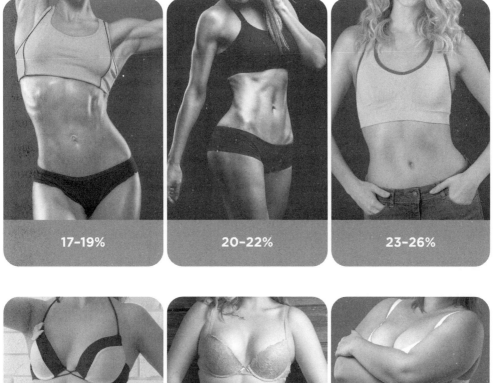

17–19%　　**20–22%**　　**23–26%**

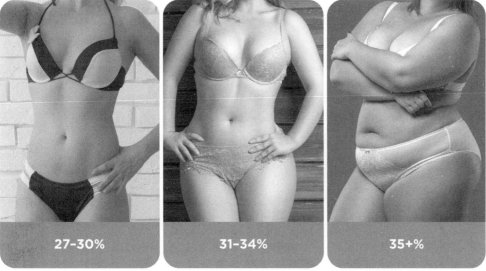

27–30%　　**31–34%**　　**35+%**

All images © Shutterstock

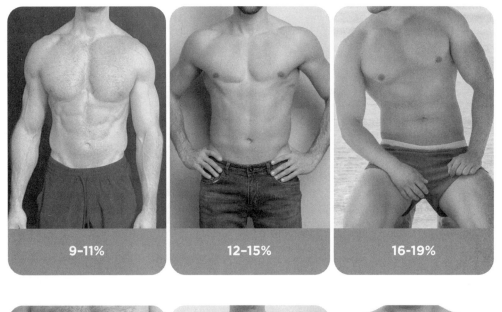

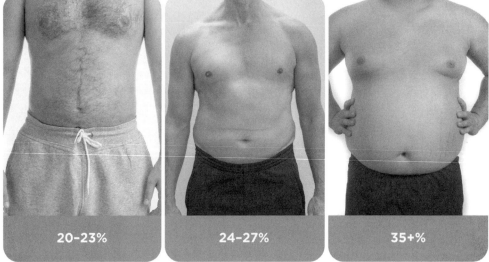

Top left: Michael Matthews; all other images © Shutterstock

As you can see, the "athletic" look begins around 25 percent body fat in women and 15 percent in men, "ripped" describes around 20/10 percent, and the leaner you get from there, the more you look like a fitness cover model.

If you want a more precise and data-driven estimate of your body composition, you can use a device called a caliper to lightly pinch and measure the thickness of the skin and underlying fat in several places on your body. The procedure of *skinfold testing* (as it's known) that's most popular among body-builders is known as the Jackson/Pollock 3-Site method, and it involves measuring in three locations—the right triceps, right thigh, and right suprailiac (just above the right hip bone) for women, and the right pec (chest muscle), abdomen, and right thigh for men—and using mathematical formulas to translate those measurements into an approximation of body fatness.

Obviously, the accuracy of this technique depends on the accuracy of the skinfold measurements, so let's review how to take them correctly, starting with the fundamentals of proper skinfold testing.

+ Take all measurements on the right side of your body while standing with your muscles relaxed (flexing will produce inaccurate measurements).
+ Pinch your skin by placing the thumb and forefinger on your body about two inches apart, firmly pushing them into your flesh and then together, and then gently pulling the skinfold away from your body.
+ Measure a pinched skinfold by placing the tips of the caliper in the middle of and perpendicular to it (between your fingertips), compress the caliper until it clicks (and no more), and note the measurement. And in case you're wondering, an example of a good

caliper that clicks when optimal pressure is applied (not all do) is one produced by the company Accu-Measure.

✦ Take each measurement three times, rotating between the different measuring sites, and calculate the average for each site. For example, if you're a woman, you'd take the first measurements of your right triceps, thigh, and suprailiac, then a second round of measurements, followed by the third, and then figure out the average number for each spot. So, if your first thigh measurement is 20 mm, your second is 24 mm, and your third is 22 mm, the average you'd use to figure out your body fat percentage would be 22 mm.

As for how to take specific measurements, here are simple instructions for each:

✦ To take a triceps measurement, standing with your right arm at your side (pointing at the floor), have someone pinch a vertical fold of skin in the center of the back side of your arm halfway between the top of your shoulder and your elbow.

✦ To take a thigh measurement, pinch a vertical fold of skin in the center of the front of your right thigh halfway between your kneecap and the spot where the top of your thigh connects with your hip.

✦ To take a suprailiac measurement, pinch a diagonal fold of skin directly above the anterior superior iliac spine, which is the bony protrusion on the front edge of your right hip bone.

✦ To take a pec measurement, pinch a diagonal skinfold halfway between your right nipple and the front edge of your right armpit.

✦ To take an abdomen measurement, pinch a vertical fold of skin one inch to the right of your belly button.

Once you have your three averages, you plug them into one of the following formulas to calculate your body fat percentage. For women, it looks like this:

Body density = 1.0994921 − (0.0009929 x sum of skinfolds) + (0.0000023 x square of the sum of skinfolds) − (0.0001392 x age)

Body fat percentage (%) = (495 / body density) − 450

And for men, like this:

Body density = 1.10938 − (0.0008267 x sum of skinfolds) + (0.0000016 x square of the sum of skinfolds) − (0.0002574 x age)

Body fat percentage (%) = (495 / body density) − 450

Chances are you'd rather skip the math, so I created a simple online calculator to do it for you, which you can find at www.muscleforlifebook.com /skinfold.

Also, before we move on, you should know that skinfold testing of any kind tends to work best for people with moderate to high levels of body fat (15 percent and higher in men and 25 percent and up in women). If you're leaner than this, it'll likely underestimate your true body fat percentage (for example, the method I just shared says I'm just over 5 percent body fat, when in reality, I'm probably closer to 9 percent).

HOW LONG SHOULD YOU CUT, LEAN GAIN, AND MAINTAIN?

How long you should cut depends on how much fat you have to lose and how quickly you lose it, and how long you should lean gain depends on how lean you are when you start and how quickly you gain fat. Here are good general directions:

+ Your cut phases should end when you're around 10 to 12 percent body fat (men)/20 to 22 percent (women). Unless you have a special reason to get leaner, don't bother, because it's not sustainable for most people. Thus, when cutting, plan to go for as long as it takes to get to your target body fat percentage (which can be higher if you prefer). This is eight to twelve weeks in most cases, but it can also take months if you have a lot of fat to lose.

+ Your lean gain phases should end when you're around 15 to 17 percent body fat (men)/25 to 27 percent (women), because if you go any further, you'll regret it once it comes time to cut. Therefore, when lean gaining, aim to go for as long as it takes to reach the body fat percentage ceiling (unless you want to end sooner for whatever reason). This is twelve to sixteen weeks for most people.

When you've finished a cutting phase, you have two options: maintenance if you're happy with your physique or just want to enjoy your new-found muscle definition before starting another round of lean gaining; and lean gaining if you have more muscle to gain and are ready to get after it.

This is the simple recipe you rinse and repeat to transform your physique—lean gaining to ~17/27 percent body fat, cutting to ~10/20 percent, assessing your figure, and proceeding accordingly. You can liken it to sculpting, where you alternate between adding clay to your creation (lean gaining) and then molding it into shapes and curves (cutting) until you're ready to bake its final form (maintenance).

When you need to cut for longer than eight weeks to reach your goal, I don't recommend you remain in a calorie deficit every day from the beginning until the end. If you have a lot of fat to lose, it may take many months to reach your body fat goal, and while you could just gut it out, a better approach is to break up the cutting phase into intermittent periods of restricting and raising your calories. An effective and evidence-based method of doing this is after every six to eight weeks of calorie restriction, increase your calories to a maintenance level for five to seven days.

These respites are known as *diet breaks* because they give your body and mind a break from the stresses of dieting. Here's how to execute a diet break properly:

1. Calculate your daily maintenance calories by multiplying your body weight by the appropriate number (as discussed in the last chapter). Fourteen calories per pound of body weight per day should work well if you're following the *Muscle for Life* program.

2. Subtract your current daily calorie intake from your maintenance calories to determine how much more you should eat every day.

3. Add food to your meal plan until you reach your maintenance calories, and for bonus points, get at least half of these extra calories from carbs, as this magnifies the benefits of the diet break.

4. Follow your modified meal plan for five to seven days.

5. Return to cutting for another six to eight weeks.

Let's see how this would work for a 200-pound man eating 2,200 calories per day to lose fat. After six weeks of cutting, his energy levels have fallen and hunger and cravings have risen—normal occurrences when dieting— and he decides to take a diet break. His maintenance calories are 2,800 per day (200 x 14), so he needs to increase his daily calorie intake by 600 calories (2,800 – 2,200). He does this by adding 150 grams of carbs to his meal plan (600 / 4 calories per gram of carbohydrate) in the form of oatmeal and fruit in the morning, pita bread at lunch, and rice at dinner. After seven days of enjoying the extra food, he removes the additional carbs from his meal plan to return to 2,200 calories per day, so he can start losing fat again. Then, six to eight weeks later, he'll consider taking another diet break.

The last issue to address before we learn how to make a meal plan is the duration of maintenance periods. How long should you maintain? Simple— for as long as you'd like.

The only downside to maintenance is not much changes with your body composition. You don't gain muscle and strength as quickly as with lean gaining, and you don't lose or gain any fat to speak of. This is why maintenance is best suited to people who have achieved a considerable amount of muscle development and definition and want to stay lean for an extended stretch of time (during the summer, for instance). Otherwise, switching between cutting and lean gaining is more productive.

All right. You now have a clear idea of where to start the *Muscle for Life* program:

1. Cutting until you reach 10 to 12 percent body fat (men)/20 to 22 percent (women), with diet breaks as needed; or
2. lean gaining until you reach 15 to 17/25 to 27 percent body fat; or
3. maintenance, until you want to lean out with cutting or accelerate muscle gain with lean gaining.

Next you need a meal plan, so let's get you one.

THE *MUSCLE FOR LIFE* MEAL PLANS

What's the easiest way to learn to ride a bike? Training wheels, right? Then, once you've built up enough confidence and skill, you can ditch the stabilizers and ride freely. This is also the best way to learn how to eat and train. You start slow and simple with clear instructions, and once you've logged enough meals and workouts, you can add more moving parts without losing control.

This section will give you one of those training wheels in the form of simple directions for creating effective meal plans you'll enjoy, and in the back of the book you'll find done-for-you examples that'll save you the time and trouble of creating your own. Then, in the next section of the book, we'll bolt on the second wheel by teaching you the rudiments of effective exercise and providing you with precise workout plans that'll put everything into immediate practice.

The *Muscle for Life* Method of Meal Planning

First, let's clarify what I mean by "meal planning," because there are many ways to define the term. In *Muscle for Life*, a meal plan is a single-day eating schedule that meets your calorie and macronutrient targets with mostly nutritional foods. You can include as little or as much variety in your meal plan as you'd like, meaning you can eat the same foods every meal, every day until you feel like switching things up; or you can include several options for one or more meals in your plan and choose between them as desired.

In my experience, many beginners think they'll need a lot of variety in their meal plan to successfully stick to it, but then are pleasantly surprised to discover they don't because when they can eat stuff they like, they don't mind eating it regularly. Further, they come to appreciate the convenience and simplicity of uniform eating.

You can also create more than one meal plan if your eating patterns will change drastically. For instance, you may want to eat fewer and different meals on the weekends than on the weekdays, and this can be easily accomplished by creating a meal plan for each scenario. In practice, most people wind up with one or two meal plans with an extra meal or two, and they follow these plans for weeks or even months before making any changes. You'll quickly discover what works best for you.

There are many ways to create meal plans, but the best ones accomplish five things:

+ They control your calories.
+ They control your macros.
+ They provide plenty of nutrition.
+ They allow you to eat foods you like.
+ They allow you to eat on a schedule you like.

The more a meal plan meets those criteria, the more likely it is to work, and when it checks all of the boxes, results are all but guaranteed. The *Muscle for Life* method does just that. The process is simple, too. All you have to do is:

1. Calculate your calories and macros.
2. Decide how many meals to eat.
3. Decide what to eat and drink.
4. Decide how much to eat and drink.

And voilà, you have a first-class meal plan and are off to the races. Let's see how to get there.

1. Calculate your calories and macros.

As you learned in the previous chapter, this is a simple matter of figuring out your calories based on your physique goals and activity level, and changing them into macros based on proportions. Let's recap calorie calculation first.

	Cutting	Lean Gaining	Maintaining
Sedentary (little or no exercise or vigorous physical activity)	8 calories per pound of body weight per day	You shouldn't be lean gaining.	12 calories per pound of body weight per day
Lightly active (1 to 3 hours of exercise or vigorous physical activity per week)	10 calories per pound of body weight per day	16 calories per pound of body weight per day	14 calories per pound of body weight per day
Moderately active (5 or more hours of exercise or vigorous physical activity per week)	12 calories per pound of body weight per day	17 calories per pound of body weight per day	16 calories per pound of body weight per day

Remember, you may need to eat slightly more or less than these guidelines indicate to actually reach your goals, but these directions provide useful jumping-off points that can be adjusted (if needed) according to how your body responds.

Stop reading for a moment, work out your daily calorie target now based on how much time you plan to give to your *Muscle for Life* workouts every week (three to six hours is ideal for most people), and write it below.

....

....

....

Next you'll need to turn your calories into macros. Let's review how to do this.

	Protein	Carbohydrate	Fat
Cutting	40 percent of daily calories	15 to 60 percent of daily calories; 30 to 40 percent is ideal for most people	20 to 55 percent of daily calories. 30 percent is ideal for most people
Lean gaining	30 percent of daily calories	15 to 60 percent of daily calories; 30 to 40 percent is ideal for most people	20 to 55 percent of daily calories; 30 percent is ideal for most people
Maintaining	30 percent of daily calories	15 to 60 percent of daily calories; 30 to 40 percent is ideal for most people	20 to 55 percent of daily calories; 30 percent is ideal for most people

And now let's pause to figure out your macros and fill them in below.

....

....

....

....

2. Decide how many meals to eat.

Raise your hand if you've heard this one before: you should eat many small meals—especially when cutting—to "stoke the metabolic fire," accelerate fat burning, and reduce hunger. When you eat, your metabolism supposedly speeds up as your body processes the food, so if you eat every few hours, your metabolism will remain in a constantly elevated state. Nibbling on food throughout the day should help with appetite control, right?

While these theories may seem plausible, they haven't panned out in scientific research. Extensive studies have found no meaningful metabolic difference between eating many small and a few large meals because small ones cause small, short metabolic gains, and large ones cause larger, longer rises. Appetite, on the other hand, can go both ways. In some people, eating more frequently has no effect on hunger levels, in others it decreases them, and in others still, it increases hunger.

So, the best meal schedule is simply the one that works best for you given your inclinations and lifestyle. Most people I've worked with enjoyed eating four to six meals per day (breakfast, lunch, and dinner, with a snack or two in between, or after dinner), but some preferred eating just two (lunch and dinner) or three (breakfast, lunch, and dinner). That said, I do recommend eating at least two meals per day, as research shows that eating just one meal per day can make it harder to gain and maintain muscle.

To help you decide how many meals to eat on the *Muscle for Life* program, here are a few things to consider:

- **Your appetite.** When are you hungriest? Probably in either the mornings or the evenings, and by taking this into account when planning your meals, you can make it significantly easier to stick to your diet and get results. So feel free to eat a large or a light breakfast—or skip it altogether if you're not hungry until around lunchtime (intermittent fasting, basically); and while I don't recommend skipping dinner (because it can produce late-night hunger that impairs sleep), it doesn't have to be a substantial amount of food—a serving of protein and vegetables is adequate.

- **Your eating preferences.** Appetite aside, are you generally a breakfast, lunch, or dinner person? Consider this when deciding how and when to eat every day. For instance, my favorite meal of the day is dinner because I most enjoy meat, vegetables, and whole grains, so I eat a large portion of my calories at the end of the day.

- **Your schedule.** Do you have time for a few sit-down meals every day or are you out the door early and on the go until dinner? If it's the latter, don't be afraid to go for long stretches of time without eating or, if you prefer, to eat smaller snack-sized meals throughout the day instead of a few squares.

Reflect on these criteria, come up with a meal schedule that makes sense to you, and write it down below.

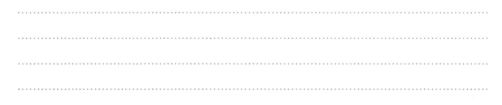

....

....

....

....

3. Decide what to eat and drink.

In this step, you'll figure out what foods to eat every day. To do this, we'll start by listing your favorite types of . . .

+ **Protein:** foods that are mostly protein, like red meat, poultry, and seafood; high-protein dairy like cottage cheese, skyr, Greek yogurt, high-protein milk, etc.; egg whites; high-protein plant foods like tofu, tempeh, seitan, etc.; and protein powders and bars.

+ **Nutritious carbs:** relatively unprocessed foods that are mostly carbohydrate, like fruits, veggies, legumes, tubers, and whole grains.

+ **Healthy fat:** relatively unprocessed foods that are mostly fat, like olive oil, avocados, nuts and nut butters, seeds, whole eggs, and most full-fat dairy like regular yogurt, cheese, butter, and milk.

+ **Treats:** relatively nonnutritious and often highly processed foods and caloric beverages, many with added sugar, like white bread and pasta, fruit juice, soda, breakfast cereal and bars, candy, and desserts.

If a food you want to eat isn't explicitly listed above, you can still include it in your meal plan—just categorize it properly. For example, my lists would look like this:

- **Protein:** chicken breast, pork tenderloin, ground beef, skyr (high-protein yogurt), New York strip steak, low-fat cottage cheese, egg whites, and whey and vegan protein powder
- **Nutritious carbs:** onions, garlic, broccoli, mushrooms, peppers, carrots, cauliflower, green beans, peas, Brussels sprouts, strawberries, bananas, blueberries, potatoes, sweet potatoes, rice, quinoa, oatmeal, and black beans
- **Healthy fat:** olive oil, avocados, pecans, walnuts, whole milk, whole eggs, and fish oil (supplement)
- **Treats:** dark chocolate, ice cream, pasta, baked goods, and pancakes

There are four important elements that need special treatment, however:

1. Recipes
2. Restaurant meals
3. Alcohol
4. Other beverages (coffee, tea, diet soda, etc.)

Let's talk about each.

Recipes

You can include recipes in your meal plans, but you must know how much protein, carbohydrate, and fat (and thus calories) are in each serving. For this reason, stick with recipes that provide the macros or simple ones with foods that fit nicely into our groups above so you can calculate the macros yourself (which you'll learn how to do soon).

The key is simplicity—ingredients you can easily measure and enhance with low- or zero-calorie spices and additions. Avoid recipes that contain ingredients, proportions, or steps that make calculating the macros difficult. Save those for later, when you're a more experienced meal planner—they're not worth the hassle right now.

So, for example, instead of eating a portion of boring boiled rice, you can add a portion of butter, a splash of lime juice, and some chopped cilantro to spice it up. Then you only need to include the portions of rice and butter in your calculations because the lime juice and cilantro contain basically no calories.

Fortunately, it's easy to find simple, delicious, and macro-friendly recipes for lean protein, nutritious carbs, healthy fat, and even desserts. The free bonus material that comes with this book (www.muscleforlifebook .com/bonus) includes twenty fitness-friendly recipes, and you can find many more of my favorites in my flexible dieting cookbook *The Shredded Chef*, and hundreds at my blog (www.muscleforlifebook.com/blog). Another fantastic resource is Gina Homolka's website www.skinnytaste.com as well as her Skinnytaste cookbooks.

Here are examples of recipes that work great with this style of meal planning:

High-Protein Breakfast Casserole

Serves 6

PER SERVING:

- ✦ 329 calories
- ✦ 34 grams of protein
- ✦ 15 grams of carbs
- ✦ 13 grams of fat

INGREDIENTS:

- ✦ 2 large sweet potatoes or red potatoes, chopped into small pieces
- ✦ 12 ounces 93% lean ground turkey
- ✦ 1 tablespoon garlic (minced or paste)
- ✦ 1 tablespoon Italian seasoning
- ✦ Sea salt and freshly ground black pepper, to taste
- ✦ 5 whole large eggs
- ✦ 10 large egg whites
- ✦ ⅓ cup skim milk
- ✦ 1 large zucchini, chopped
- ✦ 2 red bell peppers, chopped
- ✦ 1 cup chopped portobello or white mushrooms
- ✦ 1¼ cups shredded reduced-fat cheddar cheese

INSTRUCTIONS:

1. Place an oven rack in the lower third of the oven and preheat the oven to 420°F (215°C).
2. Coat a baking sheet with nonstick spray and set aside.
3. Spread the sweet potatoes evenly on the baking sheet. Bake for about 15 minutes.
4. While the sweet potatoes are baking, heat a skillet over medium-high heat and add the turkey. Season with the garlic, Italian seasoning, and

a few pinches of salt and pepper, and cook, stirring until the meat is crumbled and no longer pink on the inside (6 to 8 minutes). Remove from the heat and set aside.

5. In a medium bowl, beat together the whole eggs, egg whites, and milk.

6. In an 8 x 8-inch casserole dish or individual baking tins, add the cooked turkey, baked sweet potatoes, zucchini, bell peppers, and mushrooms. Pour the egg mixture over the other ingredients, and sprinkle the cheese on top.

7. Bake for about 25 minutes or until the cheese is browned and a knife inserted into the middle of the casserole comes out clean.

Creamy Blueberry-Banana Smoothie

Serves 2

PER SERVING:

- 228 calories
- ~10 to 35 grams of protein
- 31 grams of carbs
- 7 grams of fat

INGREDIENTS:

- 1 medium-sized ripe banana (preferably frozen), peeled and sliced
- ½ cup frozen blueberries
- ½ cup low-fat Greek yogurt
- 1 cup low-fat milk
- 1 teaspoon honey
- 1 tablespoon whole flaxseed
- 1 scoop whey or other protein powder (optional)

INSTRUCTIONS:

1. Put the banana, blueberries, milk, yogurt, honey, and flaxseed into a blender and process until smooth (about 1 minute). Pour into 2 glasses and serve!

Sweet Potato Chips

Serves 6

PER SERVING:

- 61 calories
- 1 gram of protein
- 10 grams of carbs
- 2 grams of fat

INGREDIENTS:

- 2 medium sweet potatoes (5 ounces each), peeled and thinly sliced
- 1 tablespoon extra-virgin olive oil
- ½ teaspoon salt

INSTRUCTIONS:

1. Position one rack in the center of the oven and one near the bottom. Preheat the oven to 400°F (200°C). Coat two baking sheets with cooking spray.
2. Place the sweet potatoes in a large bowl and drizzle with the oil. Toss to coat using tongs or clean hands. Arrange the potatoes on the baking sheets in an even layer.
3. Bake for 22 to 25 minutes or until the centers of the potatoes are soft and edges are slightly crispy, turning them over halfway through the baking time. Sprinkle with the salt and serve.

Raspberry-Walnut Chicken Salad Sandwich

Serves 6

PER SERVING:

+ 374 calories
+ 29 grams of protein

+ 33 grams of carbs
+ 14 grams of fat

INGREDIENTS:

+ ½ cup plain nonfat Greek yogurt
+ ¼ cup mayonnaise
+ 2 tablespoons light raspberry-walnut salad dressing
+ 1 pound chicken breast, cooked and shredded
+ 1½ teaspoons finely chopped red onion
+ ½ cup walnuts, chopped
+ ½ cup fresh raspberries
+ 12 slices whole-wheat bread

INSTRUCTIONS:

1. In a medium bowl, mix the yogurt, mayonnaise, and salad dressing together.
2. Stir in the chicken until well blended, then the onion and walnuts.
3. Gently stir in the raspberries, then spread the mixture on 6 pieces of the bread. Top with the remaining 6 pieces of bread and serve.

Creamy Herbed Chicken Salad

Serves 4

PER SERVING:

- 407 calories
- 46 grams of protein
- 25 grams of carbs
- 16 grams of fat

INGREDIENTS:

- ¼ cup fresh flat-leaf parsley leaves
- ¼ cup fresh basil leaves
- ½ cup fresh dill sprigs
- 2 oil-packed anchovies, drained
- 1 small garlic clove
- ⅓ cup mayonnaise
- ⅓ cup sour cream
- 2 tablespoons freshly squeezed lemon juice
- Freshly ground black pepper, to taste
- 1 pound chicken breast, cooked and shredded
- 2 roasted red peppers, drained and chopped
- 3 inner celery stalks with leaves, thinly sliced
- 8 cups mixed salad greens
- ½ pound tomatoes, chopped

INSTRUCTIONS:

1. In a food processor, combine the parsley, basil, dill, anchovies, and garlic until coarsely chopped. Add the mayonnaise, sour cream, and lemon juice and blend until smooth. Season to taste with the pepper.
2. In a large bowl, mix the herbed mayonnaise with the chicken, peppers, and celery. Serve on a bed of salad greens and garnish with the tomatoes.

Adobo Sirloin

Serves 4

PER SERVING:

- ✦ 237 calories
- ✦ 39 grams of protein
- ✦ 2 grams of carbs
- ✦ 7 grams of fat

INGREDIENTS:

- ✦ Juice of 1 lime
- ✦ 1 tablespoon minced garlic
- ✦ 1 teaspoon dried oregano
- ✦ 1 teaspoon ground cumin
- ✦ 2 tablespoons finely chopped canned chipotle chiles in adobo sauce plus 2 tablespoons of the sauce
- ✦ 4 (6-ounce) sirloin steaks, trimmed of fat
- ✦ Salt and freshly ground black pepper, to taste

INSTRUCTIONS:

1. In a small bowl, combine the lime juice, garlic, oregano, cumin, chiles, and adobo sauce. Mix well to combine.
2. Season the steaks with salt and pepper and place them in a large zipper-top bag with the adobo sauce. Seal tightly and shake to coat. Refrigerate for at least 2 hours and up to 8 hours, shaking occasionally.
3. Preheat a grill to high heat (about 10 minutes). Lightly coat the grill grates with cooking spray. Once the grill is hot, cook the steaks until your desired doneness, 4 to 5 minutes on each side. Let the steaks rest for 5 minutes and serve.

Lasagna with Cottage Cheese and Butternut Squash

Serves 6

PER SERVING:

- ✦ 419 calories
- ✦ 38 grams of protein
- ✦ 48 grams of carbs
- ✦ 8 grams of fat

INGREDIENTS:

- ✦ 4 cups (32 ounces) low-fat cottage cheese
- ✦ 3 cloves garlic
- ✦ 1 large egg
- ✦ Salt, to taste
- ✦ 2 (15-ounce) cans butternut squash puree
- ✦ 9 ounces (⅔ box) whole-wheat lasagna noodles
- ✦ 1 ¼ cups (5 ounces) grated part-skim mozzarella

INSTRUCTIONS:

1. Place a rack in the middle of the oven and preheat the oven to 350°F (175°C).
2. *For the cottage cheese sauce:* In a blender, process the cottage cheese, 2 of the garlic cloves, the egg, and salt until smooth.
3. *For the squash sauce:* Crush the remaining clove of garlic. In a medium-size (5-quart) bowl, combine it with the squash puree and a pinch of salt until well mixed.
4. *To assemble the lasagna:* Spread a layer of the uncooked noodles on the bottom of a 9 x 13-inch baking dish and top with half of the cottage cheese sauce. Add another layer of noodles and top with half of

the squash sauce. Repeat layering until you have used all the noodles and sauce, ending with a layer of cottage cheese sauce. Sprinkle the mozzarella cheese over the top.

5. Bake for 1 hour or until the top is lightly browned.

High-Protein Peach Cobbler

Serves 6

PER SERVING:

- 161 calories
- 12 grams of protein
- 28 grams of carbs
- 1 gram of fat

INGREDIENTS:

- 3 tablespoons blueberry, raspberry, strawberry, or mixed-fruit preserves
- 1 (15-ounce) can diced peaches in water or 100% juice, drained
- ½ cup 2% cottage cheese
- ½ cup water
- 2 scoops vanilla protein powder
- ⅓ cup Truvia or similar stevia-based sweetener
- ¼ cup all-purpose flour
- ½ cup quick-cooking oats
- 1 tablespoon honey

INSTRUCTIONS:

1. Preheat the oven to 350°F (175°C). Coat an 8 x 8-inch baking dish with cooking spray.
2. Spoon the fruit preserves into the prepared baking dish and use a spatula to spread them evenly over the bottom. Top with a layer of peaches and set aside.
3. In a medium bowl, mix the cottage cheese, water, protein powder, sweetener, and flour until well blended, then pour over the peaches.
4. In a small bowl, mix the oats and honey. Spoon over the top of the cobbler.
5. Bake until golden, about 30 minutes. Let cool for at least 20 minutes before serving.

Two-Minute Sweet Potato Brownie

Serves 1

PER SERVING:

- ✦ 207 calories
- ✦ 7 grams of protein
- ✦ 37 grams of carbs
- ✦ 8 grams of fat

INGREDIENTS:

- ✦ 2 tablespoons unsweetened cocoa powder, sifted
- ✦ 1 tablespoon coconut flour
- ✦ ¼ teaspoon baking powder
- ✦ 3 tablespoons unsweetened almond milk
- ✦ ¼ cup mashed sweet potato
- ✦ ½ tablespoon almond butter (or nut butter of choice)
- ✦ 2 teaspoons granulated sugar
- ✦ ½ teaspoon vanilla extract

INSTRUCTIONS:

1. In a small microwave-safe bowl or mug, mix the cocoa powder, coconut flour, and baking powder until well combined.
2. Add the milk and mashed sweet potato, stirring until smooth. Add the almond butter, sugar, and vanilla and stir until smooth and well blended.
3. Microwave on high for 2 to 3 minutes or until a toothpick inserted into the middle of the brownie comes out clean. If the brownie is not done after 3 minutes, continue microwaving in 30-second intervals until it's cooked through.

Restaurants

The byword of sustainable dieting regardless of your body composition goal is *versatility*, so flexible dieting must include the option of eating in restaurants, even when cutting.

The challenge with eating out is only that it's harder to control your calories and macros. For example, a palm-sized piece of meat at a restaurant often has at least 120 to 150 more calories than you'd expect because of the oil and butter absorbed during cooking. A cup of plain pasta or potato ranges from 180 to 200 calories, but when there's a sauce or another source of fat, that can easily double. Most desserts contain between 25 and 50 calories per tablespoon. Even vegetable dishes can be richer than you think because of high-fat additions like butter, oil, and cheese.

None of that means you shouldn't or can't eat out, however. You just need to make smart choices. Let's establish some simple guidelines to that end.

1. When cutting, try not to eat out more than once per week.
As calories and macros are a bit of a guessing game when eating out, by limiting yourself to one restaurant meal per week, you can minimize the chances of problematic overeating.

That said, if you can accurately estimate the macros of your restaurant meals (usually because they're simple), you can eat out more often without issue.

For instance, I used to pick up a salad with a side of rice from a local restaurant every day for lunch that contained the exact ingredients I'd use to make it myself (no hidden calories), and I had no problems. Healthier fast-food chains that allow you to build meals in layers (first rice, then beans, then protein, then veggies, etc.) can also work well for this because you can find the macros of each component online (www.cronometer.com is a good resource for this), and portions are fairly consistent.

The *Muscle for Life* Meal Plan

Some restaurants and online food databases seem to make our job easier by providing calories and macros for finished dishes, but unfortunately, many underreport these numbers. Whenever applicable, add 20 percent to the purported calories to adjust for this.

2. When lean gaining or maintaining, try not to eat out more than twice per week.

Most people pay far more attention to their calorie intake when cutting than when lean gaining or maintaining because losing weight usually feels more pressing than minimizing fat gain or stabilizing body composition.

This is understandable but counterproductive, as eating too much while lean gaining forces you to cut sooner than you'd like (before you've made much progress in gaining muscle and strength). And if you overeat too often on a maintenance phase, it no longer qualifies as maintenance and is more like lean gaining.

Therefore, if you want the best results, be mindful of your calories and macros regardless of whether you're cutting, lean gaining, or maintaining. Minimizing restaurant meals helps with this tremendously (unless you're absolutely sure of the calories and macros).

3. Try to stick to dishes that can be quantified.

When eating out, the simpler the dish, the better, because it's too difficult to estimate the calories and macros of many fancier meals like casseroles, filled pastas, and sauce-based recipes like goulash, sweet and sour chicken, salads soaked with dressing, and so forth. Thus, meals made up of individual whole foods are the ticket, such as steak with broccoli and sweet potato wedges, chicken Caesar salad with croutons and dressing on the side, or a fillet of fish with rice and grilled zucchini.

Many people like to take this a step further and come up with a handful of easily quantified meals they enjoy at the restaurants they often go to. This removes the stress of trying to figure out calories and macros at the table, or worse, of refusing to eat out because "nothing fits into the diet."

Some restaurants don't have any meals that are easy to gauge. If you look at Olive Garden's entree menu, for instance, just about everything is some kind of casserole or pasta/meat combination covered in cheese, butter, and sauce. If you can, avoid menus like these when cutting in particular—and if that's not possible, do your best to keep your calories within reason (try not to eat two baskets of bread, a mountain of creamy pasta, and a plate of dessert, for example).

Alcohol

According to some people, if you drink even sporadically, you'll always struggle with your weight. This is an odd statement considering that studies show moderate alcohol consumption is associated with lower, not higher, body weights, and can result in more weight loss when dieting, not less.

What's more, research shows that calories from alcohol itself don't affect body fat levels in the same way other calories do. Scientists at the University of São Paulo analyzed the diets of almost 2,000 adults aged 18 to 74 and were surprised to find that an increase in calories from alcohol alone didn't result in the weight gain that would normally occur if those calories had been from food. In fact, thanks to regular alcohol consumption, drinkers who took in an average of 50 to 130 more calories per day than nondrinkers and had more or less the same levels of physical activity weren't any fatter than their alcohol-free counterparts. It's almost as if the calories from the alcohol simply "didn't count."

There are two likely reasons for these findings. First, alcohol can reduce your appetite, which is conducive to weight loss and maintenance, and improve insulin sensitivity, which can positively influence fat loss. Second, and more important, the body has no way to directly convert alcohol into body fat. That is, calories provided by ethanol (alcohol) don't produce fat gain in the same way that calories from food do because they're processed differently.

We don't need to get into the chemistry here, but think of it in these terms: wood contains about 4 calories per gram, but as the human body doesn't produce the chemicals needed to digest and absorb wood, no amount of shavings on our salads can make us fatter (only sick or worse, so please don't get any ideas). Point being: not all calories matter—only those that the body can process and use—and calories in alcohol aren't handled like those in food.

Even so, alcohol does contribute to fat gain in an indirect way: it suppresses physiological mechanisms related to fat burning and increases the conversion of carbs into body fat. In other words, while alcohol doesn't provide the raw materials required for the creation of body fat (usable calories), it constipates our body's fat-burning machinery and greases the wheels of its fat-making instruments. Therefore, if you want to drink alcohol without interfering with your fitness, follow these three tips:

1. Don't have more than one serving of alcohol per day while lean gaining, or more than two servings per day while cutting or maintaining.
2. Prioritize lower-calorie wines, beers, and spirits over higher-calorie options, especially heavy beers, ciders, and fruity cocktails.
3. Consider alcohol a treat (count the calories toward your "allowance" of up to 20 percent of daily calories), and include the calories in your meal plan.

Other Beverages

Unfortunately, the calories in all of our other favorite caloric beverages, from lattes to soda to vegetable juices to sweetened teas and the rest of them, count in the same way as those in all of the foods we like to eat. And the same goes for much of the stuff we like to splash into our drinks, like milk, creamer, sugar, syrup, and so on.

Additionally, since calories from beverages aren't nearly as satisfying (or nourishing) as nutritious foods, the fewer calories you drink every day, the better your meal plan will generally work. I don't want to forbid you anything you enjoy, though, so let's make a compromise: don't drink more than 10 percent of your daily calories. That should give you plenty of room for your morning caffeine ritual and likely with some liquid calories to spare.

All right, you now have all the information you need to begin creating your meal plan! Let's start with working out what you'd like to eat every day. Write a few of your top choices in each group below.

My Favorite Proteins

Poultry, pork, beef, seafood, high-protein dairy (Greek yogurt, skyr, cottage cheese, etc.), egg whites, high-protein plant food (seitan, tofu, tempeh, etc.), and protein powders and bars

....

....

....

....

My Favorite Nutritious Carbs

Veggies, fruit, whole grains, legumes, and tubers

....

....
....
....

My Favorite Healthy Fats

Olive oil, avocados, nuts and nut butters, seeds, full-fat dairy (regular yogurt, cheese, milk, and butter), and whole eggs

....
....
....
....

My Favorite Treats

White bread, white pasta, sugary snacks, desserts, alcohol, etc.

....
....
....
....

My Favorite Recipes

....
....
....
....

My Favorite Restaurant Meals

....
....

4. Decide how much to eat.

This is where the magic happens—where we turn your favorite foods into delicious and nutritious meals that meet your calorie and macronutrient needs.

Before we examine how this process works, however, make sure you've downloaded the free bonus material that comes with this book (www.muscle forlifebook.com/bonus) because it contains digital meal plan templates as well as preprepared meal plans for cutting and lean gaining.

OVERVIEW

When I'm designing a meal plan, I like to do it in layers. First is protein; then nutritious carbs, starting with three to five portions of vegetables; then healthy fat; and finally, treats. This method works well even when meals are a combination of all categories because as I move through these layers, I subtract their calories and macros from my targets (to see how much more food I can eat), and then massage portion sizes (and possibly food choices) until I've more or less reached my daily calorie and macro targets.

You don't have to hit your numbers perfectly either—you just have to be close enough. Practically, that means within 5 percent or so of your daily calories target and 10 percent of your protein target (carbs and fats can shift however much is needed to make the meal plan you want).

There are two ways to accomplish this level of accuracy in meal planning. You can either use an online calorie and macronutrient database like www .cronometer.com (my favorite) along with a food scale and utensils to measure precise amounts of non-prepackaged foods and beverages (100 grams of dry oatmeal cooked with 50 grams of blueberries and splashed with 4 ounces of whole milk, for instance), or you can use a rough-and-ready method of eyeballing foods that doesn't require any software or hardware.

Both techniques can work, and both have advantages and disadvantages. The first technique is more precise and allows for maximum personalization, but it's also more involved and thus best suited to people who thrive on exactness, which isn't everyone. Some people also find the practice daunting and cumbersome, especially those new to flexible dieting.

If you're not sure which style will suit you best, start with the system I'll teach you in this chapter that requires only your hand, and then later, when you've made major strides toward your goals, try the more sophisticated approach if you're so inclined.

Also, to help you fully grasp each step of creating a *Muscle for Life* meal plan, I'll build one as we go for a fictitious client named Mary, who weighs 160 pounds and wants to lose fat. According to the information in the previous chapter, her daily calorie and macro targets are:

+ 1,600 calories
+ 160 grams of protein
+ 120 grams of carbs
+ 55 grams of fat

Let's start with square one: working out your (and Mary's) sources of protein.

1. Add your protein.

The goal here is to meet most (80 percent or so) of your protein needs with your preferred sources of protein. You don't need to reach 100 percent of your daily protein target because your veggies and other carbs will add protein as well (bringing you close enough to 100 percent).

In this step, then, you need to add several portions of protein to your meal plan. You can have up to three portions of protein in a single meal, but not more, because eating at least three servings of protein throughout the day is better for controlling appetite and possibly building muscle than just one or two. There are many ways to measure portions of protein, and the *Muscle for Life* method is simple:

+ **Lean meat and seafood:** If meat or seafood contains fewer than 5 grams of fat per portion, it's considered lean. One portion is a palm of cooked food (assuming it's about an inch thick) and contains about 130 calories, 25 grams of protein, 0 grams of carbs, and 3 grams of fat.

+ **Fatty meat and seafood:** If meat or seafood contains 5 or more grams of fat per portion, it's considered fatty. One portion is a palm of cooked food (assuming it's about an inch thick) and contains about 200 calories, 20 grams of protein, 0 grams of carbs, and 12 grams of fat.

+ **High-protein dairy:** If a dairy food contains 15 or more grams of protein per portion, it's considered high-protein dairy (otherwise, it's a "healthy fat"). In the case of no- and low-fat high-protein dairy (usually 2 percent fat or less), one portion is the size of your fist and contains about 150 calories, 20 grams of protein, 10 grams of carbs, and 3 grams of fat. In the case of whole-fat high-protein dairy (usually more than 2 percent fat), one portion is the size of your fist and contains 220 calories, 20 grams of protein, 10 grams of carbs, and 10 grams of fat.

- **Egg white:** One (cooked) portion is the size of your fist and contains 130 calories, 27 grams of protein, 2 grams of carbs, and 0 grams of fat.

- **High-protein plant food:** This includes seitan, tofu, and tempeh. One portion is a palm of cooked food (assuming it's about an inch thick) and contains about 150 calories, 10 grams of protein, 15 grams of carbs, and 5 grams of fat.

- **Protein supplement:** Protein supplements include protein powders and bars. One scoop of a high-quality protein powder usually contains about 100 calories, 20 grams of protein, 2 grams of carbs, and 2 grams of fat. One normal-sized protein bar (about two fingers wide and five inches long) often contains about 250 calories, 20 grams of protein, 30 grams of carbs, and 10 grams of fat. That said, the calories and macros of protein supplements can vary dramatically depending on the ingredients and serving sizes, so it's best to use the numbers given on the supplement facts panels of the specific products you want to include in your meal plan.

These figures are approximations, of course, but are accurate enough to work because individual variations in each category are slight and average out in practice. So, if you needed to eat 120 grams of protein per day, that could be a fist-sized amount of Greek yogurt at breakfast, two palms of chicken at lunch (in a salad), a "fist" of cottage cheese for a snack, and two palms of fish at dinner.

Also, to help you with building out your meal plan, here's a handy chart with many popular sources of protein categorized accordingly:

Lean Meat and Seafood	Fatty Meat and Seafood	High-Protein Dairy and Egg White	High-Protein Plant Food	Protein Supplement
Beef, ground (90/10 or leaner)	Anchovies	Cottage cheese	Seitan	Casein protein (caseinate or micellar)
Beef, round roast, trimmed of fat	Beef, ground (85/15 or fattier)	Egg white	Tempeh	Pea protein isolate
Beef, sirloin, trimmed of fat	Beef, New York strip, trimmed of fat	Greek yogurt	Tofu	Protein bar
Catfish	Beef, porterhouse, trimmed of fat	Low-fat yogurt		Rice protein isolate
Chicken, breast, skinless, boneless	Beef, ribeye, trimmed of fat	Skyr		Soy protein isolate
Clam	Beef, T-bone, trimmed of fat			Whey protein (concentrate, isolate, or hydrolysate)
Cod	Chicken, drumstick, skin removed			
Flounder	Chicken, thigh, skin removed			
Halibut	Herring, pickled or cooked			
Lobster	Lamb, ground			

Lean Meat and Seafood	Fatty Meat and Seafood	High-Protein Dairy and Egg White	High-Protein Plant Food	Protein Supplement
Mahi Mahi	Lamb, leg, trimmed of fat			
Mussels	Mackerel, canned			
Orange roughy	Pork, ribs, trimmed of fat			
Oyster, raw or cooked	Salmon, farmed			
Perch	Turkey, drumstick, skin removed			
Pollack	Turkey, thigh, skin removed			
Pork, chop, trimmed of fat				
Pork, tenderloin, trimmed of fat				
Salmon, wild-caught				
Scallop				
Shrimp				
Sole				
Swordfish				
Tilapia				
Trout				

Lean Meat and Seafood	Fatty Meat and Seafood	High-Protein Dairy and Egg White	High-Protein Plant Food	Protein Supplement
Tuna, canned in water				
Turkey breast, skinless				
Venison (deer, elk, antelope, etc.), trimmed of fat				

When you're done adding protein portions to your meal plan, subtract their calories and macros from your daily targets to see what you have left. You should have a little protein left (which will be topped off by the protein in the nutritious carbs you'll add) and plenty of fat and carbs to keep working with.

Let's see how all this would look for Mary. We recall that she weighs 160 pounds and wants to lose fat, and her daily calorie and macro targets are:

+ 1,600 calories
+ 160 grams of protein
+ 120 grams of carbs
+ 55 grams of fat

Here's how her meal plan could begin:

	Food	Portion	Calories	Protein	Carbs	Fat
Breakfast (9 a.m.)	Greek yogurt, 2% fat, plain	2	300	40 g	20 g	6 g
Lunch (12 p.m.)	Chicken, breast, skinless, boneless, grilled	1	130	25 g	0 g	3 g
Snack (3 p.m.)	Cottage cheese, 2% fat, plain	1	150	20 g	10 g	3 g
Dinner (6 p.m.)	Tilapia, cooked	2	260	50 g	0 g	6 g
Total			840	135 g	30 g	18 g
Remaining			760	25 g	90 g	37 g

As you can see, Mary has added six portions of lean protein (three portions of high-protein dairy and three portions of lean meat and seafood), totaling 840 calories, 135 grams of protein, 30 grams of carbs, and 18 grams of fat.

Now we can move to the next step and figure out what carbs to add to our meal plan.

2. Add your nutritious carbs.

This step has two parts:

1. Adding vegetables to your meal plan, which is essential for optimizing health and well-being.
2. Adding other nutritious carbs (fruits, whole grains, legumes, and tubers), which help round out a wholesome diet.

Here's another chart that shows how many popular foods fit into these carbohydrate categories:

Vegetables	Fruits	Whole Grains, Tubers, and Legumes
Artichoke	Apple	Amaranth
Arugula	Apricot	Barley
Asparagus	Banana	Beet
Beet greens	Blackberry	Black bean
Bell pepper	Blueberry	Black-eyed pea (cowpea)
Bok choy	Cantaloupe	Black rice
Broccoli	Cherry	Brown rice
Brussels sprout	Cranberry	Buckwheat
Cabbage	Date	Bulgur
Carrot	Fig	Cannellini bean
Cauliflower	Grape	Cassava (a.k.a. yuca, arrowroot)
Celery	Grapefruit	Chickpea (garbanzo bean)
Chive	Honeydew	Corn
Collard green	Kiwifruit	Cranberry bean
Cucumber	Mandarin orange (clementine, satsuma, tangerine)	Einkorn
Eggplant	Mango	Farro
Endive	Nectarine	Fava bean
Fennel	Orange	Great northern bean
Garlic	Papaya	Japanese sweet potato
Green bean	Peach	Kidney bean
Jicama	Pear	Lentils
Kale	Pineapple	Lima bean
Kimchi	Plum	Millet
Kohlrabi	Raspberry	Mung bean
Leek	Strawberry	Navy bean

Vegetables	Fruits	Whole Grains, Tubers, and Legumes
Lettuce	Watermelon	Oatmeal
Mushroom		Parsnip
Mustard green		Pea
Okra		Pinto bean
Onion		Popcorn
Pickle		Quinoa
Pumpkin		Red bean
Radish		Red potato
Rhubarb		Spelt
Sauerkraut		Sweet potato
Seaweed		Taro
Shallot		Teff
Spinach		Vitelotte potato
Squash, butternut		White potato
Squash, spaghetti		Whole-wheat bread
Squash, yellow		Whole-wheat pasta
Swiss chard		Wild rice
Tomatillo		
Tomato		
Water chestnut		
Watercress		
Zucchini		

In the first part of this step—adding vegetables—aim to include at least three portions of vegetables to your meal plan. One portion equates to a fist-sized amount of raw food and contains about 30 calories, 6 grams of carbs, 2 grams of protein, and 0 grams of fat.

There is an exception, however: dark leafy greens like spinach, lettuce, kale, and collard greens have so few calories (and macros) that they're effectively "free" (zero calories and macros). So you can add these vegetables to your plan however you'd like. Most people like to include them in lunches and dinners (salads and side dishes are popular), but do whatever works best for you (veggie omelets are great breakfasts, for instance).

Additionally, you can include multiple portions of vegetables in a single meal, up to your entire daily intake, if you prefer. There's no benefit or downside to splitting up your vegetables across different meals.

Next, add portions (or parts of portions) of the other nutritious carbs you'd like to eat up to no more than 80 percent of your daily carbohydrate target (to leave room for treats). In Mary's case, this would be about 100 grams of carbs (120 x 0.8).

As for portion size . . .

◆ **Fruits:** One portion is the size of your fist and contains about 60 calories, 15 grams of carbs, 1 gram of protein, and 0 grams of fat. (Banana, however, requires a modification: one portion is half of a large banana.)

◆ **Whole grains, tubers, and legumes:** One portion is half of a fist of cooked food or one slice of sandwich bread and contains about 120 calories, 25 grams of carbs, 3 grams of protein, and 1 gram of fat.

Once you've finished adding all of the nutritious carbs to your plan, subtract their calories and macros from your remaining amounts to see how much you have left. At this point, you should have little (if any) protein remaining and some carbs and fat.

Let's see how this step could work for Mary (the new additions are italicized).

	Food	Portion	Calories	Protein	Carbs	Fat
Breakfast (9 a.m.)	Greek yogurt, 2% fat, plain	2	300	40 g	20 g	6 g
	Banana	2	120	2 g	30 g	0 g
Lunch (12 p.m.)	Chicken, breast, skinless, boneless	1	130	25 g	0 g	3 g
	Spinach	3	0	0 g	0 g	0 g
	Tomato	1	30	2 g	6 g	0 g
	Carrot	1	30	2 g	6 g	0 g
Snack (3 p.m.)	Cottage cheese, 2% fat, plain	1	150	20 g	10 g	3 g
Dinner (6 p.m.)	Tilapia	2	260	50 g	0 g	6 g
	Brown rice	1	120	3 g	25 g	1 g
	Broccoli	1	30	2 g	6 g	0 g
Total			1,170	146 g	103 g	19 g
Remaining			430	14 g	17 g	36 g

As you can see, she still has six portions of lean protein and has added six portions of vegetables and three portions of nutritious carbs (two portions of banana and one portion of brown rice).

Now we're ready to introduce healthy fat into the plan.

3. Add your healthy fat.

Now it's time to boost your fat intake with nutritious fatty foods, with an emphasis on unsaturated fat. To do this, add portions (or fractions of portions) of healthy, fat-rich foods up to no more than 80 percent of your daily fat target (again, to leave room for treats). For Mary, this would be about 45 grams (55 x 0.8).

As the calorie and macronutrient content of fatty foods can vary substantially, portion sizes and macros depend on the food:

+ **Oils and butter:** One portion is the size of half of your thumb (roughly your knuckle to the tip of your thumb) and contains about 120 calories, 14 grams of fat, 0 grams of protein, and 0 grams of carbs.

+ **Nut butters:** One portion is the size of half of your thumb and contains about 100 calories, 8 grams of fat, 4 grams of protein, and 3 grams of carbs.

+ **Salad dressing:** One portion is the size of your thumb and contains about 100 calories, 10 grams of fat, 0 grams of protein, and 2 grams of carbs.

+ **Nuts and seeds:** One portion is the size of your thumb and contains about 80 calories, 7 grams of fat, 3 grams of protein, and 3 grams of carbs.

+ **Cheese:** One portion is the size of your thumb and contains about 120 calories, 10 grams of fat, 6 grams of protein, and 1 gram of carbs.

+ **Whole milk:** One portion is the size of your fist (about one cup) and contains about 150 calories, 8 grams of fat, 8 grams of protein, and 12 grams of carbs.

- ✦ **2% milk:** One portion is the size of your fist and contains about 100 calories, 2 grams of fat, 8 grams of protein, and 12 grams of carbs.

- ✦ **Whole egg:** One portion is the size of half of your fist and contains 70 calories, 6 grams of protein, 0 grams of carbs, and 5 grams of fat.

- ✦ **Avocado:** One portion is the size of half of your fist and contains about 120 calories, 10 grams of fat, 1 gram of protein, and 6 grams of carbs.

As usual, when you're done adding healthy fat to your meal plan, subtract its calories and macros from your remainders to prepare for the final step.

Let's see how Mary could implement this in her plan (new additions are italicized).

	Food	Portion	Calories	Protein	Carbs	Fat
Breakfast (9 a.m.)	Greek yogurt, 2% fat, plain	2	300	40 g	20 g	6 g
	Banana	2	120	2 g	30 g	0 g
	Almonds	2	160	6 g	6 g	14 g
Lunch (12 p.m.)	Chicken, breast, skinless, boneless	1	130	25 g	0 g	3 g
	Spinach	3	0	0 g	0 g	0 g
	Tomato	1	30	2 g	6 g	0 g
	Carrot	1	30	2 g	6 g	0 g
	Salad dressing	1	100	0 g	2 g	10 g
Snack (3 p.m.)	Cottage cheese, 2% fat, plain	1	150	20 g	10 g	3 g

	Food	Portion	Calories	Protein	Carbs	Fat
Dinner (6 p.m.)	Tilapia	2	260	50 g	0 g	6 g
	Brown rice	1	120	3 g	25 g	1 g
	Broccoli	1	30	2 g	6 g	0 g
Total			1,430	152 g	111 g	43 g
Remaining			170	8 g	9 g	12 g

So, she's now up to six portions of lean protein, six portions of vegetables, three portions of nutritious carbs, and three portions of healthy fat.

4. Add your treats.

As you learned in chapter 7, you can use up to 20 percent of your daily calories for less-than-nutritious foods you like to eat and drink, including alcohol, desserts, and highly processed carbohydrates such as white bread, bagels, pastries, white pasta, etc. Here's how you can incorporate these into your meal plan:

1. Determine how many lower-quality calories you can eat and drink every day.
2. Determine how many calories you have left in your plan.
3. Decide which treats you'd like to eat and drink.
4. Add treats to your plan, adjusting other meals as needed, and round off your calories and macros (if necessary).

Let's go over each step.

1. Determine how many lower-quality calories you can eat and drink every day.

To calculate 20 percent of your daily calories, multiply your daily calorie target by 0.2. You don't have to eat or drink this much "junk" every day if you don't want to, but you shouldn't be afraid to, either.

For Mary, this comes out to 320 calories (1,600 x 0.2).

2. Determine how many calories you have left in your plan.

If you've been including calories in your calculations so far, you'll know how many you have left for treats. If you've only been watching macros (which is fine), however, you can figure out how many calories you have remaining in three simple steps:

1. Multiply the number of grams of protein and carbs you have left by 4 to convert them into calories (remember, each gram of carbohydrate and protein has about 4 calories).
2. Multiply the number of grams of fat you have left by 9 to translate them into calories.
3. Add the results together.

If the amount is between 10 and 20 percent of your daily calorie target, you have enough room to continue adding treats. If the amount is less than 10 percent, however, you probably won't (one or two squares of chocolate or tablespoons of ice cream isn't exactly satisfying).

In Mary's case, we already know that she has 170 calories left for treats, but if we were dealing only with macros, here's how the math would look:

+ 8 grams of protein and 9 grams of carbs left = 68 calories
+ 12 grams of fat left = 108 calories
+ 68 + 108 = 176 calories left for treats (the result will always be slightly different this way, and that's fine)

To make more room for indulgences, simply reduce the amount of carbs and fats (but not protein, unless you're over your target) you added in the previous steps. Small adjustments add up quickly (because of the number of calories in each gram of carbohydrate and fat), so you shouldn't have to make major changes. For instance, if you only had 100 calories left for goodies, you might reduce your butter on your toast in the morning from two portions to one to free up 100 calories, and your rice at dinner from two portions to one portion to claw back another 100 calories, giving you 300 calories to play with.

3. Decide which treats you'd like to eat and drink.
Once you have enough calories for treats, pick your top three candidates from the list you created earlier, and research online how many calories they contain per serving. Based on this, decide how to proceed. Would you like to use all of your remaining calories on just one? Split them between two or all three?

If you find that your top three choices contain too many calories to satisfy, however, return to your list to find an option that works.

For example, let's suppose that Mary would like to use all 170 of her remaining calories in this step. She loves Double Stuf Oreo cookies, churros with cinnamon and sugar, and apple fritters, but learns they contain 70 calories per cookie, 220 calories per churro, and 500 calories per fritter. She could pick one for her dessert, of course, but even if she frees up 300 or so calories (20 percent of her total daily target), the portions may feel skimpy. Instead of quenching her craving, this may just leave her wanting more. And so she reviews alternatives and settles on something less calorific: light ice cream, with 200 calories per cup.

4. Add treats to your plan, adjusting other meals as needed, and round off your calories and macros (if necessary).

Work this over until you're happy with your treats and they total no more than 20 percent of your total calories. And if, in the end, you still have calories left over, adjust other meals upward as needed. For instance, if you're left with 100 calories after working out your treats to your satisfaction, you could add 25 grams of protein or carbs elsewhere in your plan (25 grams x 4 calories per gram) or 10 grams of fat (10 grams x 9 calories per gram) or a combination thereof.

Let's do this now for Mary by adding the light ice cream to her meal plan.

	Food	Portion	Calories	Protein	Carbs	Fat
Breakfast (9 a.m.)	Greek yogurt, 2% fat, plain	2	300	40 g	20 g	6 g
	Banana	2	120	2 g	30 g	0 g
	Almonds	2	160	6 g	6 g	14 g
Lunch (12 p.m.)	Chicken, breast, skinless, boneless	1	130	25 g	0 g	3 g
	Spinach	3	0	0 g	0 g	0 g
	Tomato	1	30	2 g	6 g	0 g
	Carrot	1	30	2 g	6 g	0 g
	Salad dressing	1	100	0 g	2 g	10 g

	Food	Portion	Calories	Protein	Carbs	Fat
Snack (3 p.m.)	Cottage cheese, 2% fat, plain	1	150	20 g	10 g	3 g
Dinner (6 p.m.)	Tilapia	2	260	50 g	0 g	6 g
	Brown rice	1	120	3 g	25 g	1 g
	Broccoli	1	30	2 g	6 g	0 g
	Light ice cream	1 cup	200	6 g	34 g	6 g
Total			1,630	158 g	145 g	49 g
Remaining			-30	2 g	-15 g	6 g

All right, let's review how Mary did with her meal plan.

	Target	Actual
Calories	1,600	1,630
Protein	160 g	158 g
Carbs	120 g	135 g
Fat	55 g	49 g

She ended with 1,630 calories (great), hit just about 100 percent of her protein needs (perfect), and wound up with slightly less carbs and more fat (no problem). Remember—you have as much wiggle room with carbs and fat as you'd like so long as your calories are within 5 percent and your protein is within 10 percent of your targets. In other words, by following the procedure you just learned, Mary made a meal plan that'll work like gangbusters, and now you can too!

To ensure that you understand what effective and well-designed meal plans look like, I've included examples in the back of this book for men and women of various sizes who want to cut and lean gain. You can use these meal plans as guides for building your own, or you can also just grab one that fits your needs and follow it exactly—an easy and perfectly acceptable shortcut around the math and thinking required to create a custom meal plan.

If you want to follow one of the premade plans in the back of the book, there are a few things you need to know:

1. When cutting or lean gaining, start with the plan closest to your current body weight, rounding down (if you're 227 pounds, for instance, go with the 200-pound plan and not the 240-pound one).

2. When cutting, once you're within 5 pounds of the next-lowest plan, switch to it if you want to keep losing fat (if you've cut down to 145 pounds, switch to the 140-pound plan).

3. When lean gaining, start with the plan closest to your current body weight, rounding down (if you're 180 pounds, for example, choose the 170-pound plan).

4. When lean gaining, once you're within 5 pounds of the next-highest plan, switch to it if you want to keep gaining weight (if you've lean gained up to 115 pounds, switch to the 120-pound plan).

WHAT ABOUT "CHEAT MEALS"?

Sometimes it feels great to just let go. To stop striving and stage-managing and just give in to our impulses. You know . . . to just "be human" now and then. And when it comes to dieting, that means ignoring the plan and "cheating." No counting calories, no eyeballing macros, and no minding nutrition.

There are quite a few opinions on cheating (or "free" or "normal" eating, as some experts prefer). Some people believe that even mild deviations from your meal plan can prevent you from reaching your goals. Others are of the mind that you can stray so long as you don't turn to certain forbidden foods. Still others say it's okay (or even helpful) to wallow in weekly food orgies that would kill a competitive eater.

None of these strategies are ideal. You certainly can have "off-plan" meals without ruining your progress, and you don't have to stick to a short list of "approved" foods, but you can't regularly eat yourself unconscious without paying a price.

What works well for most people is simple: you stick to your meal plan "perfectly" (well enough) for a set period of time, usually a week or so, and then enjoy something special—usually as a single "cheat meal"—even if you're not hankering for it.

Think of this approach like controlled burning, where . . . forest experts? Foresters? Silvologists? Whatever . . . burn away dead grass and trees, fallen branches, and undergrowth to prevent a raging inferno. Similarly, by regularly immolating your dietary demons when they're just cuddly little kidlets, you can avoid facing them as a gang of belligerent teenagers.

This method is preferred by most people who have achieved an elite level of fitness, and there's good scientific evidence of its effectiveness as well. For instance, studies on "diet breaks" have consistently shown that people tend to lose more fat when they alternate between periods of following a diet plan closely and loosely.

So, to anyone who says cheat meals are always bad, I say *pshaw*. God's in the details. And if you want to know how to "cheat" on your diet without ruining it, here are four points to follow:

1. Treat yourself just once or twice per week.
2. Try not to exceed your daily energy expenditure.

3. Try to keep your dietary fat intake under 100 grams for the day.

4. Drink alcohol intelligently.

Before we review each of these items, however, let's clarify what "cheating" is, because it's not merely eating sugar or dairy or some other food deemed "unclean" by some pied piper.

Let's start with the term itself—cheating—first, because it's not accurate in denotation or connotation and far too negative and loaded for what it describes. Let's reframe this discussion around treating and treat meals, which gives a proper flavor of the nature of untypical eating.

When you eat more calories in a day than you planned on eating, regardless of what foods you eat, that's treating. And when you replace a large portion of your nutritious calories with nonnutritious ones, that's treating, too. In other words, a treat meal consists of eating a lot more calories or a lot less wholesome food than you'd normally eat.

The drawbacks of treating are obvious. Eat too many calories too frequently, and you'll fail to lose weight as desired (or you'll gain weight too quickly); and disregard nutrition too frequently, and you can erode your health and face a number of problems, including bone loss, anxiety and brain fog, fatigue and muscle weakness, and cardiovascular disease.

That doesn't mean you shouldn't stray from your meal plan from time to time, however. You absolutely should if you want to, but you need to know how to do it productively. Let's learn how.

1. Treat yourself just once or twice per week.

Although treat meals don't have to result in a calorie surplus for the day, they often do, and if you do that too often, you can erase most or even all of your calorie deficit and hamstring (or even halt) your fat loss. And if you're lean bulking, you'll balloon your calorie surplus and gain too much fat too quickly.

If you treat yourself just once or twice per week, however, whether in a single meal or spread throughout an entire day, you'll be able to enjoy yourself without worrying about overdoing it.

2. Try not to exceed your daily energy expenditure.

Many people don't realize how many calories are in some of the more delightful foods they like to treat themselves with. This is especially true when eating at restaurants, because the chef's job is to make delicious—and not necessarily calorie-conscious—meals. And when that's the goal, butter, oil, and sugar are her best friends.

Consider a study conducted by scientists at Tufts University that involved the analysis of 360 dinner entrees at 123 nonchain restaurants in San Francisco, Boston, and Little Rock between 2011 and 2014. They found that the restaurant dishes contained, on average, about 1,200 calories, and among American, Italian, and Chinese restaurants in particular, the average was nearly 1,500 calories per meal.

Even more flagrant offenders can be found in an analysis of restaurant foods conducted by scientists at the Center for Science in the Public Interest. The Cheesecake Factory, for instance, makes a brûléed French toast with a side of bacon that weighs in at 2,780 calories, 93 grams of saturated fat, and 24 teaspoons of sugar. It also offers a creamy farfalle pasta with chicken and roasted garlic, which is a bit lighter at just 2,410 calories and 63 grams of saturated fat.

Let's also not forget that those are just individual entrees, which, for many people, aren't the entirety of their treat meals. Add in some bread, an appetizer, and a dessert, and the calories can soar to horrific highs. It should come as no surprise, then, that research conducted by scientists at the University of Illinois at Urbana-Champaign concluded that calorically speaking, there's not much of a difference between fast food and full-service dining.

So my point is this: If you don't pay attention to your calorie intake when having a treat meal, you can seriously set yourself back. And if you go in for an all-out treat day, you can do a number on your diet.

For example, here are the approximate calorie counts for a number of popular treat-day foods:

+ Deep-dish pizza: 480 calories per slice
+ Ice cream: 270 calories per half cup
+ Bacon cheeseburger: 595 calories per burger
+ Traditional cheesecake: 400 calories per slice
+ French fries: 498 calories per large serving
+ Chocolate chip cookies: 220 calories per large cookie
+ Creamy pasta: 593 calories per cup
+ Loaded nachos: 1,590 calories per plate
+ Pecan pie: 541 calories per slice

As you can see, just a few hearty portions of any of these is all it takes to push your calorie intake into the stratosphere.

So, all of this is why I recommend calibrating your treat meals so you don't exceed your energy expenditure for the day (your maintenance calories, or 14 to 15 calories per pound of body weight for most people). This way, you have plenty of room to eat foods you normally don't eat, especially if you're putting all those extra calories into just one or two meals.

You can also "borrow" calories from elsewhere in your meal plan to keep your calories reined in by eating more or less nothing but protein leading up to (and after) a treat meal. Suppose you have a treat meal planned at your favorite restaurant that will consist of about 1,000 calories, which is about double the calories you normally eat at dinner. To create "room" for the treat meal, you can pare down (or even eliminate) other meals by reducing or removing the carbs and fat (but not the protein). For instance, if you normally eat scrambled egg whites, oatmeal, and almonds at breakfast, you could skip the meal and eat more protein at lunch, or cut the oatmeal and nut portions in half (or more if it won't result in too much mid-morning hunger). Then, at lunch you could leave the croutons and chickpeas out of your salad with chicken, cut back on the dressing, and leave out the side of rice. Finally, you could eat the high-protein yogurt in your afternoon snack, but not the banana and granola. By making these changes, you've created a large buffer of calories to backfill at the restaurant, allowing you to eat quite a bit before reaching your daily energy expenditure.

Calorie borrowing comes with an important caveat, however: make it the exception, not the rule. I want you to develop a healthy and sustainable relationship with food, not a perverse preoccupation with meal manipulation. So try to limit calorie borrowing to when you treat yourself (once or twice per week).

3. Try to keep your dietary fat intake under 100 grams for the day.

This not only helps you keep your calories under control (remember that a gram of fat contains about 9 calories) but it also helps you minimize fat gain. So instead of doubling down on your favorite fatty foods when you treat, go high-carb instead. This will result in less immediate fat storage, and it also has other benefits when you're cutting.

One of the downsides of calorie restriction is it reduces the levels of a hormone called *leptin*, which is produced by body fat. In simple terms, leptin tells your brain that there's plenty of energy available and that your body can expend energy freely, eat normal amounts of food, and engage in normal amounts of physical activity.

When you limit your calories to lose fat, however, the drop in leptin tells your body that it's in an energy-deficient state and must expend less energy and consume more. It accomplishes this through several mechanisms, including lowering the basal metabolic rate, reducing general activity levels, and stimulating the appetite.

Raising leptin levels reverses these effects, which is one of the reasons you feel better when you stop restricting your calories and return to normal eating. To fully reverse the leptin-related negative side effects of cutting, you have to stop dieting. You can temporarily boost leptin production, however, by acutely increasing your calorie intake for a day or two, giving your metabolism a shot in the arm. Research shows that eating a large amount of carbohydrate (2 grams or more per pound of body weight per day) is particularly effective for this.

4. Drink alcohol intelligently.

As you learned earlier in this chapter, the smart way to drink alcohol is to:

1. Not drink more than one day per week.
2. Lower your carb and fat intakes that day. (Eat more protein than you normally would.)
3. Try not to eat while drinking and stay away from carb-laden drinks, like beer and fruity stuff. (Stick to dry wines and spirits.)

You now know how to use food to build muscle, lose fat, and optimize health and well-being. And that means you're ready to put your newly acquired skills into action by creating your first *Muscle for Life* meal plan (and remember that you can find a digital template for this in the bonus material).

So, let's do that now, shall we? Then, once you're happy with your plan, start using it! That's right, it's time to set your course for a fitter, leaner, and stronger you and start the program!

Then we'll keep forging ahead and learn how to incorporate effective strength and cardio workouts into your new lifestyle.

KEY TAKEAWAYS

- ✦ If you're unhappy with your body fat percentage and want to get lean, you want to cut first. If you're very overweight, you also want to cut first.
- ✦ If you're thin or lean and want to focus on gaining muscle and strength, you want to lean gain.
- ✦ If you're a man at 15 percent body fat or higher or a woman at 25 percent or higher, start by cutting down to around 10 percent body fat (men)/20 percent (women).
- ✦ If your body fat percentage is somewhere between 10 and 15 percent (men)/20 and 25 percent (women), you can choose to cut, lean gain, or maintain, based on what's most appealing to you.
- ✦ Your cut phases should end when you're around 10 to 12 percent body fat (men)/20 to 22 percent (women), unless you have a special reason to get leaner; this should take around eight to twelve

weeks in most cases, but it can take months if you have a lot of fat to lose.

+ Your lean gain phases should end when you're around 15 to 17 percent body fat (men)/25 to 27 percent (women), which should take around twelve to sixteen weeks for most people.

+ Decide how many meals to eat based on your appetite, eating preferences, and schedule.

+ Try to eat out no more than once per week while cutting, and no more than twice per week while lean gaining or maintaining.

+ If you can accurately estimate the macros of your restaurant meals (usually because they're simple), you can eat out more often without issue.

+ Don't drink more than 10 percent of your daily calories.

PART 3

THE LAST EXERCISE ADVICE YOU'LL EVER NEED

9

The Little Big Things about Building Lean Muscle (at Any Age)

Nothing in the world is worth having or worth doing
unless it means effort, pain, difficulty.
—THEODORE ROOSEVELT

Thousands of years ago, the small town of Croton in southern Italy was renowned for producing extraordinary athletes. Its crown jewel was a wrestler named Milo, who dominated the sport, winning the Olympic Games in Greece six times, the Pythian Games seven times, the Isthmian Games ten times, and the Nemean Games nine times.

Talent and technique alone weren't responsible for Milo's unprecedented success. He also possessed enormous strength that became the stuff of legend, including purported feats like carrying his own bronze statue to its place at Olympia, bracing a pillar of a collapsing building to save the inhabitants, and hoisting an adult bull onto his back before slaughtering, cooking, and eating it in a single day.

The feast in the final anecdote was also the culmination of a ritual that Milo used to develop his powerful physique. Years earlier, a calf was born near his home, and on a whim, Milo shouldered the animal and carried it around town. Despite the glares and gibes from fellow villagers, the next day he did it again, and then again, and every day thereafter for four years.

As the animal grew larger and heavier, Milo grew bigger and stronger, and eventually he was lugging around a full-grown bull and pummeling his wrestling opponents with his tremendous might. The rest, as they say, was history.

This tale illustrates one of the primary principles of strength training and muscle building—the importance of gradually increasing levels of *mechanical tension* in muscles over time, working your way up to what once seemed impossible.

Research shows that there are three primary "triggers" or "pathways" for muscle growth:

1. Mechanical tension
2. Muscle damage
3. Cellular fatigue

Mechanical tension refers to the amount of force produced in muscle fibers by stretching and contracting—in layman's terms, the strength of a muscle. *Muscle damage* refers to microscopic damage caused to the muscle fibers by high levels of tension. It's unclear whether muscle damage directly stimulates muscle growth or is just a side effect of mechanical tension, but as of now, it deserves a place on the list. *Cellular fatigue* refers to a host of chemical changes that occur inside and outside muscle fibers when they contract repeatedly. When you perform a resistance training exercise to the point of near failure (where you can no longer contract your muscles), this causes high amounts of cellular fatigue.

Studies show that mechanical tension is the most important of these three drivers of muscle growth. In other words, mechanical tension produces a stronger muscle-building stimulus than do muscle damage and cellular fatigue.

These three factors also relate to what scientists call the *strength-endurance continuum*, which works like this:

✦ Moving heavy loads produces higher amounts of mechanical tension and muscle damage and lower amounts of cellular fatigue, and primarily increases muscle *strength*.

✦ Moving lighter loads produces lower amounts of mechanical tension and muscle damage and higher amounts of cellular fatigue, and primarily increases muscle *endurance*.

Based on what you've just learned, which of those styles of training do you think is more effective for gaining muscle? That's right—the first, because moving heavy loads produces more mechanical tension than moving lighter ones, and mechanical tension activates more muscle growth than muscle damage or cellular fatigue.

Contrary to what many trainers and fitness lovers will tell you, the key to getting fit and strong isn't mixing up the stimuli your muscles are exposed to (exercises, for instance)—it's *making your muscles generate more force (tension)*. This explains why Milo's crude training regimen was so effective. Day by day, week by week, month by month, and year by year, it forced his body to handle more and more weight.

The *Muscle for Life* strength training program will do the same for you because instead of ineffective exercise methods and theories like "metabolic conditioning," "muscle confusion," and "functional training," this program revolves around progressive overload. For instance, on the beginner workout routine, you'll do two squat exercises in your first lower-body workout of the week: the bodyweight squat and bodyweight split squat. As you get stronger, your body weight alone will no longer provide enough resistance to effectively challenge your muscles. That's why the intermediate workout routine introduces you to two tougher squat exercises that use dumbbells to achieve progressive overload again: the dumbbell goblet squat and dumbbell lunge.

Now, if you're a guy, chances are you're already sold on strength training and gaining muscle. You want to get bigger, leaner, and stronger, and you're probably happy to hear that heavy resistance training is the answer. If you're a woman, however, you may have misgivings because you want to get fit and defined, not "muscular" and "bulky." If there's one mainstream misconception that causes more harm to women's fitness than any other, it's this one—the female musclehead myth.

At first glance, it seems plausible. Heavy weights are for the boys who want bulging biceps, right? Why would women who want toned and feminine muscles train in the same way? Here's the answer: it's much harder for women to build a big, bulky body than most realize. It doesn't happen by accident or overnight even for us guys—despite our significant physical advantages, we still have to work like the devil to get ripped—so women have about as much to fear from strength training as from chocolate cake.

What's more, neither men nor women can "lengthen" and "tighten" their muscles, change their shape, or specifically target the fat covering them. We can add muscle to our frame and remove body fat. Nothing more or less. Therefore, the claims that certain forms of exercise produce "long, lean" muscles, like a dancer's body, while others produce "bulging, ugly" muscles, like a bodybuilder's, are bogus, as is exercise advice for "toning," "sculpting," and "shaping" muscles. Whether you do Pilates, yoga, or strength training to develop your muscles, their shape will come out the same. The only difference is the rate at which they'll grow.

Details are important, however, because if women gain muscle willy-nilly without managing body fat levels, they can cut a blocky and bloated figure. But if they do it correctly, as they will on *Muscle for Life*, they wind up with muscle definition, curves, and lines in all the right places.

That said, there are still women out there who follow many of the training principles you'll learn in this section of the book and look bulky enough to give you pause. What you must understand, though, is that in most cases, that look is caused not by carrying around too much muscle per se, but by too much body fat.

Fat accumulates inside and on top of muscle tissue, so the more fat and muscle we have, the larger and rounder our body looks. When we reduce our body fat level, however, everything changes—instead of looking large and puffy, we look lean and athletic. Thus, for anyone (male or female) who wants to be strong and defined but not bulky, the recipe is more muscle and less body fat than average. To see what I mean, refer back to the body fat charts on pages 115 and 116.

In my experience, the figure most female fitness enthusiasts desire is around 20 percent body fat with about 15 pounds of muscle added to the right places on their bodies. As for men, the Goldilocks zone of body composition is about 20 to 35 pounds of muscle gain and 10 to 15 percent body fat. If that seems like a galaxy away because of where you're starting, don't dwell on this. Instead, focus on the initial progress you'll make on the *Muscle for Life* program, and then, as you advance further, on how far you've come from where you began. Then, as you approach the homestretch, you'll have so much momentum that motivation will take care of itself.

You may also wonder how lean both guys and gals must be to have visible abs (since you likely want to see yours in the mirror at some point). The rule of thumb is that the core muscles start to show at about 15 percent body fat in men and 25 percent in women, and they look tight and defined around 10 percent in men and 20 percent in women.

Moreover, you don't have to do a single ab exercise to get a washboard stomach. You only have to do two things:

1. Lose belly fat.
2. Develop your core muscles.

As you now know, number one is accomplished through controlling your calories and macros, and while you can accomplish number two with ab exercises, there's an easier way of developing your core muscles without ever doing a single crunch, plank, or side bend—something we'll talk more about in chapter 9.

So, to recap: *Muscle for Life* will focus on making you *strong* by exposing your muscles to larger amounts of mechanical tension (progressive overload). To do that most effectively, we'll use three exercise movements that have been the staples of strength training for over a century now:

1. Pushing
2. Pulling
3. Squatting

These categories of exercise have featured prominently in every great strength program ever devised, going all the way back to the beginning with strongman pioneers like Eugen Sandow, Katie Sandwina (who famously beat Sandow in an exhibition by pressing a 300-pound-dumbbell overhead), and George Hackenschmidt. Put simply: the stronger you are on these basic movements—the more weight you can push, pull, and squat—the better you'll look, feel, and perform. That's why most of the strength training in *Muscle for Life* falls into one of these three buckets.

Don't worry, though—that doesn't mean I plan on throwing you headlong into "extreme" weightlifting, like barbell squatting, deadlifting, and bench pressing. Instead, I'll offer you three training programs to choose from depending on your current fitness, mobility, and experience that'll provide you with challenging and productive, but not backbreaking (pun intended), workouts.

As you'll see, if you're out of shape and new to strength training, your workouts will look very different than if you're in good shape and hitting the gym regularly. I'll also give separate training programs for men and women that I hope better reflect your individual goals, as well as a variety of exercise and workout options so you can create a custom routine designed to achieve the body *you* want.

Before we get to all of that, however, let's learn about pushing, pulling, and squatting in more detail, so you can understand why they're so vital for building an outstanding body.

THE POWER OF PUSHING

Pushing against resistance is one of the best ways to develop upper-body strength and muscularity. When you push something away from your body, as you do with exercises like the push-up, dumbbell bench press, and barbell bench press, you engage some of the largest muscle groups above the waist, including your *pectorals* (chest), *deltoids* (shoulders), and *triceps* (arms).

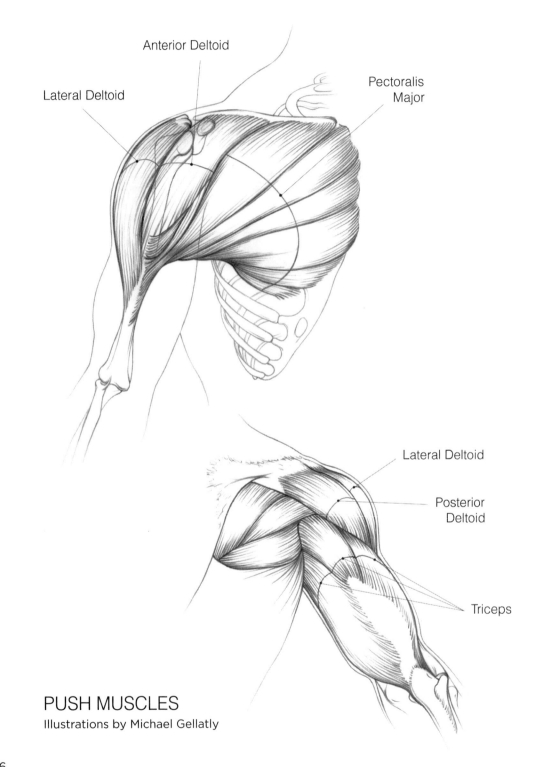

Anterior Deltoid

Lateral Deltoid

Pectoralis
Major

Lateral Deltoid

Posterior
Deltoid

Triceps

PUSH MUSCLES
Illustrations by Michael Gellatly

Push power isn't only for looking fit, either. These muscles are involved in many everyday activities like getting out of bed in the morning, opening doors and cabinets, and lifting items over your head.

THE POWER OF PULLING

Pulling against resistance is another fantastic way to gain muscle and strength in your upper body. When you pull something toward your body, as you do with exercises like the pull-up, dumbbell row, and deadlift, you activate the largest muscle group in your torso, your back muscles, and your *biceps* (arms), as well as, in some cases, your core muscles (*abs* and *obliques*) and lower body.

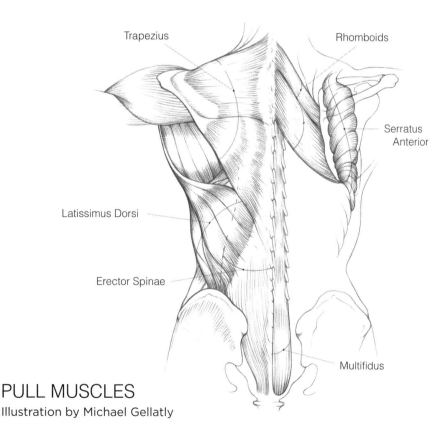

Trapezius

Rhomboids

Serratus Anterior

Latissimus Dorsi

Erector Spinae

Multifidus

PULL MUSCLES
Illustration by Michael Gellatly

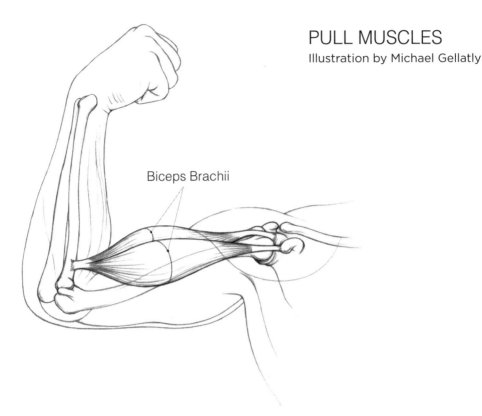

PULL MUSCLES

Illustration by Michael Gellatly

Biceps Brachii

Pulling strength is also highly functional because many routine actions rely on it, including lifting and moving heavy stuff like grocery bags, appliances, furniture, and children.

THE POWER OF SQUATTING

Squatting exercises are the absolute best way to develop a strong, athletic lower body. When you squat, as you do in popular exercises like the bodyweight squat, goblet squat, and barbell squat, you work the largest muscle group in your entire body, the *quadriceps* (front of legs), as well as every other muscle below the belt, including the *glutes* (butt), *hip flexors* (hips), *hamstrings* (back of legs), and *calves*. The squat also trains your core muscles and your upper and lower back muscles (especially your *erector spinae*).

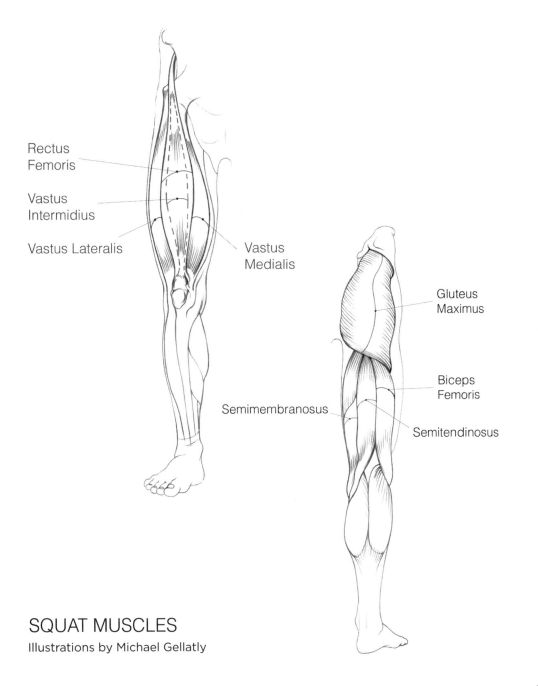

Rectus
Femoris

Vastus
Intermidius

Vastus Lateralis

Vastus
Medialis

Gluteus
Maximus

Biceps
Femoris

Semimembranosus

Semitendinosus

SQUAT MUSCLES

Illustrations by Michael Gellatly

A strong lower body that can squat well is vital for general fitness as well as for preserving our health and quality of life as we get older, because many mundane and recreational activities rely on lower-body strength and function—getting out of a chair, getting into and out of a car, and climbing a flight of stairs, for example.

You can spend hundreds of hours studying strength training and muscle building and barely scratch the surface. The biomechanics and physiology are complex and involve hundreds of functions and adaptations. Fortunately, you don't need to be a scientist to get a working understanding of the major levers for getting fitter and stronger. And this chapter has given you the three biggest ones: pushing, pulling, and squatting.

With just these movements (plus a few others we'll discuss soon), you can develop every important muscle group in your body and transform your physique. To do that, however, you'll need to understand the cardinal rules of effective strength training contained in the next chapter.

KEY TAKEAWAYS

✦ There are three primary "triggers" or "pathways" for muscle growth: mechanical tension, muscle damage, and cellular fatigue. Mechanical tension is the most important one.

✦ Simply producing high levels of tension in the muscles isn't enough to maximize growth—you must increase the amount of tension your muscles produce over time, a process known as progressive overload.

✦ The figure most female fitness enthusiasts desire is around 20 percent body fat with about 15 pounds of muscle added to the right places on their bodies, whereas for men the Goldilocks zone of body composition is about 20 to 35 pounds of muscle gain and 10 to 15 percent body fat.

✦ Pushing against resistance is one of the best ways to develop upper-body strength and muscularity, because it engages some of the largest muscle groups above the waist, including your pectorals (chest), deltoids (shoulders), and triceps (arms).

✦ Pulling against resistance is another fantastic way to gain muscle and strength in your upper body, because it activates the largest muscle group in your torso, your back muscles, and your biceps (arms), as well as, in some cases, your core muscles (abs and obliques) and lower body.

✦ When you squat, as you do in popular exercises like the bodyweight squat, goblet squat, and barbell squat, you work the quadriceps (front of legs), the glutes (butt), hip flexors (hips), hamstrings (back of legs), and calves, as well as your core muscles and your upper and lower back muscles (especially your erector spinae).

10

The 5 Commandments of Successful Strength Training

Opportunity is missed by most people,
because it is dressed in overalls and looks like work.

—UNKNOWN

f you're like most of my readers, you want a specific body. If you're a guy, you want to be muscular and lean, but not hulking. You want washboard abs; striking chest, back, and arm muscles; and strong, solid legs. And if you're a gal, you want to be toned, but not *skinny* (and definitely not "skinny fat"), with shapely legs and perky glutes; a flat, defined stomach; and a feminine but sculpted upper body.

You can have these things. You don't need top-shelf genetics or a lifetime of training to look and feel like a million bucks. You must know what you're doing, though, because you can't become an Adonis or Aphrodite by just cutting your carbs and counting your steps. Instead, you need to take a different approach to your fitness—one that's more challenging, but also more rewarding.

It begins with this: out of all the things we can do in the gym, we want to devote most of our time and efforts to the actions that produce most of the results. In other words, we want to apply the *Pareto principle* to our training, which states that in many domains, roughly 80 percent of the effects come from 20 percent of the causes.

This postulate originated with the economist Vilfredo Pareto, and we can observe it nearly everywhere we look. Research shows that around 20 percent of patients account for 80 percent of healthcare spending in the United States; 15 percent of baseball players produce 85 percent of the wins; and 20 percent of criminals commit 80 percent of the crimes.

The Pareto principle also applies to exercise, where a pocketful of training maxims and methods produces most of the progress. What are those vital principles? We can express them in a simple formula:

$$3–5 \mid 5–7 \mid 9–15 \mid 60–80 \mid 2–4$$

No, that isn't a secret code that you have to break, but it does contain the "secrets" to building the body you've always wanted. Here's the full prescription:

+ Do *3 to 5* strength training workouts per week.
+ Train major muscle groups at least once every *5 to 7* days.
+ Do *9 to 15* hard sets per workout.
+ Train with *60 to 80* percent of one-rep max.
+ Rest *2 to 4* minutes in between hard sets.

Let's go through those instructions one at a time and learn how to combine them into a workout plan that really works.

3–5

Do Three to Five Strength Training Workouts Per Week

Search the hashtag #nodaysoff on social media, and you'll find a lot of very fit people bragging about their dedication and determination. While I applaud the effort, intense training six or seven days per week is a one-way street to physical and psychological burnout (especially when cutting).

Strength training isn't easy. Your joints, tendons, and muscles take a beating, and your nervous system redlines. Although this is a healthy and necessary part of getting fitter and stronger, it also accumulates fatigue that leads to reductions in speed, power, and technique. Some research shows that this response to training may be more of a mental or emotional state, rather than a purely physical phenomenon, but it's real, and you need to know how to deal with it.

If you ignore your body's signals and keep pressing on, you can develop symptoms related to overreaching, including:

+ Soreness, fatigue, and weakness that don't go away with rest
+ Trouble sleeping
+ Reduction in appetite and unintended weight loss
+ Irritability, anxiety, impatience, and restlessness
+ Irregular heart rate
+ Inability to focus
+ Depression

Therefore, I recommend three to five days of strength training per week, which is enough to achieve your fitness goals without putting your health or well-being at risk. This is why all of the *Muscle for Life* workout routines entail three strength training workouts per week and encourage up to two hours of cardiovascular exercise per week as well. There's a time and place for more strength training—up to five workouts per week—but chances are you're new to my approach to fitness and therefore don't need to do more than three sessions of strength training per week to make fantastic progress (so why spend more time in the gym than you need to?).

A caveat, though: as you gain experience on this program (and start seeing results), you'll probably begin to feel like your "rest days" are wasted opportunities to build a little more muscle or lose a little more fat. Remember, however, that downtime is vital component of *Muscle for Life* because it allows you to relax and recharge and give your all to your workouts every week.

5-7

Train Each Major Muscle Group at Least Once
Every Five to Seven Days

How frequently you should train each *major muscle group* (the primary muscles involved in pushing, pulling, and squatting that you learned about in the previous chapter) depends on your schedule, your goals, and the difficulty of each workout. A good rule of thumb, however, is to train all the muscles you most want to develop at least once per week.

For instance, if you're training three days per week and are most interested in developing your upper body, you'd want to emphasize your push and pull muscles over your squat muscles by, let's say, using sessions one and three for both pushing and pulling, while training your lower body in session two. Similarly, if you most want to develop your lower body, you'd want to spend more time squatting than pushing or pulling.

How many push, pull, squat, and other strength training workouts you can do every week depends on how difficult they are, and the difficulty of strength training workouts mostly depends on their *intensity* (the amount of resistance used in exercises) and *volume* (the amount of work done). The more weight (resistance) you use on exercises, and the more sets you do in a session, the harder the workout is to do and recover from. Therefore, the higher the intensity and volume of individual workouts, the less frequently you can do them. This means, for instance, that you could do two or even three squat or push workouts per week, but they could only be so difficult— you could only use so much weight and do so many sets in each one.

(And in case you're not familiar with the term *set*, it's a group of consecutive *repetitions* or *reps*, which are individual complete motions of an exercise. If you do ten push-ups before resting, that's 1 set of 10 reps.)

The key, then, is striking a balance between working out too hard and not hard enough, which brings me to the next point . . .

9–15

Do 9 to 15 Hard Sets Per Workout

Each *Muscle for Life* workout will entail warming up and performing 12 *hard sets* (meaning your difficult muscle- and strength-building sets), which will take you about one hour. That means I'm asking for as little as three hours of your time each week—or about as much time as the average American spends in front of the TV or on social media every day.

This is probably less effort and time than you expected, given the results I'm promising, especially if you've seen popular strength training workouts that call for 25 to 30 hard sets or more per session. Such workouts are popular but often inefficient and even counterproductive, because you can only train an individual muscle group so much in a single workout before reaching the point where further effort fails to produce further muscle growth. Research shows that this threshold is likely between 8 and 10 hard sets, depending on how much resistance you're using and how fit you are.

Just as the number of hard sets per muscle group *per workout* is important, so is the number of hard sets per muscle group *per week*. A growing body of evidence shows that someone new to proper strength training needn't do more than 10 hard sets per major muscle group per week to gain considerable muscle and strength, and intermediate and advanced trainees need to do upward of 15 to 20 hard sets per week to continue making progress.

60–80

Train with 60 to 80 Percent of Your One-Rep Max

In *Muscle for Life*, you'll use weights that are between 60 and 80 percent of your *one-rep max*, which is the most weight you can move on an exercise for one rep. This will mean doing anywhere from 8 to 15 reps per set before stopping to rest—much harder than many people who do resistance training are used to, because a lot of fitness programs involve light weights and many reps, which is an inefficient way to train. While training with lighter loads can cause muscle growth, research shows that it only results in significant improvements when sets are taken to or close to *muscle failure* (the point where you can no longer complete a full repetition).

There are two problems with this style of training: first, doing 20+ reps per set is *extremely* unpleasant (sets take longer, feel harder, and cause more fatigue than lower-rep, higher-load training); and second, training to muscle failure regularly isn't optimal because it can increase the risk of injury.

By increasing the weight and doing fewer reps per set, however—as you will on this program—you can produce a powerful muscle-building stimulus without having to bust a gut or extend yourself to muscle failure.

Now, you may be hoping it's easy to calculate your one-rep maxes to ensure you use the proper amount of weight in your workouts. You may also be concerned that this system will be complicated or that you'll mess it up. Fear not, because no math will be required. Instead, I'll give you a simple and intuitive method for figuring out your starting weights and then properly progressing to heavier loads. But first, let's discuss the final strength training precept on our list.

2-4

Rest Two to Four Minutes in Between Hard Sets

Since most people go to the gym to move and sweat, sitting around in between sets seems like a waste of time, so they keep rest periods short or even skip them, preferring to always stay in motion. This is fine when you just want to burn calories, but if you want to gain muscle and get stronger, it's a mistake.

Strength training involves pushing your muscles to their limits and then backing off, and resting enough between sets is a vital step because it gives your heart time to settle down and gets you ready to give maximum effort in your next hard set.

Science agrees, too. A study conducted by scientists at the State University of Rio de Janeiro found that resting three to five minutes between sets allowed participants to do more reps, use heavier weights, and get in more total training (volume). Similar findings were demonstrated in another study conducted at Eastern Illinois University. In this case, researchers concluded that when training with heavy weights, two to four minutes of rest between sets produces the best results.

In practice, you can rest slightly less (two minutes) between hard sets for smaller muscle groups, like the biceps, triceps, and shoulders, and slightly more (up to four minutes) between hard sets for your larger muscle groups, like your back, chest, and legs.

Don't be surprised if that much rest feels strange to you at first. You may even feel guilty, as if you're sitting around more than working out. Trust the process, however, watch how your body responds to the workouts, and rest easy (literally) knowing that the lulls are contributing significantly to the whole.

As for what to do while resting between sets, most important is actually *resting* so your body is ready for another round of intense exertion. That means you should mostly be sitting or standing, not doing plyometrics or cardiovascular exercise. Another must is keeping track of time so you don't accidentally under- or overrest. The stopwatch app on your phone is a simple tool for this.

Beyond that, whatever you do or don't do while resting is up to you, but most people find they enjoy their training more if they stay off the Internet, social media, and e-mail, and instead focus on how their workout is going, how their body is feeling, and what they hope to accomplish in their next set (in fact, studies show that envisioning the successful completion of a resistance training set beforehand can increase performance!).

––––––––––

Now that we've gone through the entire formula I introduced you to at the beginning of this chapter, let's discuss other aspects of strength training that are vital for optimizing your results.

HOW TO ACHIEVE PROGRESSIVE OVERLOAD

One of the most important parts of strength training is progressive overload. No matter how much thought you put into frequency, intensity, volume, or any other factor related to workout programming, if you don't get progressive overload right, you won't make it very far. It's the key to avoiding stagnation and breaking through training plateaus when they inevitably occur.

There are a couple of practical ways to achieve progressive overload in strength training, but one of the best methods is known as *double progression*. In double progression, you work with a weight in a *rep range* (a minimum and maximum number of reps to strive for in a set, like 10 to 12 reps, for instance), and once you hit the top of that rep range for a certain number of hard sets in a row, you increase the weight. Then, if you can finish your first hard set with the new, heavier weight within at least a rep or two of the bottom of your rep range, you continue working with that weight until you can hit the progression target again. So, with this approach to progressive overload, you work to increase your reps, and then "cash in" that progress to increase your weights. Hence, *double progression.*

To see how this works in action, let's say you're following one of the men's intermediate programs, which has you working in the rep range of 8 to 10 reps for many exercises and requires 3 hard sets of 10 reps in a row on an exercise before increasing the weight. You start your pushing workout, which begins with 3 sets of the dumbbell bench press. So far, you've worked up to 50 pounds on this exercise, and this time, you get 10 reps on all 3 sets. Hooray! Time to progress!

That means the following week, when you do this workout again, you'll use 55 pounds on the dumbbell bench press. Since you're working in the 8 to 10 rep range, your goal is to get at least 6 reps on your first hard set (within at least 2 reps of 8, the bottom of your rep range). If you can do this, your progression has succeeded, and you'll now work with 55 pounds until you can do 3 hard sets of 10 reps in a row, and so on. And what if you can't get at least 8 reps in your first hard set with 55 pounds? We'll talk more about progression in this program, including this point and others, in chapter 12.

HOW TO USE A PROPER RANGE OF MOTION

Range of motion refers to how much you *flex* or *extend* a joint during an exercise. *Flexion* occurs when you reduce the angle between two parts of your body—shortening the angle between your forearm and upper arm when curling a dumbbell, for instance. *Extension* occurs when you increase the angle between two parts of your body, like when you stand up from a chair, which increases the angles between your thighs and torso and your thighs and shins.

When you perform a strength training exercise, there's a limit to how much you can safely and comfortably flex and extend the major joints involved (your knees and hips in the squat, elbows in the barbell curl, shoulders and elbows in the bench press, and so forth). A proper range of motion in a strength training exercise is a *full* one, which involves moving the major joints to their natural limits of flexion and extension (beyond which, injury could occur).

For example, with the push-up, a full range of motion requires that you lower your chest until it touches the floor (elbow flexion), and then press upward until your arms are straight (elbow extension). And with the pull-up, you must raise your body until your chin is above the bar (elbow flexion), and then lower yourself until your arms are straight (elbow extension).

Using a full range of motion when strength training is important because it increases muscle and strength gain, and may also reduce the risk of injury because when you use a partial range of motion, the stress produced by the exercise is concentrated on smaller areas of your joints.

When doing a partial squat (only lowering your butt a foot or two), for instance, much of the stress is concentrated on the tendons at the front of your knee. As you keep lowering your body, though, the burden shifts to other tendons and ligaments. By using a full range of motion, then, you allow your entire joints to share the strains of strength training, and this reduces the chances of localized irritation and inflammation.

HOW TO USE PROPER FORM

Along with a full range of motion, you also need to control how your body and the weight are moving in each rep. You should always feel like you're using your muscles to execute the movements, not gravity or momentum.

For example, when doing push-ups, instead of relaxing your chest and arms and allowing your torso to drop toward the floor, you want to keep your upper-body muscles tight as you lower your chest. Similarly, on the chin-up, instead of swinging your knees to help you ascend and then allowing your body to drop downward, you want to keep your legs motionless as you pull yourself up and then smoothly lower yourself down.

To use a full range of motion and proper form in your workouts, you need to know how to do exercises properly, of course, but you also need to use the right amount of weight. We'll talk about how to determine your training weights later in this section of the book, but know this for now: if you use too much weight, you won't be able to complete your workouts as prescribed without shortening the range of motion or spoiling your form, which compromises the effectiveness and safety of your training.

So, in summary, proper form is achieved when an appropriate weight is moved through the right range of motion with the right technique.

HOW HARD YOUR "HARD SETS" SHOULD BE

To get the most out of double progression, you must ensure that your hard sets are hard enough to produce high levels of tension in your muscles. Here's how to do this:

+ End all hard sets of bodyweight exercises 1 rep shy of muscle failure, which is the point where you fail to complete a rep. That is, continue hard sets of bodyweight exercises until you feel you have 0 good reps left in the tank.
+ End all hard sets of machine, dumbbell, and barbell exercises 2 to 3 reps shy of muscle failure (1 to 2 good reps left).

Why the difference in difficulty? You can work harder in bodyweight exercises because failure is less exhausting and dangerous than with machines, barbells, and dumbbells. So, if your workout calls for push-ups, you'd end each hard set at the point where you feel you can't complete another rep. And with, let's say, the barbell bench press, you'd push your hard sets to where you feel you can do 1 or 2 more reps.

And how do you gauge how close you are to muscle failure? It's mostly a matter of trial and error, but once you start training, you'll quickly become attuned to your proximity to failure. An easy way to develop this intuition faster is, as you're approaching the end of a hard set, to ask yourself, "If I absolutely had to, how many more reps could I get with good form?" Your instinctive answer will often be accurate, especially as you become more experienced.

It may not seem like it, but you've just learned one of the unsung keys to successful strength training: knowing how hard to train in your workouts. Many people don't work hard enough and wonder why nothing changes, and many others work too hard and wonder why they're always stuck in a rut and hurting. You now know how to thread this needle effectively.

HOW USE A PROPER REP TEMPO

Rep tempo refers to how quickly you do an exercise when strength training, and there are two schools of thought here: slowly and fairly quickly. People who advocate for a slow tempo often say that "muscles don't know weight, only tension," and the longer muscles remain under tension, the more effective the training. Thus, by slowing down your reps, they claim you can produce more muscle growth than with faster reps. But research shows otherwise—slow-rep training has been put to the test in quite a few studies, and in each instance, a faster rep tempo produced better results.

Time under tension isn't important enough to warrant special attention because if you perform an exercise slowly, you have to reduce either the load or the number of reps, or both, compared to a faster tempo. As load and reps are major factors in how much muscle and strength you gain from training, reducing either (and especially both) is detrimental.

Therefore, I recommend that you follow a "1-0-1" rep tempo for all strength training exercises. This means the first part of each rep should take about one second, followed by a momentary pause, followed by the return to starting position in about one second. If we apply this to a simple exercise like the bodyweight squat, it would mean sitting down in about one second ("one, one thousand"), pausing for an instant, and standing up at the same pace.

Don't worry about trying to achieve this tempo perfectly. You're doing it right when you're moving through the first part of an exercise in a swift but controlled manner, barely pausing, and finishing the rep as quickly as possible while maintaining good technique.

HOW TO AVOID INJURY

Many strength training injuries aren't caused by training too hard in any individual workout, but by failing to recover from previous workouts. Here's a common scenario: Your knee feels stiff the day after a lower-body workout, and you shrug it off. A few weeks later, it's starting to hurt while you squat. "No pain, no gain," you say, and keep going. A few more weeks and . . . well, now your knee doesn't want to knee anymore.

These are called *repetitive stress injuries* (RSIs), and they're the bane of every athlete—not painful enough to put you on the sidelines, but troubling enough to hinder your performance. Fortunately, a bit of rest is all it usually takes to eliminate RSIs. In fact, that's the only way to do it—once an RSI has set in, you must avoid the activity that caused it (and will continue to aggravate it), along with any other activities that prolong the problem. This often means avoiding specific exercises, but sometimes also forces you to stop training a muscle group altogether until the injury has healed.

Strength training isn't nearly as dangerous as many people think, but as with any strenuous physical activity, if you do it enough, you'll probably experience at least a mild RSI of one kind or another along the way. That doesn't mean you can't take preventive actions to stave them off for as long as possible, though. Let's learn how.

If It Feels Bad, Don't Do It

The rule here is simple: if something hurts or feels "off" while you're doing a set, stop immediately. I'm not talking about muscle soreness or the burning sensation that occurs as you approach failure, but pain or "strange" sensations (especially in or around your joints).

If a rep hurts enough to make you wince, for example, it's a warning that something is wrong, and if you don't listen to it, you're looking for trouble. RSIs can be insidious, and the early symptoms don't always manifest as pain. Instead, your elbow feels "weird" on the last few reps of dumbbell pressing; your knee feels "funny" during a squat workout; or your back feels "tight" when deadlifting. While such sensations aren't always a sign of an RSI, they should get your attention, like a weird noise while driving.

So, when you hit pain or strange, stop, rest for a couple of minutes, and try the exercise again. If it's no better the next time around, do another exercise (that feels fine), and then come back to the problematic one in your next workout and see how it goes. If it's still an issue, substitute a different one again and stay away from the offender until it's no longer bothersome.

If you aren't sure whether what you're feeling qualifies as worrisome or as the normal discomfort of training, ask yourself these two questions:

1. Is the pain on both sides of my body or just one? When you perform exercises correctly, both sides of your body are subjected to stress fairly equally. Thus, if one side hurts more than the other, it's more likely a sign of trouble rather than of muscle burn or fatigue.

2. Is the pain concentrated around a joint or other specific spot? These are the pains you're most likely to encounter. Muscle and joint aches and stiffness usually go away while you warm up, but genuine problems won't and can get worse.

Progress Gradually

One of the easiest ways to get hurt in strength training is through zeal. Maybe you're feeling strong one day or you want to impress someone in the gym or just progress faster, so you load the bar with a weight that makes your Spidey sense tingle. This is almost always a bad idea. It increases the likelihood that your form will break down, and it can place too much stress on your joints and ligaments and impair recovery.

A slow and steady philosophy is much smarter—and ultimately more effective. For instance, if you're new to strength training and you can increase the weight for most exercises every week or two for the first several months, you're doing great. And as you become more experienced, gaining just 1 rep per week on your most difficult exercises (and thus adding weight every few weeks) is respectable.

A winning motto for strength training is "progress is progress," understanding that sometimes you'll advance quickly and other times slowly, but so long as you're moving forward, you're playing the game well.

Be a Stickler for Good Form

Bad form can allow you to move more weight, but it also reduces the quality of the training and increases the risk of injury. This runs counter to the purpose of strength training: controlling heavy loads through full ranges of motion with good technique, not haphazardly lifting as much weight as possible. This is especially important with the most effective push, pull, and squat exercises because, while they're not dangerous, they involve the heaviest weights and most technical skill.

So, don't sacrifice form for the sake of progress or convenience. Instead, learn proper form for every exercise you do and stick to it.

You now possess a powerful plan for long-term fitness success: a moderate dose of relatively short, invigorating strength training workouts that produce consistent results and never leave you feeling agonized, exhausted, or burned out—workouts that you'll delight in rather than dread.

Although simple, my strength training strategy has enough horsepower to radically transform your body and health and enough latitude to accommodate just about all bodies and biases. So, if you've had a falling-out (or five) with fitness, here's your chance to fall back in love with it; and if this is your first foray, you're in for a good time.

Before you can begin your *Muscle for Life* workouts, however, we need to discuss another element of the training methodology: exercise selection.

KEY TAKEAWAYS

+ How frequently you should train each major muscle group (the primary muscles involved in pushing, pulling, and squatting) depends on your schedule, your goals, and the difficulty of each workout, but a good rule of thumb is to train all the muscles you most want to develop at least once every five to seven days.

+ You should rest slightly less (two minutes) between hard sets for smaller muscle groups, like the biceps, triceps, and shoulders, and slightly more (up to four minutes) between hard sets for your larger muscle groups, like your back, chest, and legs.

+ In double progression, you work with a weight in a rep range (a minimum and maximum number of reps to strive for in a set, such as 10 to 12 reps), and once you hit the top of that rep range for a certain number of hard sets in a row, you increase the weight.

+ Proper form is achieved when the right weight is moved through the right range of motion with the right technique.

+ End all hard sets of bodyweight exercises 1 rep shy of muscle failure, which is the point where you fail to complete a rep, and end all hard sets of machine, dumbbell, and barbell exercises 2 to 3 reps shy of muscle failure (2 to 3 good reps left).

+ Use a "1-0-1" rep tempo for all strength training exercises.

+ If something hurts or feels "off" while you're doing a set, stop immediately and rest for a couple of minutes, before trying the exercise again. If it's no better the next time around, do something else, then come back to the problematic exercise in your next workout and see how it goes. If it's still a problem, substitute a different exercise once again and stay away from the offender until it's no longer bothersome.

+ A winning motto for strength training is "progress is progress," understanding that sometimes you'll advance quickly and other times slowly, but so long as you're moving forward, you're playing the game well.

11

The Best Strength Exercises for Building Your Best Body Ever

There is no reason to be alive if you can't do the deadlift!
—JÓN PÁLL SIGMARSSON

O f all the strength training exercises you can do, a few dozen stand head and shoulders above the rest in terms of easiness to execute, measurable effects, and overall impact. And of those, a handful are the real breadwinners, proving the Pareto principle yet again.

This is great news for us because it means we can disregard most of what we see people doing in magazines, social media, and the gym, and focus instead on getting strong on a short list of exercises. In fact, constantly changing exercises to challenge your body in new ways is a poor strength training strategy. The more often you make a switch, the harder it is to become proficient at any of the exercises you're doing, and this slows down your progress. If you stick with a relatively small selection of highly effective exercises that allow you to safely overload your muscles, however, you can get fit and strong faster than you ever thought possible.

In this chapter, I'll share those superior exercises with you, separated into two categories:

1. Primary exercises

2. Accessory exercises

Primary exercises will be responsible for the lion's share of your results because they train (and develop) the most muscle mass and produce the most whole-body strength. As effective as the primary exercises are, however, some muscles are particularly stubborn and slow to respond to training, and others aren't adequately trained by primary exercises alone. We'll use *accessory exercises* to address these issues—further training muscle groups that need more stimulation than primary exercises alone can provide—and also to help prevent and correct muscle imbalances and weaknesses that can limit your progress on your primary exercises.

The *Muscle for Life* exercises will also be divided into pushing, pulling, and squatting movements, and the primary exercises will be labeled as beginner, intermediate, or advanced (there isn't a big enough difference in difficulty between the accessory exercises to require the same designations).

The beginner exercises are for people new to strength training, and they establish a foundation of strength, balance, and coordination that prepares them for more challenging training. Many of the beginner exercises use only your body weight for resistance (bodyweight exercises), while others use weights, like the leg press (machine exercise). Someone who has conquered the beginner exercises is ready for the intermediate exercises, which are similar but with a twist: added weight in the form of dumbbells, barbells, and more machines. Finally, when intermediate exercises are no longer difficult enough, there are the advanced exercises, which are mostly tougher versions of the intermediate-level barbell and dumbbell exercises.

Following is a chart showing all of the exercises included in *Muscle for Life* classified by type and difficulty. No matter where you begin, the ultimate goal is mastering the advanced exercises, which may take a year or longer depending on your current level of fitness.

	Pushing Exercises	Pulling Exercises	Squatting Exercises
Beginner Primaries	Push-up	Bodyweight Row	Bodyweight Squat
	Machine Chest Press	Dumbbell Deadlift	Bodyweight Split Squat
	Machine Shoulder Press	One-Arm Dumbbell Row	Bodyweight Lunge
	Triceps Dip		Bodyweight Step-up
			Leg Press
Intermediate Primaries	Dumbbell Bench Press	Trap-Bar Deadlift	Dumbbell Goblet Squat
	Incline Dumbbell Bench Press	Seated Cable Row	Dumbbell Lunge
	Seated Dumbbell Overhead Press		Dumbbell Split Squat
			Dumbbell Romanian Deadlift
Advanced Primaries	Barbell Bench Press	Barbell Deadlift	Barbell Back Squat
	Incline Barbell Bench Press	Chin-up	Barbell Romanian Deadlift
	Chest Dip	Pull-up	
Accessories	Cable Triceps Pushdown	Lat Pulldown	Leg Extension
	Dumbbell Triceps Overhead Press	Machine Row	Leg Curl
	Machine Cable Fly	Alternating Dumbbell Curl	Glute Bridge
		Cable Biceps Curl	

Although the lingo can make these movements sound formidable, you can rest assured that they're simple enough in practice for anyone to pick up, regardless of their athletic aptitude.

Let's examine these exercises, then, including the major muscle groups involved. Also, to help you visualize each of the movements, I've included links to video demonstrations of them in the free bonus material that comes with this book (www.muscleforlifebook.com/bonus).

THE *MUSCLE FOR LIFE* PUSHING EXERCISES

Pushing exercises involve moving your hands away from your torso either horizontally (in front of your body) or vertically (above your head). In some cases, you use your arms to push your torso away from your hands, as in the push-up (horizontal) and handstand push-up (vertical); and in others, you push a weight away from you, such as a dumbbell or barbell, as with the barbell bench press (horizontal) and seated dumbbell overhead press (vertical).

We recall from chapter 9 that pushing exercises primarily train three major muscle groups:

1. Pectoralis
2. Triceps
3. Deltoids

Together, these muscles are responsible for straightening the elbows, pushing the arms out from and above the body, and rotating the arms.

THE PRIMARY PUSHING EXERCISES

The *Muscle for Life* primary pushing exercises will build much of your upper-body strength and muscle definition, including your chest, shoulders, and arms. Let's go over each of them.

The Beginner Primary Pushing Exercises

Push-up

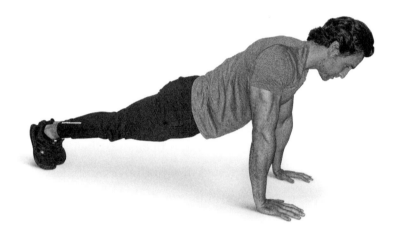

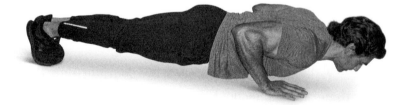

There are three push-up variations included in the *Muscle for Life* program (and in the next chapter, you'll learn why):

1. Regular push-up. Get into the starting position shown opposite. Keeping your back straight, lower your chest to the floor, and then push your body up and return to the starting position.
2. Knee push-up. The knee push-up works exactly like the regular push-up, except instead of resting your weight on your toes and hands, you're on your knees and hands.
3. Feet-elevated push-up. The feet-elevated push-up is identical to the regular push-up, except instead of resting your feet on the floor, you place them on a surface that's about knee-height off the floor.

Machine Chest Press

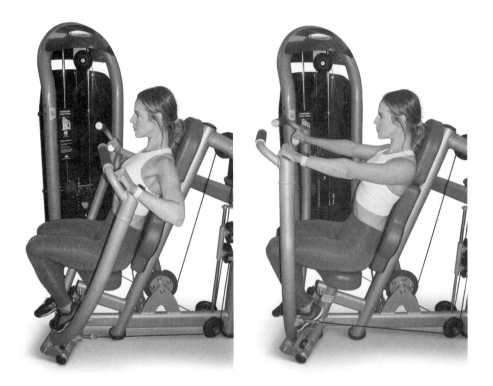

Adjust the handles and seat so the handles are in line with your shoulders and just a few inches from your chest. Grip both handles, press forward until your arms are straight, then bring the handles backward and return to the starting position.

Machine Shoulder Press

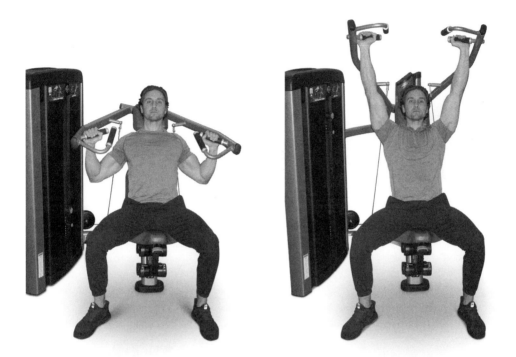

Adjust the handles and seat so the handles are in line with your shoulders and about three to six inches directly above your shoulders. Grip both handles, press them upward until your arms are straight, then lower the handles and return to the starting position.

Triceps Dip

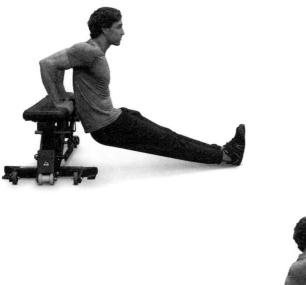

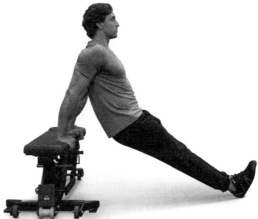

Get into the starting position shown above by facing forward and placing your palms behind you on a chair seat, bench, or other flat surface about knee-height off the floor, and pushing your feet out in front of you and resting on your heels.

Keeping your legs straight and heels on the floor, push your torso upward until your arms are straight. Then reverse the motion until your upper arms are roughly parallel with the floor, push yourself back up again, and return to the starting position.

The Intermediate Primary Pushing Exercises

Dumbbell Bench Press

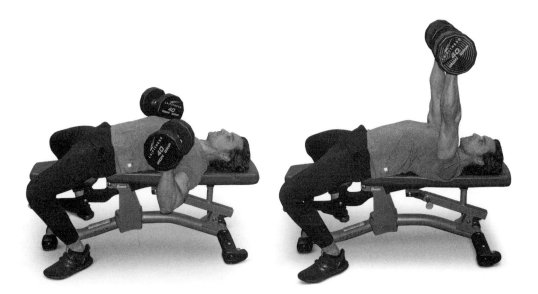

Sit on the edge of the bench with the dumbbells on your thighs. Then get into the starting position shown above by leaning back slowly and gently kicking your thighs (and the dumbbells) toward your chest. Continue to roll back onto the bench until you're lying flat with the dumbbells at either side of your chest.

Pull your shoulder blades together and toward your butt (imagine you're "putting your shoulder blades into your back pockets"), and position your elbows six to ten inches from your ribs.

Then, keeping your shoulder blades and elbows tucked, push the dumbbells straight up until your arms are locked, and finally, lower the dumbbells by reversing the motion (maintaining the position of your shoulder blades and elbows) and return to the starting position.

When you're finished with a set of the dumbbell bench press, you can either lower the dumbbells to your chest and then drop them to the floor, or bring your legs up and toward you into a sitting position, shift the dumbbells onto your thighs, and then sit up by swinging your legs and dumbbells downward and your torso upward. I prefer the latter method—it's slightly more difficult but ensures I don't damage the equipment.

Incline Dumbbell Bench Press

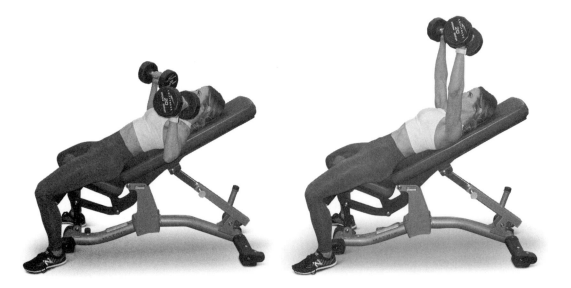

The incline dumbbell bench press works just like the dumbbell bench press, except you first adjust the bench to roughly a 45-degree angle.

Seated Dumbbell Overhead Press

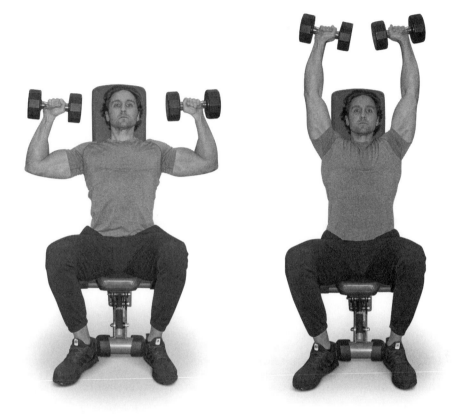

Adjust a bench to an upright position (most people prefer a slight incline, around 75 degrees or so), and get into the starting position shown above by lifting or kicking the dumbbells up with your knees. Then tuck your shoulder blades back and down, push the dumbbells straight up until your arms are locked, lower them, and return to the starting position.

The Advanced Primary Pushing Exercises

Barbell Bench Press

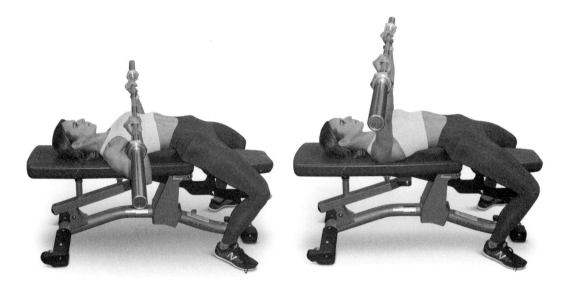

Position yourself on a bench so your eyes are directly under the bar, tuck your shoulder blades back and down, and grab the bar. Your hands should be slightly wider than shoulder-width apart, your fingers and thumbs should be wrapped around the bar, and your wrists should be slightly bent backward, not folded back at a 90-degree angle.

Plant your feet solidly on the floor about shoulder-width apart, squeeze the bar as hard as you can, and move it from the pins or hooks to directly over your chest. Lower the bar until it touches your chest, keeping your elbows six to ten inches from your torso. Then, keeping your shoulder blades and elbows tucked, push the bar straight up, lower it, and return to the starting position.

When you're on the last rep of a set of the barbell bench press, finish it fully, and then bump the bar back into the upright metal bars, and lower it onto the pins or hooks. Don't try to press the bar directly back into the pins or hooks because if you miss, it can fall on your face.

Incline Barbell Bench Press

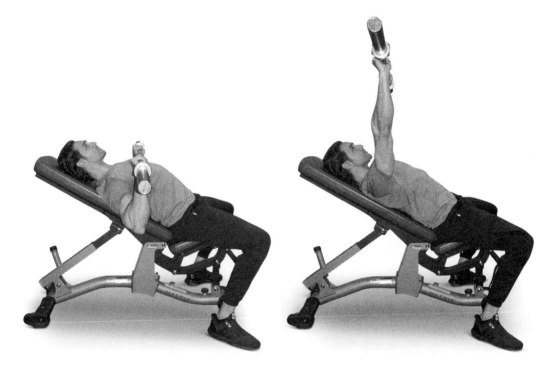

The incline barbell bench press works the same way as the barbell bench press, except you first adjust the bench to roughly a 45-degree angle.

Chest Dip

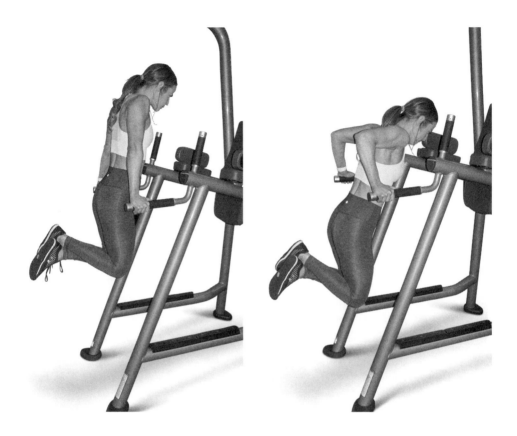

Get into the starting position shown above, with your hands underneath your shoulders. Lower your body until your arms are at a 90-degree angle, then push upward and return to the starting position.

The Accessory Pushing Exercises

Many people struggle to fully develop their chest and shoulders with primary pushing exercises alone or find their triceps definition lacking. Accessory exercises are the solution because they allow us to give these muscle groups extra attention.

Cable Triceps Pushdown

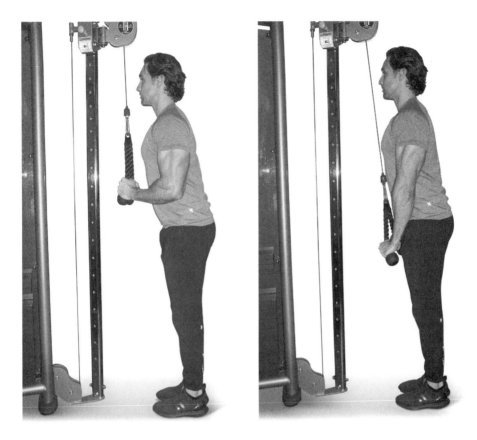

Several handles can work for this exercise, but my favorite is the rope because it's the most comfortable. If your gym doesn't have a rope handle, use either the straight handle or EZ-bar handle (the zigzag one), depending on which you like most.

Attach a handle to a cable machine in its highest position (closest to the ceiling), and get into the starting position shown above. Stand tall, grab the handle, and, keeping your elbows at your sides, push down until your arms are straight. Then, with your elbows remaining fixed to your sides, raise your hands and return to the starting position.

Dumbbell Triceps Overhead Press

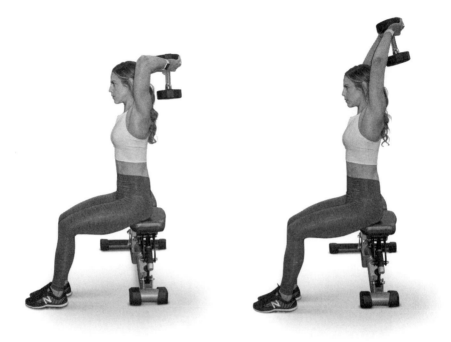

Get into the starting position shown above, look at a spot on the floor six to ten feet in front of you, press your back into the bench, and lower the dumbbell behind your head. Go as far as your flexibility allows, then push the dumbbell toward the ceiling, and return to the starting position. Try to minimize your upper-arm movement during the exercise, as shifting your arms increases the chances of knocking your noggin with the dumbbell.

Machine Cable Fly

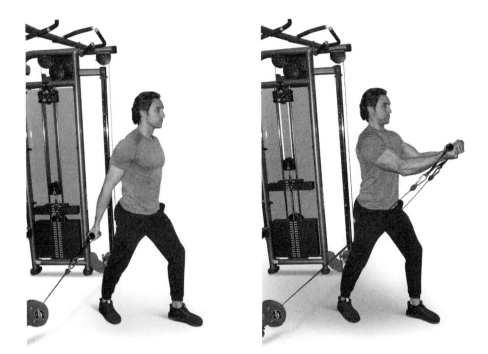

Several handles can also work for this exercise, but my favorite is the strip of nylon with a metal ring on one end and straight plastic handle on the other. If you don't have plastic handles, however, metal ones work as well.

Attach two handles to a cable machine in their lowest position (closest to the floor). This is known as the *low* cable fly, and I prefer it over higher positions because it minimizes stress on the shoulders. If you find this height uncomfortable, however, you can raise the handles to find a level that works better for you.

Get into the starting position shown above and, keeping your arms slightly bent, bring your hands toward each other, squeezing your chest muscles, until your hands are three to six inches apart. Then move your hands away from each other and return to the starting position.

THE *MUSCLE FOR LIFE* PULLING EXERCISES

Pulling exercises involve pulling toward your torso, either horizontally (perpendicular to your torso) or vertically (parallel with it). In a horizontal pulling exercise, you pull directly toward the middle of your torso, usually from beneath or in front of you; and in a vertical exercise, you pull from the floor by standing up or from above toward your chest, or you pull your chest up toward your hands.

Pulling exercises primarily train four major muscle groups:

1. Latissimus dorsi
2. Upper back muscles
3. Lower back muscles
4. Biceps

Collectively, these muscles are responsible for pulling the hands toward the torso; stabilizing the shoulder blades, neck, and spine; and assisting with back extension (going from a hunched position to an upright one).

THE PRIMARY PULLING EXERCISES

The *Muscle for Life* primary pulling exercises will complete your base of upper-body strength and power and prevent imbalances between pushing and pulling muscles (which can lead to aesthetic and functional problems).

The Beginner Primary Pulling Exercises

Bodyweight Row

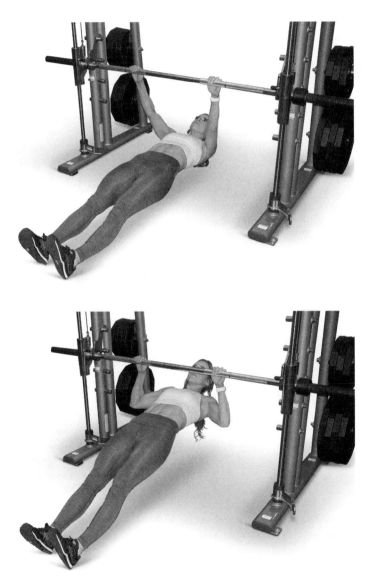

Find a surface to lie under that's more than arm's length off the floor (such as a table, tall bench, or dip station). Get into the starting position shown above, and, keeping your back and legs straight and your butt high, pull your chest upward until it touches the bar (or your nose touches the surface, if using a table, bench, etc.). Then lower yourself and return to the starting position. To increase or decrease the difficulty of this exercise, lower or raise whatever you're holding on to (making your body less or more upright).

Dumbbell Deadlift

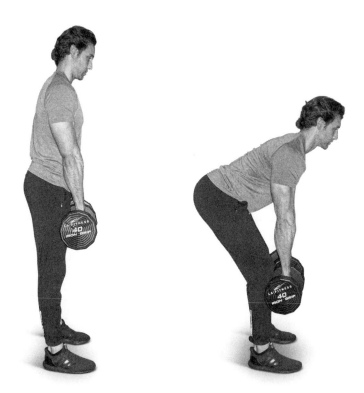

Get into the starting position shown above, holding one dumbbell in each hand. Position your feet slightly narrower than shoulder-width apart, and turn your toes out slightly. Stand up tall with your chest out and arms at your sides, and take a deep breath into your stomach (as opposed to your chest), bracing your abs as if you were about to get punched in the gut.

Squeeze the dumbbells as hard as you can, press your upper arms into your sides (imagine you're crushing oranges in your armpits), and start the descent by pushing your hips backward and bending at the knees. Don't allow your lower back to round as you move downward—instead, arch it slightly. Also, keep your arms straight and locked, and the dumbbells directly beneath (or slightly behind but not in front of) your shoulders. Allow your knees to bend slightly more as the dumbbells pass them, and keep going until the dumbbells are six to eight inches from the floor.

To stand up, drive your body upward by pushing through your heels, keeping your arms straight, lower back slightly arched (no rounding!), and core tight. Also, ensure that your hips and shoulders rise together and at the same rate. Don't make the common mistake of shooting your hips up and then using your back like a lever to raise the dumbbells upward. If your hips are moving up, your shoulders should be as well, and neither should be moving faster than the other.

Once the dumbbells pass your knees, push your hips forward as you return to the starting position. When you're fully upright, your chest should be out and shoulders down, and you shouldn't lean back, hyperextend your lower back, or shrug the dumbbells up.

One-Arm Dumbbell Row

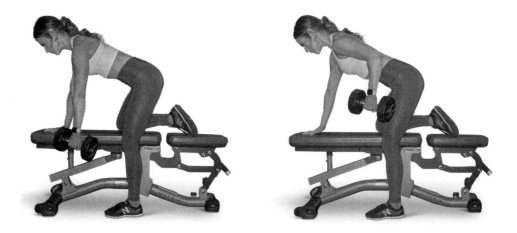

Get into the starting position shown above, and with your right knee and arm firmly planted on the bench and your left foot on the floor a foot or two from the bench, pull the dumbbell toward your torso. As the dumbbell moves upward, it should drift backward toward your abdomen, which should remain more or less motionless and parallel with the floor. Keep pulling until the dumbbell touches the side of your belly or the bottom of your rib cage, then lower it and return to the starting position.

Also, as this is the first single-limb exercise I've given you, a quick note: one set of a single-limb exercise entails training both limbs. For instance, you've completed 1 set of 10 reps of the one-arm dumbbell row when you've done 10 reps for *each arm*.

The Intermediate Primary Pulling Exercises

Trap-Bar Deadlift

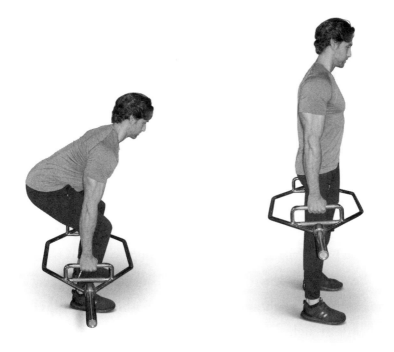

Load the trap-bar with plates. If you aren't strong enough (yet!) to use at least one 45-pound plate on either side of the bar, you'll need to create a platform to ensure that the bar is about eight to ten inches off the floor. To do this, create two stacks of plates to rest the loaded trap-bar on (one on either side of it).

Position your feet about shoulder-width apart inside the center of the trap-bar, and turn your toes out slightly. Stand up tall with your chest out and arms at your sides, take a deep breath into your stomach, and brace your abs. Then get into the starting position shown above by pushing your hips backward and bending at the knees. Don't allow your lower back to round as your hands approach the bar. Instead, arch it slightly.

You'll notice that the trap-bar has high handles, which I'm holding in the pictures above, but also low handles underneath, which you can use by flipping the bar over before loading it (so the high handles are pointing toward the ground). The low handles make the exercise more difficult (especially for the lower back), so if you're new to trap-bar deadlifting, you may want to start with the high handles.

With your arms straight and locked, squeeze the handles as hard as you can, and press your upper arms into your sides. As with the dumbbell deadlift, stand up by pushing through your heels, keeping your arms straight, lower back slightly arched, and core tight. Also, remember to ensure that your hips and shoulders rise together and at the same rate, and when you're fully upright, your chest should be out and shoulders down. And there should be no leaning back, hyperextending your back, or shrugging the weight up.

To lower the bar to the floor, begin by pushing your hips backward, not bending at the knees, and, with your lower back slightly arched and core tight, let the bar move straight down. Continue pushing your hips back, lowering the bar in a straight line down to the ground until you return to the starting position. Don't try to lower the bar slowly or quietly—the entire descent should take just one to two seconds.

Once the bar is on the floor, without releasing your grip on it or standing up, adjust your body as needed to get into the proper starting position for the next rep.

Seated Cable Row

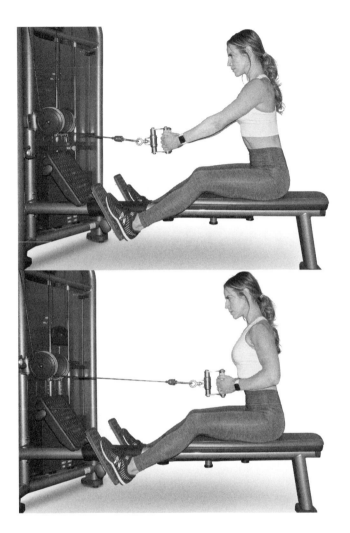

Attach a narrow-grip handle to the cable row machine, and get into the starting position shown above. Keeping your back upright, pull the handle to your abdomen, allowing your torso to move backward just enough to help you finish the rep, but no more. Once the handle touches your torso, straighten your arms and return to the starting position.

The Advanced Primary Pulling Exercises

Barbell Deadlift

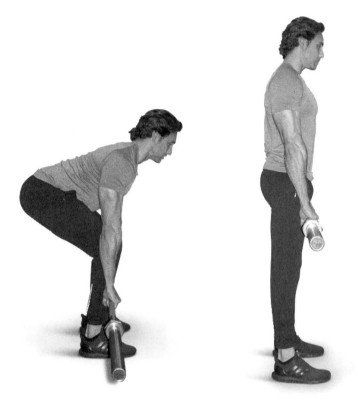

Load the bar with plates, stand in front of the middle of it, position your feet slightly narrower than shoulder-width apart, turn your toes out slightly, and move the bar toward you until it's over the middle of your feet.

Stand up tall with your chest out and arms at your sides, take a deep breath into your stomach, and brace your abs. Then get into the starting position shown above by pushing your hips backward and bending at the knees. Don't allow your lower back to round as your hands approach the bar. Instead, arch it slightly.

Grip the bar just outside your shins with both palms facing down, squeeze it as hard as you can, and press your upper arms into your sides. The bar should be over (or slightly behind but not in front of) the middle of your feet, and your arms should be straight and locked, with enough room on the sides for your thumbs to clear your thighs as you ascend and descend.

As with the trap-bar deadlift, stand up by pushing through your heels, and keep your arms straight, lower back slightly arched, and core tight. Also, ensure that your hips and shoulders rise together and at the same rate. Once the bar passes your knees, push your hips into it as you continue to stand up, and when you're fully upright, your chest should be out and shoulders down. Don't lean back, hyperextend your lower back, or shrug the weight up.

To lower the bar to the floor, push your hips backward and, keeping your lower back slightly arched and your core tight, let the bar slide straight down your thighs until it clears your knees. Then, maintaining your grip on the bar, allow it to drop to the floor, and adjust your body as needed to get into the proper starting position for the next rep.

Chin-up

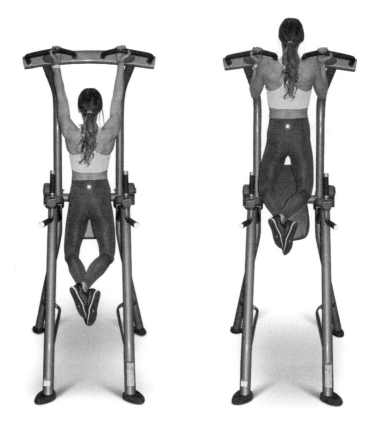

Get into the starting position shown above, with your palms facing you and about shoulder-width apart and your arms straight. Without swinging your feet or your knees, pull your body upward until your chin rises above your hands, then lower yourself and return to the starting position.

Pull-up

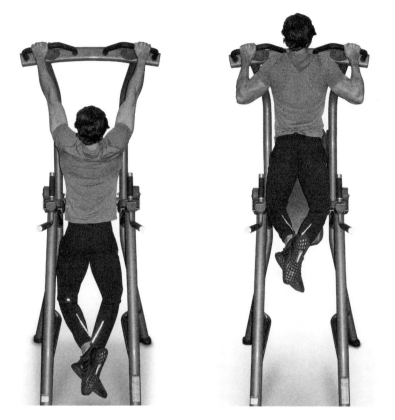

The pull-up works just like the chin-up, except you begin with your hands facing away from you and about shoulder-width apart.

The Accessory Pulling Exercises

There are two reasons to do accessory pulling exercises:

1. Some of the back muscles and the biceps are stubborn and take their sweet time to grow.
2. The many muscles in your back are difficult to fully develop with primary exercises alone because of how they attach to your skeleton.

Lat Pulldown

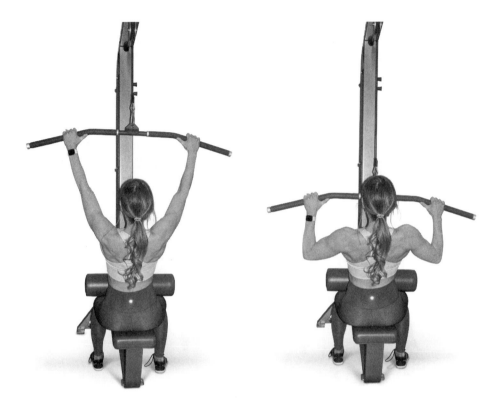

Adjust the seat so you can get a full grip on the bar when your butt is about one to two inches above the seat, then adjust the thigh pad so it settles snugly against your legs when seated and prevents your butt from rising off the seat when you pull the bar down.

Stand in front of the seat, grab the bar with your palms facing away from you, and sit down, wedging your legs underneath the thigh pad, and fully straighten your arms. Then, pull the bar down until it's a few inches from your collarbone, then raise it and return to the starting position.

Machine Row

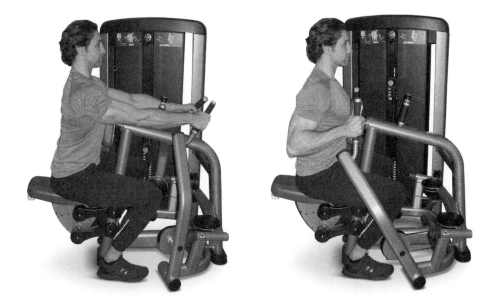

Adjust the seat so the handles are around chest height when seated, and then the chest pad so the handles are barely out of reach when seated. Then reach forward and grab the handles, and sit down with your chest against the pad. Pull the handles toward your torso until they're about level with your chest, then straighten your arms and return to the starting position.

Alternating Dumbbell Curl

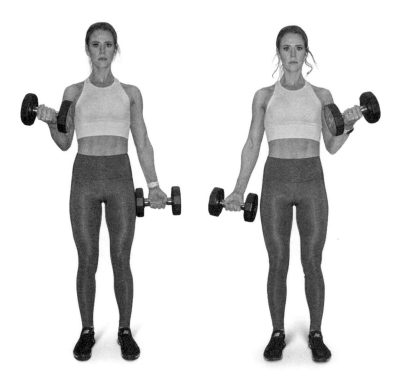

Stand tall with the dumbbells at your sides and then, as shown above, curl one hand toward your shoulder until your forearm is roughly perpendicular to the floor. Allow your elbow to move forward slightly as the dumbbell rises. Then lower the dumbbell and return to the starting position.

Cable Biceps Curl

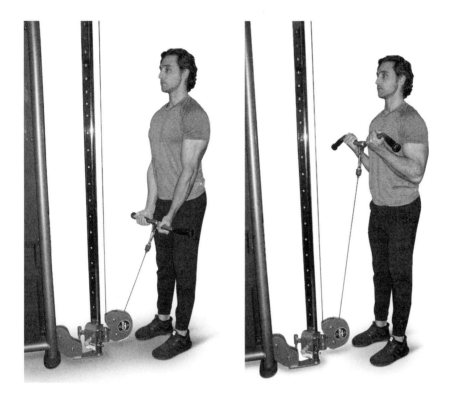

The cable biceps curl is similar to the alternating dumbbell curl, except you use a straight bar or EZ-bar (whichever is most comfortable for you) attached to a cable machine in its lowest position (closest to the floor).

THE *MUSCLE FOR LIFE* SQUATTING EXERCISES

Squatting exercises involve lowering your butt to the floor by bending at your knees and hips simultaneously, often with resistance provided by bands, dumbbells, or a machine or barbell. These exercises primarily train five major muscle groups:

1. Quadriceps
2. Glutes
3. Upper and lower back
4. Hamstrings
5. Calves

THE PRIMARY SQUATTING EXERCISES

The Beginner Primary Squatting Exercises

Bodyweight Squat

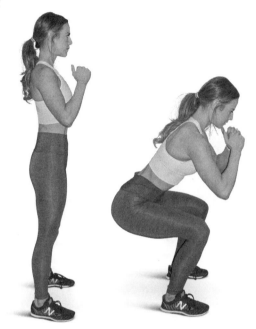

Stand up straight with your feet around shoulder-width apart and your toes pointing out at about 20 to 25 degrees (around one and eleven o'clock). Take a deep breath into your stomach, brace your abs, and sit straight down by pushing your hips backward and bending your knees at the same time.

As you lower your butt toward the floor, keep your spine straight, core tight, and chest up (imagine you're trying to show someone a logo on your T-shirt). You should feel like you're dropping your torso between your heels, and if you have trouble maintaining your balance as you descend, keep your arms extended straight out in front of you.

Once your thighs are parallel with the floor (or slightly lower, but not higher), stand up and return to the starting position.

Bodyweight Split Squat

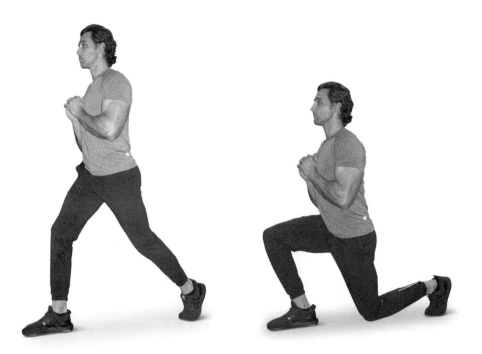

Get into the starting position shown above and, keeping your right foot firmly planted on the floor, lower your butt by bending both knees at the same time. Keep descending until your left knee touches the floor, and then stand up and return to the starting position. When you've reached your rep target, repeat with the other side.

Bodyweight Lunge

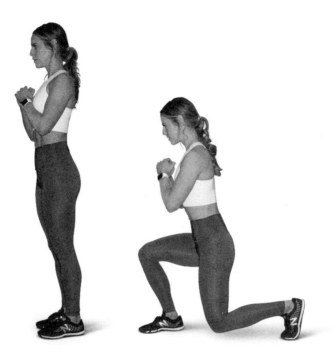

Stand up straight with both feet about shoulder-width apart. Take a long step forward with your right foot—about two to three feet—and, with most of your weight on your front foot, lower your body until your left knee touches the floor. Then reverse the motion by pushing off the floor with your front foot and leaning slightly backward, allowing your legs to straighten. Once you're standing, bring your right foot back to the starting position, and then repeat the pattern with your other foot (to complete one full rep).

This is known as the *in-place lunge*, which is ideal for when you have limited space. There are two other versions of the lunge worth learning, though, as they challenge your muscles in slightly different ways:

1. The *reverse lunge*, which is the in-place lunge in reverse (stepping backward instead of forward)
2. The *forward lunge*, which has you walk forward in a sequence of steps instead of remaining in place

To do the reverse lunge, start in the same position as the in-place lunge, but instead of taking a long step forward with your right foot, take a long step backward. With most of your weight on your front foot, kneel until your right knee touches the floor, then reverse the motion by pushing off the floor with your back foot and straightening your legs. Once your legs are straight, bring your right foot back to the starting position, and then repeat the pattern with your other foot (to complete one full rep).

The forward lunge works the same way as the in-place lunge, but instead of returning to the starting position by bringing your front foot to your back one, you bring your back foot to the front (moving you forward).

Bodyweight Step-up

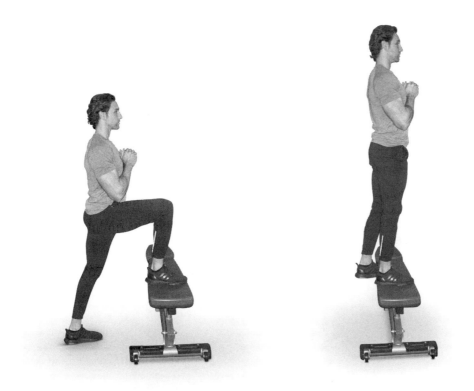

Get into the starting position shown above, and place your right foot on a box, stool, or other surface about knee-height off the floor. Keeping your weight on your right foot, fully straighten your right leg. Then lower your left foot toward the floor and return to the starting position. When you've reached your rep target, repeat with the other side.

Leg Press

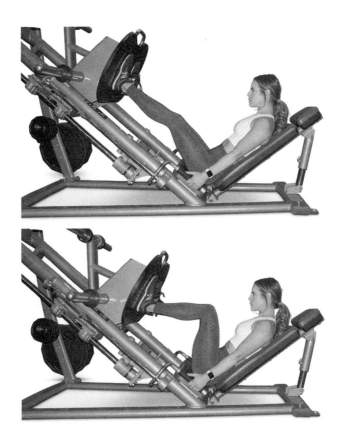

Load a leg press with plates and adjust the seat to its lowest position (with the backrest closest to the floor, at about a 30-degree angle). Then get into the starting position shown above, and wedge your butt down into the base of the seat.

Bend your knees slightly, use the safety handles to release the weight, and, ensuring your butt remains firmly in place and your lower back doesn't round, lower the footplate toward your chest until your thighs are twelve to sixteen inches from your torso. Finally, push the footplate upward until your legs are almost but not completely straight (knees slightly bent at the top of the rep).

The Intermediate Primary Squatting Exercises

Dumbbell Goblet Squat

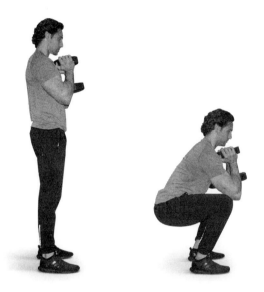

The dumbbell goblet squat works the same way as the bodyweight squat, except you hold a dumbbell directly in front of your chest as shown in the images above.

Dumbbell Lunge

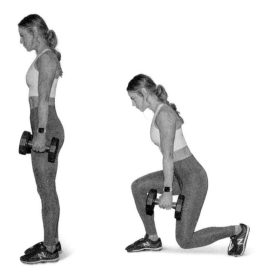

All three variations of the dumbbell lunge (in-place, reverse, and forward) work the same way as their bodyweight counterparts, except you hold a dumbbell in each hand.

Dumbbell Split Squat

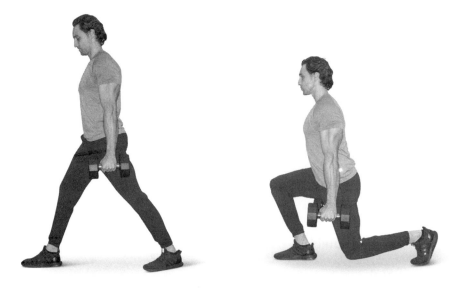

The dumbbell split squat works the same way as the bodyweight split squat, except you hold a dumbbell in each hand.

Dumbbell Romanian Deadlift

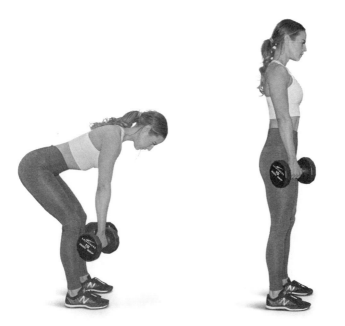

The dumbbell Romanian deadlift works the same way as the dumbbell deadlift, but there are two important differences:

1. Instead of lowering the dumbbells six to eight inches from the floor, you lower them to just below your knees (where your wrists are directly in front of your kneecaps).
2. Instead of continuing to push your hips backward and bend your knees as the dumbbells pass them, your legs remain slightly bent until the end of the movement (which places more stress on the hamstrings).

The Advanced Primary Squatting Exercises

Barbell Back Squat

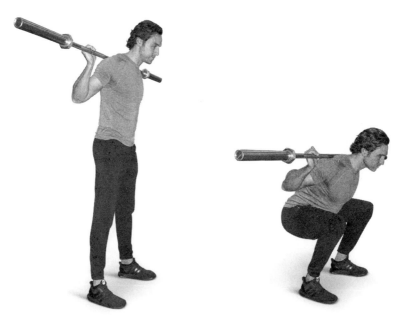

Adjust the hooks or pins in a squat rack so the bar is at your midchest, and load it with plates (or not, if the bar alone is enough weight). Grip the bar with your palms facing forward and your hands three to six inches wider than shoulder-width apart. Holding on to the bar for balance, place your feet underneath it about shoulder-width apart, and then move under the bar and place it across your upper-back muscles, directly across your shoulder blades. Tuck your shoulder blades back and down, and gently adjust the bar until you feel it resting on the "shelf" created by the bony protrusions of your shoulder blades and surrounding back muscles. This is the position the bar must remain in throughout the entire exercise.

Next, narrow your grip to tighten your upper-back muscles, and get your hands as close together as you comfortably can while keeping the bar solidly on your back muscles, not in your hands or on your spine. Get into the starting position shown opposite by unracking the bar and taking one step back with each foot (one at a time). Then adjust your feet so they're shoulder-width apart and your toes are pointing out at about 20 to 25 degrees (around one and eleven o'clock). Stand tall with your chest out, take a deep breath into your stomach, and brace your abs.

As with the bodyweight squat, to descend, sit straight down by pushing your hips backward and bending your knees at the same time. Your gaze should be forward (not down at your toes or up at the ceiling), and keep your spine straight, core tight, and chest up. Feel like you're dropping your torso between your heels in a swift but controlled manner, not simply falling as quickly as you can, because this greatly increases the amount of force placed on the joints. Also, as you descend, keep your knees pointed at your toes to prevent your knees from collapsing inward (into a knock-kneed position), which can irritate them. To help with this, you can imagine you're pushing the floor apart with your feet. Keep sitting down until your thighs are parallel to the floor (or slightly lower, but not higher), and then stop your descent and prepare to stand up.

Start the ascent by driving through your heels and the middle of your feet (not your toes), ensuring your shoulders move upward at the same rate as your hips. Your lower back should remain in a neutral position; your core should stay tight and your gaze forward (not down at your toes or up at the ceiling). Around the halfway mark, begin exhaling, and push your hips forward and underneath the bar by squeezing your glutes, and return to the starting position.

When you're on the last rep of a set of the barbell back squat, finish it fully (legs locked) and then move the bar back to the pins or hooks. Don't try to squat the bar directly back into the pins or hooks because if you miss, you can fall.

Barbell Romanian Deadlift

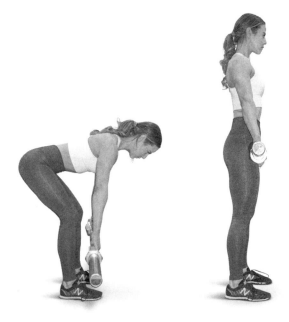

Adjust the pins or hooks in a squat rack so the bar is at your midthigh, and load it with plates (or not, if the bar alone is enough weight). If you don't have access to a squat rack, load the bar on the floor instead, and then stand in front of the middle of it with your feet slightly narrower than shoulder-width apart. Get into the starting position shown above by gripping the bar just outside of your thighs with your palms facing you, lifting it off the rack (or floor), taking one step back with each foot (one at a time), and turning your toes out and bending your knees slightly.

Stand up tall with your chest out and arms at your sides, take a deep breath into your stomach, and brace your abs. Squeeze the bar as hard as you can, press your upper arms into your sides, and, with a flat back, lower the bar toward the floor in a straight line, allowing your butt to move backward as the bar descends. Once you feel a stretch in your hamstrings, bend your knees slightly more, and continue lowering the bar until your lower back begins to round—just below the knees for most people, and about midshin for those who are particularly flexible. Then, stop descending, and bring the bar upward by driving your hips toward it, keeping your arms straight, lower back slightly arched, and core tight, and return to the starting position.

When you're on the last rep of a set of the barbell Romanian deadlift, finish it fully (legs locked), and then move the bar back to the pins or hooks. Don't try to deadlift the bar directly back into the pins or hooks because if you miss, you can fall.

The Accessory Squatting Exercises

As great as primary squatting exercises are, they don't adequately train each of the major muscle groups in the lower body. Dumbbell and barbell squat exercises are phenomenal for training the quadriceps, for instance, but not the hamstrings, and many people struggle to get the glutes they want with primary exercises alone. Accessory exercises allow you to target and further develop these and other muscles that need extra emphasis.

Primary squatting exercises are also some of the most difficult strength training movements to perform and recover from, so you can only profitably do so much of them every week. Accessory exercises, on the other hand, are less demanding, allowing you to train your lower body more without compromising your form or recovery.

Leg Extension

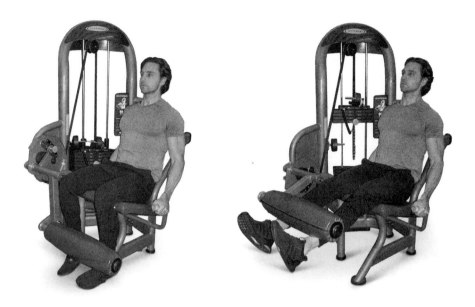

Adjust the back pad so your knees are just in front of the edge of the seat when you're seated, then adjust the leg pad closest to the floor so it touches your shins right above your ankles and puts your feet as close to your butt as possible. If the machine has a leg pad across your thighs as well, adjust it so it's snug when seated but not painful. Grab the handles, push your feet toward the ceiling until your legs are straight, then lower your feet and return to the starting position.

Leg Curl (Lying and Seated)

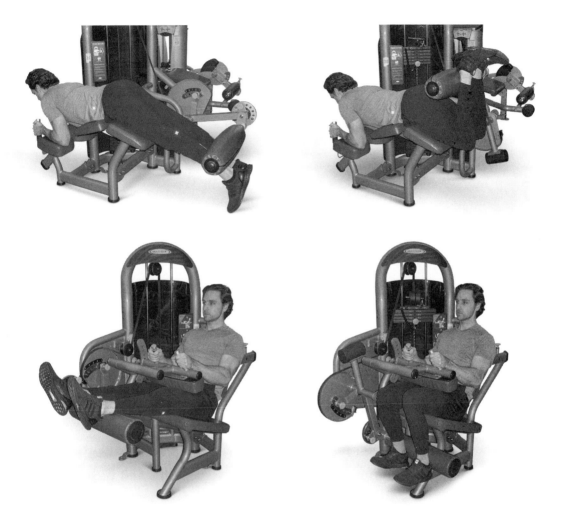

Adjust the heel pad so it's across your Achilles tendons when you're on the machine, and if you're seated, with your kneecaps a couple of inches off the pad supporting your body. Grab the handles, press your heels toward your butt until your shins are at least perpendicular to your thighs (it's fine to go slightly further), then lower your heels and return to the starting position.

Glute Bridge

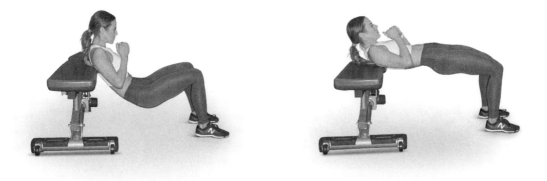

Get into the starting position shown above, and lift your butt off the floor by pressing your shoulders into the bench and heels into the floor. Raise your butt and squeeze your glutes until your shoulders, butt, and knees form a straight line, then lower your butt and return to the starting position.

You now have all the know-how you need to start the *Muscle for Life* strength training workouts! You understand how volume, intensity, and progressive overload relate to getting fit and strong, the anatomy of effective strength training, and the exercises that athletes and bodybuilders have been using for over a century to develop powerful and beautiful bodies.

In other words, you now have the ingredients, and all you need next is the recipe—the instructions on how to transform everything you've learned into a workout program—and that's exactly what I'll give you in the next chapter.

KEY TAKEAWAYS

✦ *Primary exercises* will be responsible for the lion's share of your results because they train (and develop) the most muscle mass and produce the most whole-body strength.

✦ *Accessory exercises* are used to develop muscles that are particularly stubborn and slow to respond to training, and muscles that aren't adequately trained by primary exercises alone.

✦ Pushing exercises involve moving your hands away from your torso either horizontally (in front of your body) or vertically (above your head), and primarily train three major muscle groups: the pectoralis (major and minor), triceps, and deltoids.

✦ Pulling exercises involve pulling toward your torso, either horizontally (perpendicular to your torso) or vertically (parallel with it), and primarily train four major muscle groups: the latissimus dorsi, upper back muscles, lower back muscles, and biceps.

✦ Squatting exercises involve lowering your butt to the floor by bending at your knees and hips simultaneously, often with resistance provided by bands, dumbbells, or a machine or barbell.

12

The *Muscle for Life* Workout Program

Our greatest weakness lies in giving up.
The most certain way to succeed is always to try just one more time.
—THOMAS EDISON

n chapter 10, you learned the following strength training formula:

✦ Do *3 to 5* strength training workouts per week

✦ Train major muscle groups at least once every *5 to 7* days

✦ Do *9 to 15* hard sets per workout

✦ Use *60 to 80* percent of one-rep max

✦ Rest *2 to 4* minutes in between sets

And in this chapter, we'll turn that blueprint into beginner, intermediate, and advanced strength training programs for losing fat, gaining lean muscle, and getting strong. Then we'll discuss cardiovascular exercise and how to incorporate it into your training regimen without overextending yourself.

You could use everything you've learned so far to create your own strength training plan, but I recommend you follow one of mine for at least three months before going off on your own. Workout programming can be difficult because there are several layers that must work together—phases, routines, and workouts—and numerous interdependent factors to consider, including goals, intensity, frequency, volume, and recovery, among others. It also helps to have a bit of experience under your belt before creating strength training plans because you'll better understand what is and isn't likely to work in actual practice.

Also, if you like my programming and want to continue with it, you'll find spreadsheets and printable templates for an entire year's worth of *Muscle for Life* strength training workouts in the free bonus material available at www.muscleforlifebook.com/bonus.

So, let's start our review of my strength training system with the first of the three layers I just mentioned: the training phase.

THE *MUSCLE FOR LIFE* STRENGTH TRAINING PHASE

A training phase is a block of training designed to accomplish a specific goal, like increased power, strength, muscle growth, endurance, or recovery. In *Muscle for Life*, our primary aims for all training phases are to increase strength and muscle size and definition.

A training phase can last a number of weeks or even months. In this program, a training phase lasts nine weeks and consists of two parts:

1. Hard training. Each training phase begins with eight weeks of challenging workouts designed to increase strength and muscularity.
2. Deloading. Each training phase ends with one week of deloading to facilitate recovery.

Each year, then, can be divided roughly into six training phases.

THE *MUSCLE FOR LIFE*
STRENGTH TRAINING ROUTINES

Whereas a training phase delineates the goals and duration of a training block, a training routine outlines what you'll do in that time to achieve those goals—how often you'll train and what you'll do in each workout.

In *Muscle for Life*, you have six different workout routines to choose from depending on your sex and fitness level—there are beginner, intermediate, and advanced routines for men and for women. Each routine consists of three workouts per week, and you'll notice the men's and women's routines are similar, but the men's emphasize upper-body development and the women's have a lower-body bias. This reflects the fact that most guys especially want to develop their "beach muscles," whereas most gals want to point up their legs and glutes. If you're not one of those men or women, however—if you're a woman more interested in gaining upper-body definition or a man chasing a great set of wheels—feel free to follow the other routine.

The beginner workout routines will introduce you to proper strength training, teaching you the fundamentals of proper technique and greatly enhancing your strength, balance, and coordination. By mastering a beginner routine, you'll make your first major step toward your new lean, defined, and healthy body.

The intermediate routines increase the difficulty of your workouts by incorporating more challenging exercises, including more dumbbell exercises. Once you've licked an intermediate routine, you'll have a lot to be proud of—you'll be markedly fitter, leaner, and stronger and well on your way to your ideal physique.

The advanced routines are the most difficult in the *Muscle for Life* program. They introduce you to barbell exercises, which offer more bounce for the ounce in terms of strength and muscle gain. When you conquer an advanced routine, you'll be a shining example of conditioning and vitality—a true outlier in strength, definition, and function who embodies the power of smart, science-based fitness.

Although the details of the workouts differ, all of the routines follow the same template: They entail three workouts per week, with one or two for the upper and lower body depending on the routine. These workouts are labeled A or B (simply to differentiate them), with the upper-body training focused on pushing and pulling and the lower-body on squatting.

The Men's Strength Training Routine

Workout 1	Workout 2	Workout 3
Upper Body A	Lower Body A	Upper Body B

The Women's Strength Training Routine

Workout 1	Workout 2	Workout 3
Lower Body A	Upper Body A	Lower Body B

If you're new to strength training or haven't done it consistently in at least a year, start with the beginner routine. It's a demanding but approachable introduction to the *Muscle for Life* style of training.

If you dabble in strength training (a weekend warrior, for instance), start with the intermediate routine if you meet or exceed the following strength standards. (Otherwise, start with the beginner routine.)

Men's Strength Standards	Women's Strength Standards
1 set of 15 feet-elevated push-ups	1 set of 10 push-ups
1 set of 15 bodyweight rows*	1 set of 10 bodyweight rows*
1 set of 15 bodyweight squats	1 set of 15 bodyweight squats

*With your body as close to parallel with the ground as possible (the most difficult variation of the exercise)

The advanced routine involves the most difficult exercises and heaviest weights and is meant for experienced weightlifters. Start with it if you meet or exceed the following strength requirements (men and women):

+ Dumbbell bench press: 25 percent of your body weight (both dumbbells combined) for at least 1 set of 5 reps
+ Trap-bar deadlift: 75 percent of your body weight for at least 1 set of 5 reps
+ Dumbbell goblet squat: 25 percent of your body weight for at least 1 set of 5 reps

THE *MUSCLE FOR LIFE* STRENGTH TRAINING WORKOUTS

You learned earlier in this chapter that there are six phases of training per year, and each phase comprises eight weeks of hard training and one week of deloading. The workouts shared here are your first eight weeks of *Muscle for Life* training ("phase one"), followed by a one-week deload.

When you've completed phase one of a beginner or intermediate routine, you can repeat it if you don't qualify for an intermediate or advanced routine yet, modify it based on what you're learning in this book, or follow my phase two (and three and beyond) programming in the back of this book (as well as the bonus material available at www.muscleforlifebook.com/bonus).

THE BEGINNER STRENGTH TRAINING WORKOUTS

The Women's Beginner Strength Training Routine
Phase One

Workout 1 Lower Body A	Workout 2 Upper Body A	Workout 3 Lower Body B
Bodyweight Squat 3 hard sets of 12–15 reps	Push-up 3 hard sets of 12–15 reps	Dumbbell Deadlift 3 hard sets of 12–15 reps
Dumbbell Deadlift 3 hard sets of 12–15 reps	Lat Pulldown 3 hard sets of 12–15 reps	Bodyweight Lunge 3 hard sets of 12–15 reps
Bodyweight Split Squat 3 hard sets of 12–15 reps	Machine Chest Press 3 hard sets of 12–15 reps	Leg Press 3 hard sets of 12–15 reps
Triceps Dip 3 hard sets of 12–15 reps	Bodyweight Row 3 hard sets of 12–15 reps	Leg Curl 3 hard sets of 12–15 reps

The Men's Beginner Strength Training Routine
Phase One

Workout 1 Upper Body A	Workout 2 Lower Body A	Workout 3 Upper Body B
Push-up 3 hard sets of 12–15 reps	Bodyweight Squat 3 hard sets of 12–15 reps	Machine Shoulder Press 3 hard sets of 12–15 reps
Lat Pulldown 3 hard sets of 12–15 reps	Dumbbell Deadlift 3 hard sets of 12–15 reps	Bodyweight Row 3 hard sets of 12–15 reps
Machine Chest Press 3 hard sets of 12–15 reps	Leg Press 3 hard sets of 12–15 reps	Machine Chest Press 3 hard sets of 12–15 reps
Bodyweight Row 3 hard sets of 12–15 reps	Leg Curl 3 hard sets of 12–15 reps	Cable Biceps Curl 3 hard sets of 12–15 reps

THE INTERMEDIATE
STRENGTH TRAINING WORKOUTS

The Women's Intermediate Strength Training Routine
Phase One

Workout 1 Lower Body A	Workout 2 Upper Body A	Workout 3 Lower Body B
Trap-Bar Deadlift 3 hard sets of 10–12 reps	Dumbbell Bench Press 3 hard sets of 10–12 reps	Dumbbell Lunge 3 hard sets of 10–12 reps
Dumbbell Split Squat 3 hard sets of 10–12 reps	Lat Pulldown 3 hard sets of 10–12 reps	Dumbbell Romanian Deadlift 3 hard sets of 10–12 reps
Leg Curl 3 hard sets of 10–12 reps	Seated Dumbbell Overhead Press 3 hard sets of 10–12 reps	Leg Press 3 hard sets of 10–12 reps
Dumbbell Goblet Squat 3 hard sets of 10–12 reps	Seated Cable Row 3 hard sets of 10–12 reps	Leg Curl 3 hard sets of 10–12 reps

The Men's Intermediate Strength Training Routine
Phase One

Workout 1 Upper Body A	Workout 2 Lower Body A	Workout 3 Upper Body B
Dumbbell Bench Press 3 hard sets of 10–12 reps	Trap-Bar Deadlift 3 hard sets of 10–12 reps	Seated Dumbbell Overhead Press 3 hard sets of 10–12 reps
Lat Pulldown 3 hard sets of 10–12 reps	Dumbbell Goblet Squat 3 hard sets of 10–12 reps	Seated Cable Row 3 hard sets of 10–12 reps
Machine Chest Press 3 hard sets of 10–12 reps	Leg Curl 3 hard sets of 10–12 reps	Machine Chest Press 3 hard sets of 10–12 reps
Seated Cable Row 3 hard sets of 10–12 reps	Dumbbell Split Squat 3 hard sets of 10–12 reps	Alternating Dumbbell Curl 3 hard sets of 10–12 reps

THE ADVANCED
STRENGTH TRAINING WORKOUTS

The Women's Advanced Strength Training Routine
Phase One

Workout 1 Lower Body A	Workout 2 Upper Body A	Workout 3 Lower Body B
Barbell Back Squat 3 hard sets of 8–10 reps	Barbell Bench Press 3 hard sets of 8–10 reps	Dumbbell Lunge 3 hard sets of 8–10 reps
Barbell Deadlift 3 hard sets of 8–10 reps	Lat Pulldown 3 hard sets of 8–10 reps	Barbell Romanian Deadlift 3 hard sets of 8–10 reps
Leg Curl 3 hard sets of 8–10 reps	Incline Barbell Bench Press 3 hard sets of 8–10 reps	Leg Press 3 hard sets of 8–10 reps
Dumbbell Lunge 3 hard sets of 8–10 reps	One-Arm Dumbbell 3 hard sets of 8–10 reps	Leg Curl 3 hard sets of 8–10 reps

The Men's Advanced Strength Training Routine
Phase One

Workout 1 Upper Body A	Workout 2 Lower Body A	Workout 3 Upper Body B
Barbell Bench Press 3 hard sets of 8–10 reps	Barbell Back Squat 3 hard sets of 8–10 reps	Seated Dumbbell Overhead Press 3 hard sets of 8–10 reps
Lat Pulldown 3 hard sets of 8–10 reps	Barbell Deadlift 3 hard sets of 8–10 reps	One-Arm Dumbbell Row 3 hard sets of 8–10 reps
Dumbbell Bench Press 3 hard sets of 8–10 reps	Dumbbell Split Squat 3 hard sets of 8–10 reps	Dumbbell Bench Press 3 hard sets of 8–10 reps
One-Arm Dumbbell Row 3 hard sets of 8–10 reps	Leg Curl 3 hard sets of 8–10 reps	Alternating Dumbbell Curl 3 hard sets of 8–10 reps

HOW TO PROGRESS
IN YOUR STRENGTH TRAINING

In *Muscle for Life*, you'll progress in your strength training in two ways: by increasing the loads (weight) and difficulty of the exercises.

In chapter 10, you learned about double progression for increasing loads—the system of working to increase reps with a weight until you can do a number of sets at the top of a given rep range and then increasing the weight.

Here's how it works in *Muscle for Life*:

+ On a beginner routine, you're working in the 12-to-15 rep range, and once you can do 3 hard sets of 15 reps in a row, switch to a harder exercise variation (bodyweight exercise) or increase the weight by 10 pounds (5 pounds per dumbbell). Also, if you find that you can't do 3 hard sets of at least 12 reps in a row of a bodyweight exercise, switch to an easier variation.

+ On an intermediate routine, you're working in the 10-to-12 rep range, and once you can do 3 hard sets of 12 reps in a row, increase the weight by 10 pounds (5 pounds per dumbbell). And the weight is too heavy if you can't do 3 hard sets of at least 10 reps in a row, so when this happens, decrease the weight in 5- or 10-pound (total) increments until you can get at least 10 reps for 3 hard sets in a row. One exception worth mentioning again, however, is when you first move up to a heavier weight. If you can finish your first hard set with the new, heavier weight within at least a rep or two of the bottom of your rep range, continue working with that weight until you can hit the progression target again.

+ On an advanced routine, you're working in the 8-to-10 rep range, and once you can do 3 hard sets of 10 reps in a row, you increase the weight by 10 pounds (5 pounds per dumbbell). And if you can't do 3 hard sets of at least 8 reps in a row, decrease the weight in 5- or 10-pound increments until you can.

To better understand how this works, let's go through some examples. On a beginner routine, once you can do 3 sets in a row of at least 15 push-ups, you should upgrade to feet-elevated push-ups. If, however, you do 15 regular push-ups in your first set followed by 14 and 13 reps in the next 2 sets, you're not ready to progress yet, so you should keep doing them until you can do 15 in each set (and then switch to the feet-elevated push-up).

What if you do 11 regular push-ups in your first set, followed by sets of 10 and 9? You're not reaching the bottom of your rep range (12), so you should switch to knee push-ups until you can do three sets of 15 in a row. Then you can go back to regular push-ups.

Another scenario: on an intermediate routine, once you can do three sets in a row of 12 reps of the trap-bar deadlift, you should add 10 pounds to the bar (5 on either side) and work with that new weight until you can do 3 sets of 12 reps with it. And what if you added 10 pounds, then did sets of 9, 8, and 7 reps? You need to make the exercise a little easier so you can do 3 sets of at least 8, 9, or 10 reps, so you should take 5 pounds off the bar.

The second method of progression in *Muscle for Life* is proceeding from the beginner to intermediate and intermediate to advanced routine.

✦ To graduate to the intermediate routine, you must meet the strength standards you learned a moment ago: if you're a man, you must be able to do 1 set each of at least 15 feet-elevated push-ups, bodyweight rows, and bodyweight squats; and if you're a woman, at least 1 set each of 10 push-ups and bodyweight rows and 1 set of 15 bodyweight squats.

+ To graduate to the advanced routine, you must be able to dumbbell bench press 25 percent of your body weight for at least 1 set of 5 reps, trap-bar deadlift 75 percent of your body weight for at least 1 set of 5 reps, and dumbbell goblet squat 25 percent of your body weight for at least 1 set of 5 reps.

Once you qualify for the next routine, finish your current workouts for the week and begin your new ones the following week. Remember, however, to deload when you would've on the easier routine. For example, if you switch from the beginner to intermediate routine on week six, you'd do two weeks of intermediate training, deload, and carry on with your intermediate workouts.

How to Warm Up for Your Workouts

What many people do to warm up for their strength training is rather silly—twenty minutes on the treadmill, followed by another twenty of stretching, foam rolling, hopping around, and so forth. One reason they do this is to raise the temperature of their muscles in the belief that it reduces the risk of a pull or tear. Fortunately, however, when you work out, your body isn't whistling Dixie while you load it with heavier weights until it breaks. It has a complex system to manage how its muscles contract that involves a lot more than muscle temperature. In other words, it's not clear that heating up our muscles before loading them makes injury less likely. Some studies show it does, while others have found otherwise.

Warming up properly is an important part of successful strength training, however. The best way to warm up for strength training is with the exercises you'll be doing in your workouts. If you've ever done any strength training, you know how hard it can be to maintain proper form as you approach failure. You've probably felt your knees cave in while squatting, your wrists go crooked while pressing, and your lower back bend while pulling. By doing warm-up sets before your hard sets, you can help protect against these mistakes by troubleshooting your form and "grooving in" proper movement patterns. Think of your warm-up sets as practice—the more times you perform an exercise correctly, the more that becomes your default way to move.

This is particularly important for beginners. When you first start strength training, you can get away with bad technique because the weights are light. It's hard to get hurt when you're squatting just the bar (or your body weight). As you get stronger, though, that changes. Weights get heavier, and poor form becomes more dangerous.

Studies also show that a short warm-up routine that I'll give you can boost performance levels by raising the temperature of muscle cells and increasing blood flow, which can translate into more muscle and strength over time.

So, to ensure that each of the major muscle groups you'll train in a workout is ready for optimum performance, I'll have you do a couple of warm-up sets with the first exercises in the workout for each, except in the case of a bodyweight exercise. For bodyweight training, you don't need to warm up and can just begin with your first hard set because the load (your body) isn't heavy enough to require warm-up sets, and the technique isn't demanding enough to benefit from additional practice.

When you're doing barbell, dumbbell, or machine exercise, however, you need to include warm-up sets in your workout. Specifically, I recommend 2 warm-up sets before your hard sets. On the first, do 10 reps with about 50 percent of your hard-set weight, and rest for a minute. On the second, do 5 reps with about 70 percent of your hard-set weight, and rest for a minute. So, if your hard-set weight for squats is 135 pounds, your first warm-up set would be 10 reps with 65 to 75 pounds. Then you'd rest for a minute, and do 5 reps with 90 to 100 pounds. And that's it. You're now ready to do your hard sets.

Now, I said you need to warm up each major muscle group you'll train in a workout, but that doesn't mean you need to do warm-up sets before every barbell, dumbbell, or machine exercise. To understand how this works, let's say you're following the Women's Intermediate Program, which calls for a lower-body workout that goes like this: dumbbell lunge, dumbbell Romanian deadlift, leg press, and leg curl, in that order. You'd first warm up for the dumbbell lunge (squat muscles) and then do your hard sets. Next is the dumbbell Romanian deadlift, but you won't need to warm up for it because it trains the same major muscle groups as the dumbbell lunge (squat muscles). The same goes for the leg press and leg curl, too—your quads and hamstrings will be ready. Therefore, in this case, your warm-up sets for the dumbbell lunge serve as a warm-up for the entire workout.

That's not always the case, though. Let's say you're following the Men's Advanced Program and are about to do the following upper-body workout: seated dumbbell overhead press, one-arm dumbbell row, dumbbell bench press, and alternating dumbell curl. Here, you'd warm up on the seated dumbbell overhead press first (push muscles), followed by your hard sets. Then you'd warm up on the one-arm dumbbell row (pull muscles), followed by your hard sets. And last you'd do your hard sets for the dumbbell bench press and alternating dumbell curl without warm-up sets because the (push and pull) muscles trained by these last two exercises were readied by the first two exercises.

How to Find Your Starting Weights

It's all well and good to know you should work in a specific rep range, but how do you figure out how much weight to use? Simply start light on an exercise, try it out, and increase the weight for each successive hard set until you've figured it out. That said, the following chart will make the process easier and faster:

Exercise	Male Starting Weight (lb.)	Female Starting Weight (lb.)
Machine Chest Press	30	15
Machine Shoulder Press	20	10
Dumbbell Bench Press	30 (per dumbbell)	15 (per dumbbell)
Incline Dumbbell Bench Press	20 (per dumbbell)	10 (per dumbbell)
Seated Dumbbell Overhead Press	20 (per dumbbell)	10 (per dumbbell)
Barbell Bench Press	95	45
Incline Barbell Bench Press	65	45
Cable Triceps Pushdown	30	15
Dumbbell Triceps Overhead Press	20 (per dumbbell)	10 (per dumbbell)
Machine Cable Fly	20 (per handle)	10 (per handle)
Dumbbell Deadlift	10 (per dumbbell)	5 (per dumbbell)
One-Arm Dumbbell Row	30 (per dumbbell)	15 (per dumbbell)
Trap-Bar Deadlift	95	65
Seated Cable Row	40	20
Barbell Deadlift	135	95
Lat Pulldown	30	15
Machine Row	30	15
Alternating Dumbbell Curl	10 (per dumbbell)	5 (per dumbbell)
Cable Biceps Curl	20	10

Exercise	Male Starting Weight (lb.)	Female Starting Weight (lb.)
Leg Press	90	50
Dumbbell Goblet Squat	30 (per dumbbell)	15 (per dumbbell)
Dumbbell Lunge	20 (per dumbbell)	10 (per dumbbell)
Dumbbell Split Squat	20 (per dumbbell)	10 (per dumbbell)
Dumbbell Romanian Deadlift	30 (per dumbbell)	15 (per dumbbell)
Barbell Back Squat	95	65
Barbell Romanian Deadlift	95	65
Leg Extension	40	20
Leg Curl	40	20

HOW TO DELOAD

Dialing back your workouts every so often is an effective way to boost recovery and prevent injuries, and the best way to do this is by reducing your workout intensity or volume for a period, usually a week.

This technique is known as deloading, and it's based on research on how the body deals with physical stress. Here's the basic outline:

1. You provide a stimulus (exercise).

2. You remove the stimulus (rest and recovery).

3. Your body adapts (gets bigger, stronger, faster, etc.).

Like maintaining good sleep hygiene and managing your energy balance properly, deloading is a tool that falls under number two above (removing stimulus), and its purpose is to help with number three (adaptation).

There's no one-size-fits-all answer to how often you should deload because some people's bodies can take more stimulus than others' before needing a break. That said, in *Muscle for Life*, every ninth week, you'll do the following:

1. Do the previous week's workout but instead of 3 hard sets per exercise, do 2.
2. Warm up and use heavy weights as usual, but end hard sets 2 reps short of the bottom of your normal rep range. For example, if you're following an intermediate routine, you'd do 8 reps per set with your normal heavy weights when deloading (instead of 10 to 12), and if you're working on an advanced routine, 6 reps per set (instead of 8 to 10).

How to Include Cardio in Your Regimen

Strength training is more important than cardio for maintaining health, vitality, and function, so if you have time for just one, pick strength training. When combined, however, strength training and cardio unlock your full fitness potential, so I recommend doing both if you can.

Fortunately, cardio is much easier to incorporate into your routine than strength training, and you don't have to do much to make a difference. Here are the ground rules:

1. Do one to three hours of cardio per week.
2. Do only low- and moderate-intensity cardio (for now).
3. Do the types of cardio you most enjoy.

If you follow those three simple principles, you'll enjoy most of the benefits cardio has to offer with none of the potential downsides. Let's review each.

1. Do one to three hours of cardio per week.

The only reason to do a lot of cardio is to improve your cardiovascular endurance, so if you don't enjoy it, feel free to do just as much as it takes to achieve your health and body composition goals and no more. If you do like cardio, though, you can do more than the bare minimum, but not so much that it impairs your strength training, recovery, or health.

How much cardio is just enough and too much? On the low end, one hour per week is a reasonable "minimum effective dose" for improving cardiovascular and metabolic health. You can break this hour up into several sessions, but try to ensure that each is at least fifteen minutes long. As for the high end, limit your cardio to no more than the amount of time you spend training your muscles. For instance, if you do three hours of strength training per week (like you will on this program), don't do more than three hours of cardio in the same period. And again, you can split this time up into multiple workouts so long as each is at least fifteen minutes long (and ideally, none would be longer than forty-five minutes or so).

Why the upper time limit to a cardio session? Because while cardio isn't "bad" for gaining muscle and strength per se, doing too much is. There are three primary reasons for this:

1. A lot of cardio wears you out physically and mentally, making it harder to progress in your strength training. This systemic fatigue can be insidious, setting in slowly and imperceptibly.

2. Cardio can cause a fair amount of muscle damage and soreness that hinders performance in the gym. Your body has to work hard to recover from intense strength training, and if you also do a lot of cardio, it can struggle to keep up.

3. Research shows that cardio causes adaptations at a cellular level

that are fundamentally at odds with the adaptations produced by strength training. This is known as the *interference effect* and it boils down to this: our body (and muscles in particular) can't fully adapt to both strength and endurance training at the same time.

By limiting your cardio to a couple of hours per week, however, you can more or less neutralize these disadvantages.

2. Do only low- and moderate-intensity cardio (for now).

Broadly, there are three types of cardio: low-intensity, moderate-intensity, and high-intensity. Cardio is low-intensity when you can talk in full sentences while you do it, like a stroll around the neighborhood or a leisurely bike ride. You're doing moderate-intensity cardio when you can talk in only a few short sentences before catching your breath, like with jogging or swimming. And in high-intensity cardio you can't talk in full sentences (or at all), like with sprints of any kind.

You've probably heard that high-intensity cardio can produce the most fat loss and health benefits, and that's somewhat true. It can burn more than twice as many calories per unit of time as low-intensity cardio and provide some of the same health benefits in a fraction of the time.

It also causes more fatigue, soreness, and muscle damage than lower-intensity cardio, however, which makes it more likely to interfere with your strength training (especially when cutting, which impairs post-workout recovery). High-intensity cardio comes with a higher risk of injury, too—especially if you do several sessions per week—and requires a good deal of focus and mental energy.

Thus, unless you're already an experienced endurance trainee, I recommend you stick with low- and moderate-intensity cardio while on the *Muscle for Life* program and save high-intensity work for later in your fitness journey.

3. Do the types of cardio you most enjoy.

Exactly what you do for your cardio workouts isn't important—only that you do them consistently. So, feel free to pick whatever you like, including activities that aren't properly "exercise"—playing a sport, taking a walk in the evening with your significant other, or going for a bike ride or hike on the weekend, for example. Those types of exercise are just as effective as hitting the treadmill or elliptical machine (and more enjoyable!).

That said, it's best to stick with low-impact types of cardio, such as cycling, elliptical, rowing, walking, hiking, cross-country skiing, and swimming. Research shows that these kinds of exercise cause little muscle damage or soreness and don't interfere with strength training, and sometimes (as with cycling), they may even enhance muscle and strength gain.

Higher-impact forms of cardio, like running, tennis, or basketball, aren't verboten, but they shouldn't make up more than half of your total cardio. If you do two hours of cardio per week, then, no more than one hour should be high-impact activities.

Finally, if you aren't sure what kind of cardio to do, try my favorite: cycling. It's basically all pros and no cons:

+ It's easy on your joints, tendons, and ligaments.
+ It causes little muscle damage and soreness, and thus doesn't hamper your strength training (and some research even shows it can enhance lower-body muscle growth).
+ It burns a lot of calories.

- ✦ It's something you can do indoors when the weather is bad and outdoors when it's nice.
- ✦ When indoors, you can pair it with another activity you enjoy, such as reading, watching TV or movies, or listening to podcasts, audiobooks, music, etc. (or with something you need to do anyway, like work calls, which is what I usually do).

With the workout routines I've just given you, it won't be a matter of *if* you can get fit, lean, and strong but *when*. It won't take long to see real progress, either—in just a couple of months, you can lose 10 to 15 pounds of fat and gain noticeable muscle definition.

What's more, if you're like the tens of thousands of people I've spoken and worked with over the years, strength training in particular will give you a lot more than a new body—it'll give you a new lease on life. You'll feel strong, confident, and competent as you make strides toward more muscle, strength, and vitality. You'll lose fat and experience less fatigue. People will start noticing and asking for your "secrets."

To get there, however, you need to add one more tool to your repertoire: tracking your progress.

The *Muscle for Life* Workout Program

KEY TAKEAWAYS

+ If you're new to strength training or haven't done it consistently in at least a year, start with the beginner routine.

+ Start with the intermediate routine if:
    + You're a man and can do at least 1 set of 15 feet-elevated push-ups, 1 set of 15 bodyweight rows, and 1 set of 15 bodyweight squats.
    + You're a woman and can do at least 1 set of 10 strict push-ups, 1 set of 10 bodyweight rows, and 1 set of 15 body-weight squats.

+ Start with the advanced routine if you're a man or woman and can dumbbell bench press 25 percent of your body weight for at least 1 set of 5 reps, trap-bar deadlift 75 percent of your body weight for at least 1 set of 5 reps, and dumbbell goblet squat 25 percent of your body weight for at least 1 set of 5 reps.

+ On a beginner routine, you're working in the 12-to-15 rep range, and once you can do 3 hard sets of 15 reps in a row, switch to a harder exercise variation (bodyweight exercise) or increase the weight by 10 pounds (5 pounds per dumbbell), and if you can't do 3 hard sets of at least 12 reps in a row of a bodyweight exercise, switch to an easier variation.

+ On an intermediate routine, you're working in the 10-to-12 rep range, and once you can do 3 hard sets of 12 reps in a row, increase the weight by 10 pounds (5 pounds per dumbbell), and if you can't do 3 hard sets of at least 10 reps in a row, decrease the weight in 5- or 10-pound (total) increments until you can (except when you first move up to a heavier weight—in this case, if you can finish your first hard set with the new, heavier weight within at least a rep or two of the bottom of your rep range, continue working with that weight until you can hit the progression target again).

+ On an advanced routine, you're working in the 8-to-10 rep range, and once you can do 3 hard sets of 10 reps in a row, increase the weight by 10 pounds (5 pounds per dumbbell), and if you can't do 3 hard sets of at least 8 reps in a row, decrease the weight in 5- or 10-pound increments until you can.

+ To graduate to the intermediate routine, you must meet the following strength standards: if you're a man, you must be able to do 1 set each of at least 15 feet-elevated push-ups, bodyweight rows, and bodyweight squats; and if you're a woman, at least 1 set each of 10 push-ups and bodyweight rows and 1 set of 15 bodyweight squats.

+ To graduate to the advanced routine, you must be able to dumbbell bench press 25 percent of your body weight for at least 1 set of 5 reps, trap-bar deadlift 75 percent of your body weight for at least 1 set of 5 reps, and dumbbell goblet squat 25 percent of your body weight for at least 1 set of 5 reps.

+ For bodyweight training, you don't need to warm up and can just begin with your first hard set.

+ To warm up before a barbell, dumbbell, or machine exercise, do 2 warm-up sets before your hard sets: do 10 reps with about 50 percent of your hard-set weight for the first warm-up set, rest for a minute, then do 5 reps with about 70 percent of your hard-set weight for the second, followed by a one-minute rest.

- The *Muscle for Life* deload protocol is simple:
  - Every ninth week, do the previous week's workout, but instead of doing three hard sets for each exercise, do two.
  - Warm up and use heavy weights as usual, but end hard sets 2 reps from the bottom of your normal rep range (for example, if you're following an intermediate routine, and normally do sets of 10 to 12 reps, do 8 reps per set with your normal heavy weights when deloading).
- Do between one and three hours of cardio per week, ensuring it's no more than the amount of time you spend training your muscles.
- Feel free to pick whatever type of cardio you like, including activities that aren't properly "exercise"—playing a sport, taking a walk in the evening with your significant other, or going for a bike ride or hike on the weekend, for example.

13

The Right (and Wrong) Ways to Track Your Progress

When you can measure what you are speaking about,
and express it in numbers, you know something about it.
—SIR WILLIAM THOMSON

S ir William Thomson (also known as Lord Kelvin) was a brilliant nineteenth-century physicist, and his insight on the importance of measuring applies to many things in life, including exercise and diet. Only when you can measure your progress (or lack thereof) and express it in real numbers can you know whether you're headed in the right direction. If you don't have any consistent, objective way to assess progress, however, you're working blind and hoping for the best. This is one of the major reasons so many people fail to achieve their fitness goals.

Monitoring the wrong things or the right ones incorrectly can also mislead you. For example, many people use electronic devices or smartphone apps to estimate calories burned in workouts and track their body composition. Research shows that these gadgets and software are notoriously inaccurate, however, and while body weight is important to watch, daily fluctuations aren't important, so cursing or cheering them is counterproductive.

To correctly track your fitness progress, you only need to do two things:

1. Track your body composition.
2. Track your training.

Let's learn how to do each.

HOW TO TRACK YOUR BODY COMPOSITION

Even when you do everything right, it takes time to see marked changes in your appearance. And when the fleshy parts don't firm up as quickly as you'd like, it's easy to lose heart because all your work can feel like it's for naught. If you learn to track your body composition properly, however, you'll always know what is or isn't happening with your physique and will be able to adjust your diet and training accordingly. This process has three steps:

1. Weigh yourself every three days and calculate the average every two weeks.
2. Take body measurements every two weeks.
3. Take progress pictures every two weeks.

If that sounds like a lot of work, don't worry—it takes but five minutes a week, and as your body responds to your training, you'll come to enjoy it. Games are more fun when you keep score, and recording your physical results is how you do that in the "building a better body" contest. Furthermore, if your numbers aren't moving in the right direction, you want to know as soon as possible so you can take corrective actions.

1. **Weigh yourself every three days and calculate the average every two weeks.**

Your weight can change daily for reasons that have nothing to do with fat or muscle loss or gain, including fluid retention, glycogen levels, and bowel movements (or the lack thereof), so expect regular ups and downs, and don't fret over sudden increases.

To get an accurate picture of what's happening with your weight, weigh yourself every three days and calculate the average every two weeks (fourteen days). If these averages are moving down over time, you're losing weight, and if they're moving up, you're gaining weight. Simple and clean. Here's the procedure:

1. Weigh yourself every third day first thing in the morning, naked, after relieving yourself and before eating or drinking anything, and record the numbers somewhere accessible like a fitness journal, an Excel file or a Google spreadsheet, or the notepad app in your phone. If you want to take this tracking a step further, you can also graph the numbers in a spreadsheet.

2. Every two weeks, add your weigh-ins together and divide the sum by the number of weigh-ins to get your average daily weight for the period. Record this as well.

Here's an example of how this could look for someone cutting:

Monday: 163 pounds
Thursday: 164 pounds
Sunday: 162 pounds
Wednesday: 161 pounds

Saturday: 161 pounds

Tuesday: 160 pounds

Average daily weight: 971 (pounds) / 6 (weigh-ins) = 162 pounds

This method of tracking your weight keeps you focused on the bigger picture instead of fussing over meaningless day-to-day variances, which can cause unnecessary frustration and confusion. Also, for women, as your weight can shoot up a few pounds during your period, focus on the biweekly averages of the weeks before and after your period weeks.

2. Take body measurements every two weeks.

Your weight alone doesn't tell you how your body composition is changing because it doesn't show whether you're gaining or losing muscle or fat. "Newbie gains" also render weight less important because if you're new to strength training and have fat to lose, you can expect to gain muscle and lose fat at the same time. When this "recomposition" happens, weight may not change as much as one would expect. I've seen some dramatic one- and even two-year transformations, for instance, where weight only changed by 5 pounds (women) to 15 pounds (men).

So, in addition to your weight, measure and record at least one body measurement every two weeks: your waist circumference. The size of your waist is a reliable indicator of fat loss or gain, and by monitoring it, you can quickly assess whether your body fat level is changing.

To take this measurement, first thing in the morning, naked, after relieving yourself and before eating or drinking anything, wrap a tape measure around your bare stomach, right at your navel. Make sure the tape is parallel to the floor (not slanted) and snug to your body, but not so tight that it compresses the skin. Take a deep breath in, exhale gently until your lungs are mostly empty, and, without sucking in your stomach, note the number and record it somewhere handy.

If you're the type of person who loves data, here are a few more measurements you can take every two weeks:

- ✦ Your upper-leg circumference. Wrap a tape measure around the widest part of one leg's thigh and hamstrings. Then do your other leg.

- ✦ Your flexed arms. Flex one of your arms and wrap a tape measure around the largest part (the peak of your biceps and middle of your triceps). Then do your other arm.

- ✦ Your chest circumference. Stand upright with your arms comfortably at your sides (no flaring your elbows or spreading your lats). Then have a friend place a measuring tape at the fullest part of one of your pecs and wrap it around you, under your arms (in your armpits), across your shoulder blades, and back to the starting point.

- ✦ Your shoulder circumference. Stand upright with your arms comfortably at your sides (again, no flaring your elbows or spreading your lats). Then have a friend wrap a measuring tape around your shoulders and chest right around the top of your armpits.

- ✦ Your flexed calves. Flex one of your calves (raise your heel off the ground), and wrap a measuring tape around the largest part. Then do your other calf.

3. Take progress pictures every two weeks.

In principle, taking pictures is even better than measurements because ultimately what we see in the mirror matters far more than the numbers. Revealing pictures can be a source of frustration and guilt, however—especially early on—because they're stark reminders of how far we are from where we want to be.

This reaction is perfectly normal, but it can be reframed in a positive light. Instead of viewing the shots as intimate and immutable reflections of *you*—your essence and identity—regard them merely as part of a growing collection of data about how your body is changing that'll help you calibrate your diet and exercise efforts for better results. Plus, before long, you'll be downright shocked by how much your body has improved.

Remember too that nobody else needs to see these pictures—but don't be surprised if, after some time, you're itching to share your "before" and "after" shots with at least a few people in your life.

So, even if you're feeling camera-shy, let's take your "before" pictures now (if you haven't already), and then snap progress pictures every two weeks. Here's how to do it right:

+ Take pictures from the front, side, and back.
+ Show as much skin as you feel comfortable with—the more the better, because it gives you the best idea of how your body is changing.
+ Use the same camera, lighting, and background for each picture. If this isn't possible, make sure the pictures are clear.
+ Take the pictures at the same time of day, preferably in the morning, after using the bathroom, and before breakfast.
+ Take both flexed and unflexed pictures to better see how your muscles are developing.

I also recommend saving all your progress photos in an individual album on your phone or computer so you can easily scroll through them like a flip-book and see how your body is evolving.

HOW TO TRACK YOUR STRENGTH TRAINING

Tracking your strength training is just as important as tracking your body composition because it's the only way to ensure you're progressively overloading your muscles. At first, your strength will shoot up by leaps and bounds, but in time, progress will slow, and the details get hazy if you don't have a training journal. You won't remember what you did in your previous workouts and thus won't know if your strength is going up or down.

Remember that as you become more experienced, a successful workout is one where you beat your last performance by even a little—a rep or two with the same weight on just one exercise, for instance. With double progression, you build muscle and strength one rep at a time, so when you step up to a barbell, dumbbell, or machine, you want to have a clear goal in mind for each set, not a fuzzy inkling of what you did the last time. For example, if you know your first hard set of squats in your previous lower-body workout was 135 pounds for 8 reps, in this next workout, all you should have on your mind is hitting 9 or 10 reps with that same weight.

If you don't track your strength training, however, you won't be able to train with this level of focus and intentionality. Your workouts will get sloppy and eventually turn into lifting random amounts of weight for random numbers of reps. This is better than nothing and can produce satisfactory results in beginners, but it won't cut it in the long run. You need to work from real data to achieve a real transformation. Just as failing to track your body composition can cause you to miss the positive or negative changes occurring in your physique, leading to confusion, anxiety, and demotivation, if you don't track your workouts, you'll eventually stop gaining muscle and strength, which can be just as distressing.

Plus, tracking your training makes it more exciting—you get to watch hard data change for the better and, as time passes, review old records and see how much progress you've made.

To track your *Muscle for Life* strength training, the two easiest options are a pen and paper or the notepad app in your smartphone. In both cases, the process is the same: all you do is write out a workout and then record your performance of it. Specifically, put down the exercises, rep ranges, and number of hard sets for a workout, and then note the weight and reps of each set as you do them.

Here's a simple way to lay this out:

Phase 1
Week 1
Workout 1
Monday 8/23/2021

UPPER BODY A

Push-up
12–15 REPS

Set 1:
Set 2:
Set 3:

Lat Pulldown

12–15 REPS

Set 1:

Set 2:

Set 3:

Machine Chest Press

12–15 REPS

Set 1:

Set 2:

Set 3:

Bodyweight Row

12–15 REPS

Set 1:

Set 2:

Set 3:

When you do this workout, you can fill it out like this:

Week 1

Workout 1

Monday 8/23/2021

UPPER BODY A

Push-up
12-15 REPS

Set 1: 13
Set 2: 13
Set 3: 12

Lat Pulldown
12-15 REPS

Set 1: 15
Set 2: 14
Set 3: 14

Machine Chest Press
12-15 REPS

Set 1: 30 x 13
Set 2: 30 x 13
Set 3: 30 x 12

Bodyweight Row
12-15 REPS

Set 1: 12
Set 2: 12
Set 3: 12

You can also include notes like if you felt strong or weak on a set or exercise, experienced an ache or pain, didn't sleep well the night before, etc. These observations can help you better understand your numbers when you're reviewing them later. Many people like to record their body measurements in the same place (an app or a notebook, usually) as well for an extra boost of motivation.

Just writing everything down isn't enough, though. You have to use the data to inform your training. To do that, before you do a workout again, look back at what you did the previous times around to see what you'd like to achieve in this week's performance. For instance, in the workout example just listed, you got 13 reps in your first set of push-ups, which is in spitting distance of your goal of 15 reps. Therefore, the next time you do this workout, you could strive for 14 or 15 reps in your first set and at least 13 reps in both your second and third sets, which would be an improvement.

If you'd prefer a more technologically savvy approach to planning and tracking your training, there are many good apps for this (I have a free one called Stacked, which you can get at www.getstackedapp.com), and Excel and Google Sheets are popular as well. You can find spreadsheets with an entire year's worth of *Muscle for Life* strength training workouts for men and women in the free bonus material that comes with this book (www.muscleforlife book.com/bonus).

This is a big moment for us. You've digested the key principles and strategies for both diet and exercise. If I've done my job well, you've gained a whole new perspective on exercise and fitness and are ready to start your *Muscle for Life* workouts.

To make this as smooth as possible, in the next chapter I'll share with you a quickstart guide that'll walk you through the whole process.

KEY TAKEAWAYS

+ To track your body composition, weigh yourself every three days and calculate the average every two weeks, and take body measurements and progress pictures every two weeks.

+ Your weight can change daily for reasons that have nothing to do with fat or muscle loss or gain, including fluid retention, glycogen levels, and bowel movements (or the lack thereof), so expect regular ups and downs, and don't fret over sudden increases.

+ Measure and record your waist circumference every two weeks, because the size of your waist is a reliable indicator of fat loss or gain.

+ If you're the type of person who loves tracking data, you can also measure your upper-leg circumference, your flexed arms, your chest circumference, your shoulder circumference, and your flexed calves every two weeks, and record the data.

+ Tracking your strength training is just as important as tracking your body composition because it's the only way to ensure you're progressively overloading your muscles.

+ To track your *Muscle for Life* strength workouts, the two easiest options are a pen and paper or the notepad app in your smartphone, though in both cases, the process is the same: all you do is write out a workout and then record your performance of it.

14

The *Muscle for Life* Workout Quickstart Guide

We are what we repeatedly do. Greatness, then, is not an act, but a habit.
—WILL DURANT

To make your first phase of *Muscle for Life* training as smooth as possible, I've prepared a comprehensive checklist that breaks the process down into five steps:

1. Buy your supplies.
2. Join or set up a gym.
3. Create your workout schedule.
4. Do your first week of training.

Let's go through each.

1. Buy Your Supplies

You don't need much in the way of gear and gadgets to do your *Muscle for Life* workouts. The only items you truly need are a measuring tape and a bathroom scale for tracking your transformation. There are other items that can be useful, however:

1. A pair of workout gloves for preventing calluses.

2. A pair of training shoes for steadier squatting and deadlifting (intermediate and advanced strength routines).

3. A pair of lifting straps for deadlifting when the weights get heavy (intermediate and advanced strength routines).

4. A pair of shin guards or a few pairs of knee-high socks for protecting your shins while deadlifting (advanced strength routines).

5. A cheap wristwatch or stopwatch if your phone or current wristwatch doesn't have a stopwatch function.

6. If you're going to run or walk for cardio, a comfortable pair of running shoes. Affordable and high-quality brands include Asics, Brooks, Saucony, Adidas, and Mizuno. You can ignore more or less all of their marketing puffery, by the way, and just pick whatever feels the best on your feet as you walk or jog around.

7. Equipment for your home gym (we'll talk specifics below).

Also, if you're interested, you can find links to my specific product recommendations in the free bonus material that comes with this book (www.muscleforlifebook.com/bonus).

2. Join or Set Up a Gym

Some people are turned off by gyms, and understandably so. Sweaty, smelly guys groaning and gawking; wannabe Instagram celebrities snapping selfies; and stony-faced bodybuilders laying claim to most of the equipment can make a trip to the gym seem about as appealing as a tray of gas station sushi.

Fortunately, now that working out is more mainstream than ever before, it's easy for most people to find a clean, pleasant, and inviting gym that more resembles an upscale community center than a dingy dungeon.

The most important things to consider when picking a gym are:

1. Does it have the equipment you'll need for your workouts? Just about any gym that's well stocked with free weights and machines will do. So long as it has a few bench presses and squat racks, a full set of dumbbells, and some basic machines, and it allows deadlifting (an important point if you're starting with the intermediate or advanced routines)—you're golden.

2. Is it close enough that you won't have any trouble going consistently? I've found that if going to the gym requires more than about forty minutes of driving (there and back), compliance declines. So, if you can, minimize the commute by finding a gym that's close to your home or workplace.

3. Does it fit your budget? Don't spend more on a gym than you can afford, but it's a good idea to invest in one that's clean and has nice equipment, friendly staff, and other perks you may want to use, such as showers, towels, cardio machines, a pool, etc. Most entry-level gym memberships will cost you anywhere from $10 to $50 per month, depending on where you live. Higher-tier gym memberships will cost anywhere from $100 to $300 per month, and often offer fitness classes you may want to attend for cardio instead of the more conventional options. For entry-level gyms, your best bets will be Gold's Gym, 24 Hour Fitness, LA Fitness, and Anytime Fitness. For premium gyms, Equinox and Life Time Fitness are my favorite choices.

You can also work out at home with a home gym, and this comes with pros and cons in terms of cost effectiveness, convenience, and privacy. On the pro side:

+ You can't beat the convenience, and this may make it easier to stick to the plan.
+ You can train whenever you want and don't need to work around holiday hours or other limitations.
+ You never have to wait for equipment.
+ You don't have to worry about the cleanliness of the facilities.
+ You won't receive unwanted attention.
+ You can blare your favorite music, decorate the walls however you like, and create your own little fitness playground.
+ You save the time and money you'd spend on dues and getting to the gym.

On the other hand:

+ If you want new equipment, you'll need a couple hundred dollars' worth for the beginner program, a bit more for the intermediate program, and $1,000 to $1,500 in hardware for the advanced program. If you're willing to look for deals on used equipment online, websites like craigslist or eBay are good resources for getting what you need for quite a bit less.
+ You'll also need at least 100 to 200 square feet to set everything up (for reference, the average two-car garage is about 650 square feet).
+ You'll be fairly limited in the exercises you can do, and if you want to do cardio on a machine, you'll need to buy that too.

- You may enjoy your workouts less, since you'll likely be doing them alone. A friendly training partner can improve consistency by enhancing accountability and making training more fun.
- You have to clean, maintain, repair, and replace your equipment.
- You may get distracted by chores, kids, pets, your spouse or partner, etc.

All things considered, I recommend a commercial gym if you're starting with the beginner strength routine, which includes more machine exercises than the intermediate and advanced routines. However, it's possible to swap out these machine exercises for "approved" bodyweight and free-weight alternatives given in chapter 11 that you can do at home.

For example, you could do the feet-elevated push-up instead of the chest press machine, the one-arm dumbbell row instead of the lat pulldown, and the bodyweight squat or dumbbell goblet squat instead of the leg press (technically, the goblet squat is an intermediate-level exercise, but most beginners can do it without issue).

Bear in mind, however, that free-weight exercises are harder to learn and execute than bodyweight and machine ones, which partially defeats the purpose of a beginner routine. If you're a beginner and your only option is home workouts, however, don't despair. You'll do just fine.

Beginner Routine Workout Equipment

If you'll be training at home and starting with one of the beginner strength training routines, you'll want the following:

- **Set of dumbbells**
  You have two options here:

1. Regular dumbbells (where each dumbbell is a fixed amount of weight)

Regular dumbbells are the most comfortable to handle, but they also take up a lot of space, which makes them unworkable for many people who don't have much room for their home gym. If that's not an issue for you, however, start with a set that ranges from 10 to 50 pounds per dumbbell in 5-pound increments. You can add more dumbbells later, as you get stronger. If you're already an experienced trainee and need heavier weights, consider buying in 10-pound increments over 80 pounds if you need to save money or space. Fractional plates (small plates ranging from 0.25 to 1.25 pounds that can be attached to dumbbells) can be useful in this case as well.

2. Adjustable dumbbells (where you can change the weight of each dumbbell)

Adjustable dumbbells are more unwieldy than regular dumbbells, but they're plenty usable and take up very little space, making them an ideal fit for many home gyms. Choose a set that goes up to at least 50 pounds per dumbbell, and if the product doesn't allow you to further extend its weight incrementally (Bowflex, for instance), you may want to consider getting a model that goes up to 90 to 100 pounds or choose another product that you can augment gradually as you get stronger (PowerBlock dumbbells, for example), so you don't have to buy a whole new set of dumbbells in six or twelve months.

- **Adjustable bench**

  An adjustable bench is a padded bench with wheels that can be set completely flat or upright. It allows you to do many seated and lying exercises, like the dumbbell bench press, seated dumbbell overhead press, flat and incline bench and dumbbell presses, as well as other exercises, like the one-arm dumbbell row and split squat.

- **Dip stand (also called a *dip bar* and *dip stand station*)**

  A dip stand is a metal frame for bodyweight dips and rows.

Intermediate Routine Workout Equipment

If you'll be training at home and starting with one of the intermediate strength training routines, you'll want all of the equipment for the beginner routines as well as the following:

- **Trap-bar**

  You'll need this for the trap-bar deadlift, although you can make do with a barbell (by doing the conventional deadlift instead of trap-bar variation) if you don't want to buy both a trap-bar and a barbell.

- **Weight plates**

  If you're a woman, start with at least two 2.5-, 5-, 10-, 25-, and 45-pound plates, and if you're a man, two 2.5-, 5-, 10-, and 25-pound plates, as well as four to six 45-pound plates depending on how strong you are. (If you're starting with the beginner routine, four is fine; if the intermediate or advanced, go with six.) Then you can add to your collection as you get stronger (most people like to add extra 10- and 45-pound plates).

Also, make sure you get round plates and not multisided ones, which shift out of position when you deadlift.

✦ **Rubber flooring**

These are thick tiles of rubber that link together so you can deadlift without damaging your floor or equipment or making too much noise.

Advanced Routine Workout Equipment

If you'll be training at home and starting with one of the advanced routines, you'll want all of the equipment for the beginner and intermediate routines plus the following:

✦ **Power rack**

A power rack, also called a squat rack, is a sturdy metal frame usually about eight feet tall, four feet wide, and three to six feet deep, with adjustable hooks to hold a barbell and safety bars to enhance safety when alone. With this piece of equipment, you can do the barbell back squat, barbell Romanian deadlift, and incline and flat barbell bench press.

✦ **Barbell**

Many of the exercises in the advanced routines require a barbell, so this is a must-have.

✦ **Pull-up bar or power tower**

A pull-up bar is a bar you can install in a doorway that allows you to do pull-ups and chin-ups. A power tower is a metal frame for pull-ups, chin-ups, and dips, and thus it replaces the dip stand and pull-up bar.

There are countless other tools, toys, and machines you can buy, but you'll be able to do almost all the exercises in the *Muscle for Life* workouts with these setups. For the exercises you can't do—the leg press, machine shoulder press, machine chest press, and leg curl, for example—simply swap them for approved exercises listed in chapter 11 that you can do.

Here's a chart that'll help you make the right choices:

Exercise	Substitution #1	Substitution #2
Machine Chest Press	Dumbbell Bench Press	Push-up
Machine Shoulder Press	Seated Dumbbell Overhead Press	Incline Dumbbell Bench Press
Machine Cable Fly	Push-up	Chest Dip
Cable Triceps Pushdown	Triceps Dip	Dumbbell Triceps Overhead Press
Seated Cable Row	One-Arm Dumbbell Row	Bodyweight or Dumbbell Row
Lat Pulldown	Bodyweight or Dumbbell Row	Chin-up or Pull-up
Machine Row	One-Arm Dumbbell Row	Bodyweight or Dumbbell Row
Cable Biceps Curl	Alternating Dumbbell Curl	Bodyweight or Dumbell Row
Leg Press	Dumbbell Goblet Squat	Bodyweight or Dumbbell Lunge

Exercise	Substitution #1	Substitution #2
Leg Extension	Bodyweight or Dumbbell Split Squat	Bodyweight Step-up
Leg Curl	Dumbbell Romanian Deadlift	Romanian Deadlift

In terms of where to set up your home gym, pick a room that has a concrete floor if you can, like a garage or unfinished basement, and that's on the first floor or in the basement because working out on an upper floor—deadlifting in particular—can scare others in the house or even damage your floor.

3. Create Your Workout Schedule

First, let's decide which days of the week you'll do your strength training. Here are some helpful considerations:

+ Try to evenly space your strength training workouts throughout the week.
+ Try to include at least one day of no strength training between your strength training workouts.
+ Many people, including myself, enjoy doing their strength training workouts during the week and keeping the weekends free for cardio and other activities.

As for your cardio workouts, here are a few scheduling guidelines:

1. Don't do more than one cardio workout per day.
2. Try to schedule cardio workouts on days with no strength training.

3. When doing strength training and cardio workouts on the same day, try to do your strength training first followed by your cardio.

4. When doing strength training and cardio workouts on the same day, try to schedule cardio on days with upper-body strength training.

5. Make sure your week includes at least one and up to two rest days (no workouts or vigorous physical activity).

Here are examples of well-designed workout routines:

	Mon.	Tue.	Wed.	Thu.	Fri.	Sat.	Sun.
Morning	Lower Body A	Cardio	Upper Body A		Lower Body B		
Afternoon/ Evening				Cardio			

	Mon.	Tue.	Wed.	Thu.	Fri.	Sat.	Sun.
Morning	Lower Body A		Upper Body A		Lower Body B	Cardio	Cardio
Afternoon/ Evening							

	Mon.	Tue.	Wed.	Thu.	Fri.	Sat.	Sun.
Morning	Lower Body A	Cardio		Upper Body A		Lower Body B	
Afternoon/ Evening			Cardio	Cardio			

	Mon.	Tue.	Wed.	Thu.	Fri.	Sat.	Sun.
Morning	Upper Body A		Lower Body A			Upper Body B	
Afternoon/ Evening	Cardio	Cardio		Cardio			

	Mon.	Tue.	Wed.	Thu.	Fri.	Sat.	Sun.
Morning	Upper Body A		Cardio	Lower Body A		Upper Body B	
Afternoon/ Evening	Cardio				Cardio	Cardio	

	Mon.	Tue.	Wed.	Thu.	Fri.	Sat.	Sun.
Morning	Upper Body A	Lower Body A	Cardio		Upper Body B		Cardio
Afternoon/ Evening					Cardio		

So, are you ready to create your plan? Let's begin:

1. Decide when and where you'll do your workouts (strength or cardio or both). Write your schedule in the chart that follows.

2. Next, review your plan and consider what else must occur for you to follow it. For example, if you want to do your workouts first thing in the morning, what time will you need to be in bed to ensure you're well rested (including Fridays and Saturdays, if applicable)? Or if your plan is to train after work, what time will you need to leave the office? Create what–when–where statements for any important preconditions and write them below.

3. Then consider your what–when–where statements and look for

ways things can go awry. What will you do if you miss a workout? (Can you do it on another day, or do you need to skip it?) What'll you do if you're running late to the gym? (Can you leave the gym later, or do you need to cut your workout short?) What if you need to travel? (Can you do your regular workouts on the road, or will you need to do something else like a dumbbell-only or bodyweight routine? Or will it be cardio only?) Create if–then statements to address the obstacles you're likely to face from time to time, and write them below.

	Mon.	Tue.	Wed.	Thu.	Fri.	Sat.	Sun.
Morning							
Afternoon/ Evening							

....

....

....

....

....

....

....

....

....

....

4. Do Your First Week of Training

During your first week of *Muscle for Life* workouts, your main goals are to get comfortable with the strength exercises and to determine your starting weights (or exercise variations, in the case of the beginner routines).

Here are key points to remember:

+ Do exercises one at a time and complete all of the hard sets for one exercise before moving on to another.
+ Don't do warm-up sets for bodyweight exercises.
+ Do two warm-up sets with the first exercises for each major muscle group in a workout. On the first, do 10 reps with about 50 percent of your hard-set weight, and rest for a minute. On the second, do 5 reps with about 70 percent of your hard-set weight, and rest for a minute.
+ Rest three to four minutes between hard sets of primary exercises and two to three minutes between hard sets of accessory exercises.
+ For all exercises, use double progression to first increase the reps and then the weight or difficulty of the exercise. To do this, increase the weight (weighted exercises) or graduate to a more difficult exercise variation (bodyweight exercises) when you hit the top of the rep range you're working in for three hard sets in a row. Then the next time you do the exercise, if you can finish your first hard set with the new, heavier weight or harder exercise variation within at least a rep or two of the bottom of the rep range you're working in, continue until you can do three hard sets at the top of the range in a row, and progress again.
+ You'll generally lose 2 to 4 reps for every 10 pounds you add to an

exercise (5 per dumbbell), and gain 2 to 4 reps for every 10 pounds you remove.

✦ End all hard sets of bodyweight exercises 1 rep shy of muscle failure (0 good reps left), and end all hard sets of machine, dumbbell, and barbell exercises 2 to 3 reps shy of muscle failure (2 to 3 good reps left).

✦ Use a "1-0-1" rep tempo for all exercises, which means the first part of each rep should take about one second, followed by a momentary pause, followed by the final part of the rep, which should also take about one second.

✦ Expect to be sore for your first week or two, even if you're not new to strength training. Your body will be challenged in new and taxing ways on this program and must adapt. This will happen quickly, however, so by the end of the second or third week, you shouldn't experience much soreness after your workouts.

✦ If you want to boost your body's ability to recover, aim for an additional thirty to sixty minutes of sleep each night of week one. This may improve your workout performance too!

Also, don't be surprised or discouraged if week one is a bit of a brute. I remember my first week clearly: I felt weak, awkward, and out of place, but I also knew that was an unavoidable and temporary phase. The initial difficulty isn't a sign that it's probably not worth it—it's a signal of its worth. Nor is struggling at the start evidence that you don't belong in the arena—it's a chance to prevail and prove you're worthy.

Consider: transforming your body is much more than merely building muscle and losing fat—you're sacrificing who you are for who you want to be. You're using iron and steel to forge your new form—a mystical act of heat and fire, hammer and anvil. It's not changing your underwear or cutting your nails. It's supposed to be hard. Fortunately, though, it's not *that* hard. It's not shaving with an axe or combing your hair with a broom. It's picking up stuff and putting it down until your muscles burn and your body aches. That doesn't mean you'll enjoy every workout—you won't—but you'll always dig *having worked out.*

Early on, I explained that this isn't a book you just read, but one you *do*. And we've reached the jumping-off point. It's time to screw up the courage and start the program. You can keep reading as well, of course, because there's more to learn and implement to further enhance your body composition and health, but as the rest of the material in this book is meant to support your efforts in the kitchen and gym, the sooner you begin those activities, the sooner you'll be able to benefit from what else I have to teach to you.

So, are you ready? Maybe a little nervous or uncertain? Good! That's exactly how you should feel—the "pre-event nerves" that even professional athletes regularly experience. Contrary to popular belief, research shows that such feelings aren't a sign that something is wrong or that you need to "calm down" or "stop stressing." Rather, this uneasiness can be reframed and harnessed for better performance by simply telling yourself "I am excited" instead of trying to suppress the sensation. This shifts your attitude from an unproductive one (anxious and reluctant), what scientists call a *threat mindset*, to a constructive one (fired up and ready to roll)—an *opportunity mindset*. So, does the thought of beginning your journey make your heart beat a little faster? Your blood pump a little harder? Your breathing a little stronger? Perfect! Let's go! Show me what you've got!

PART 4

THE LAST SUPPLEMENT ADVICE YOU'LL EVER NEED

15

The Smart Supplement Buyer's Guide

To begin is easy, to persist is an art.
—GERMAN PROVERB

Most of your results with *Muscle for Life* will come from following your diet and exercise plans, and no pills, powders, or potions will change that. Supplements just aren't as important as most fitness folk believe.

While some can speed up results and improve health, many (if not most) are duds. For instance, branched-chain amino acids are hugely popular and said to aid muscle growth, but a growing body of evidence shows they don't. *Garcinia cambogia* is one of the most popular weight loss supplements of all time, but studies show that it's a flop. The same goes for the go-to supplement for boosting testosterone, *Tribulus terrestris*.

If you have the budget, however, there are supplements you should consider because the few that work can enhance many meaningful aspects of your body composition and physiology, including muscle growth, fat loss, strength, inflammation, heart health, mood, brain and gut health, insulin sensitivity, energy levels, immunity, and more.

There are seven supplements that can make a marked difference in your health and fitness:

1. Protein powder
2. Multivitamin
3. Vitamin D
4. Fish oil
5. Creatine
6. Joint support
7. Vitality support

That's also their order of importance. Protein powder is at the top because it makes eating enough protein easy. The second important supplement is a high-quality multivitamin because many people don't get enough of certain key nutrients through their diets (including those who "eat healthy"). Then there's vitamin D and fish oil, because maintaining adequate D and omega-3 intake is tricky with food alone and these benefit your health and performance in many ways. Next is creatine, an amino-acid-like molecule, because it's the single best supplement you can take for boosting strength, muscle growth, and post-workout recovery. After that are supplements to help your joints, because aches and pains kill progress and motivation (if you're having joint issues, this may be the most important category for you), and vitality supplements that increase energy and well-being, because the livelier you feel, the better your workouts are, not to mention everything else in life.

Let's review each of these types of supplements and learn how to choose and use them properly.

PROTEIN POWDER

Whey and casein and soy, oh my! The selection of protein powders can be overwhelming because there are dozens of popular brands and products.

Should you choose an animal-based protein powder like whey, casein, or collagen? Or maybe a plant-based protein powder like rice, soy, hemp, or pea? Or maybe a blend?

A good protein powder meets a few criteria:

1. It tastes good and mixes well. If you have to choke it down, you'll have trouble eating it every day.
2. It's high in protein and low in carbohydrate and fat. This keeps calories to a minimum and allows you to eat more food (more satisfying).
3. It's rich in essential amino acids and absorbed well by the body. This determines its quality as a source of protein and how good it is for improving body composition.
4. It's affordable and offers good value (a reasonable cost per serving).

I also prefer all-natural protein powders (and other supplements) that don't contain artificial sweeteners, food dyes, or other synthetic junk because I take six to eight servings of supplements per day and wouldn't want to regularly ingest that many chemicals. Such substances may not be as dangerous as alarmists would have you believe, but studies do show that they can cause adverse reactions in some people.

So, which popular protein powders meet my requirements and which don't? Let's find out.

The Scoop on Whey Protein

Whey protein is the pooh-bah of protein powder for good reason: it provides a lot of protein per scoop and dollar, it tastes good, and it's rich in amino acids and highly bioavailable.

Pretty good for a translucent liquid that remains after curdling and straining milk to make cheese—one that was once considered a worthless by-product of dairy processing. Whey became valuable, however, when scientists discovered its high-protein content in the late 1800s. Investment into technology for turning whey into a food followed, and an industry was born.

Researchers later discovered that whey is digested and absorbed quickly and is flush with the amino acid *leucine*, which plays a vital role in stimulating protein synthesis. This put whey at the top of the list for bodybuilders, and as methods of refining the raw ingredient improved, so did the palatability and popularity of the final product.

So, whey is an excellent all-around choice for protein supplementation, and you have three types to choose from:

1. Whey concentrate. This is the least-processed form of whey protein, ranging from 25 percent protein (bad) to 80 percent (good) by weight depending on the quality, and it contains dietary fat and lactose.
2. Whey isolate. This is whey protein processed to remove the fat and lactose, and it's at least 90 percent protein by weight.
3. Whey hydrolysate. This is whey protein (concentrate or isolate, but usually isolate) processed to be more easily digested and absorbed.

Whey isolate and hydrolysate are often marketed as better for muscle building than whey concentrate, but this isn't always true. Isolate and hydrolysate have advantages—more protein by weight, no lactose, better mixability and digestibility, and some would say better taste—but as far as bottom-line results go, a high-quality whey concentrate works just fine.

One rule to keep in mind when choosing a whey protein powder, however, is you'll generally get what you pay for. If a product costs a lot less than the going rate, that's probably because it's made with low-quality ingredients. But high prices aren't always indicative of top quality. For example, some disreputable supplement companies will add small amounts of whey isolate and hydrolysate to a base of low-quality concentrate to create a "blend" and then call special attention to just the isolate and hydrolysate on their packaging and in their marketing.

Fortunately, there's an easy way to sniff out obvious clunkers: checking ingredient lists and serving sizes relative to protein per serving.

Ingredients are listed in descending order according to predominance by weight, meaning there's more of the first ingredient than the second, more of the second than the third, and so on. Therefore, if a protein powder bills itself as a whey isolate but has whey concentrate as the first ingredient, it contains more of that than anything else. In fact, it may be mostly concentrate and contain very little isolate. Worse are "whey" protein powders that list milk protein (a cheap alternative) before any form of whey.

You should also look at the amount of protein per scoop relative to the scoop (serving) size. They'll never match exactly because even the "cleanest" protein powders have sweetener, flavoring, and other minor but requisite ingredients besides the protein powder itself, but a large discrepancy between the two is a red flag that something isn't right. For instance, if a serving weighs 40 grams but contains just 20 grams of protein, don't buy the product unless you know that the other 20 grams are stuff you want.

So, in summary, a high-quality whey protein is easy to spot:

1. Whey concentrate, isolate, or hydrolysate is the first ingredient.
2. Whey isolate or hydrolysate is the first ingredient if either is emphasized on the packaging or in the marketing.

3. The serving size is fairly close to the amount of protein per serving.

The Scoop on Casein Protein

Like whey, casein protein comes from milk and is highly effective for muscle building. Unlike whey, however, casein digests slowly, resulting in a steadier, more gradual release of amino acids into the blood—a property that makes it no better or worse for our purposes. Most people who pick casein just prefer its taste and mouthfeel over whey's.

You have two types of casein protein supplements to choose from:

1. Calcium caseinate
2. Micellar casein

Calcium caseinate is casein processed to improve mixability, and micellar casein is a higher-quality form processed to preserve the small bundles of protein (*micelles*) responsible for its slow-digesting properties. For that reason, research shows that micellar casein is digested more slowly than calcium caseinate, but both are equally effective for meeting protein needs, so choose whichever you like better.

As with whey, when buying a casein protein, make sure to look at the amount of protein per scoop relative to the scoop size.

The Scoop on Soy Protein

Soy is an all-around effective source of protein and essential amino acids, but it's also the subject of ongoing controversy, especially among men. According to some research, soy can have feminizing effects in men because of estrogen-like molecules in soybeans called *isoflavones*. On the other hand, other studies have found that normal levels of soy and isoflavone intake don't alter male fertility or hormones.

What gives? There isn't a simple answer yet. Studies show that these effects can vary depending on the presence or absence of certain intestinal bacteria, for instance, which exist in 30 to 50 percent of people, but more research is needed to understand the significance of this phenomenon.

So, while soy protein is a viable option comparable to whey and casein in terms of quality and effectiveness, if you're a man, just choose one of the other options discussed in this chapter. If you're a woman, however, soy protein is a wonderful plant-based source of protein with no known risks or downsides.

You have two types of soy protein to choose from, too—soy concentrate and isolate—and since an isolate has more protein by weight (and less carbohydrate and fat), that's my recommendation.

The Scoop on Collagen Protein

Collagen is the main protein in connective tissues in animals, and collagen protein is all the rage at the moment. Unfortunately, it doesn't even deserve a spot on the stage, let alone the spotlight.

As you know, the amount of essential amino acids a source of protein provides is very important, especially for improving body composition. The fewer essential amino acids per serving, the less nourishing the protein is.

Collagen protein gets low marks in this regard because while it's rich in the nonessential amino acids *glycine*, *proline*, and *alanine*, it's lacking in the essential amino acids most related to muscle growth: *leucine*, *isoleucine*, and *valine*. Collagen protein is low in sulfur as well, which is involved in many bodily functions such as blood flow, energy production, and protecting cells from oxidative damage.

One thing collagen protein has going for it, however, is its abundance of glycine, which may improve the quality of your skin, hair, and nails. That said, glycine is dirt cheap (and tastes good), so you can buy it as a stand-alone supplement if you want to see if it can make you look prettier.

The Scoop on Rice Protein

You may not think much of the protein in rice or even realize it contains any protein, but it has a high *biological value* (a measurement of how efficiently the protein is absorbed and utilized by your body) of about 80 percent (similar to beef's) and a robust amino acid profile (similar to soy's).

Rice protein powder also has a mild taste and pleasant texture, making it an all-around winner for plant-based protein supplementation (and if you want to make it even better, you can mix it with the next option).

As far as forms go, rice protein isolate is best.

The Scoop on Pea Protein

When's the last time you heard a meathead say he's eating a lot of peas to bulk up? As it happens, he could because pea protein also has a high biological value (about the same as that of rice) and a large amount of leucine, making it effective in promoting muscle gain.

People also often mix pea protein powder with rice protein powder because they taste great together and have complementary amino acid profiles, combining into a mixture that's chemically similar to whey. In fact, this blend is often referred to as the "vegan's whey."

Pea protein powder comes in two forms—concentrate and isolate—and both are created by drying and grinding peas into a fine flour, mixing it with water, and removing the fiber and starch, leaving mostly protein with a smattering of vitamins and minerals. Pea protein isolate needs to be at least

90 percent protein by weight, however, whereas pea protein concentrate can be anywhere from 70 to 90 percent protein by weight.

Thus, I prefer pea isolate over concentrate (more protein and less carbohydrate and fat per serving).

The Scoop on Hemp Protein

Hemp protein is nutritious but only about 30 to 50 percent protein by weight, which means it contains more carbs and fat per serving than all the other protein powders we've discussed so far. Furthermore, hemp protein isn't absorbed as well as soy, rice, or pea protein and is lower in essential amino acids, making it even less useful as a protein supplement.

Therefore, I look at a hemp powder as a food rather than a protein supplement and don't recommend it for protein supplementation.

How to Take Protein Powder

To boost protein intake, most people like to take a scoop of protein powder before or after workouts because it's quick and convenient and then another scoop or two during the day as a snack (midafternoon is popular). This works well.

Some people get most of their daily protein from powders, but this can cause gastrointestinal distress. We can have only so much protein powder in a day before something just doesn't feel right, especially with milk-derived powders like whey and casein. Tolerance varies from person to person, but for me, any more than 70 to 80 grams of whey or casein in a day will upset my stomach.

The primary reason for this is powders are digested faster than foods, so if you gulp down a large amount of protein powder in one sitting, protein molecules can make their way into the large intestine only partially digested, resulting in gassiness and discomfort. This problem is unique to protein powder because it's so easy to eat, whereas sources of protein that require chewing are more filling and harder to overconsume. A protein shake with a couple of chicken breasts' worth of protein can be downed in a matter of seconds, for instance, placing an immediate and intense demand on your digestive system.

Whey protein can be particularly troublesome in this regard because many people can't comfortably digest a large amount of dairy protein in one sitting. This is less of an issue with whey isolate protein, which doesn't contain lactose, but it can still occur.

So, all things considered, here are my recommendations for protein powder:

1. Don't get over 50 percent of your daily protein from protein powders.
2. Don't eat more than 40 to 50 grams of protein from powder in one sitting.

MULTIVITAMIN

According to research conducted by scientists at Colorado State University and published in 2005, at least half of the US population doesn't get enough vitamin B6, vitamin A, magnesium, calcium, and zinc, and 33 percent of the population doesn't get enough folate. A more recent study conducted by scientists at Tufts University and published in 2017 found that over 30 percent of the US population was deficient in calcium, magnesium, and vitamins A, C, D, and E. Other research shows that average vitamin K and D intake levels may be suboptimal as well, which is particularly detrimental as we get older, since these vitamins play an important role in bone growth and repair, blood vessel and immune function, cancer prevention, joint health, and more.

Thus, a high-quality multivitamin can help you in a few ways:

1. It can plug nutritional "holes" in your diet, which are common even among people who eat well.

2. It can boost your intake of certain vitamins and minerals that improve health and wellness at higher doses, like B vitamins, zinc, and chromium.

3. It can provide beneficial ingredients that are difficult or impossible to obtain from food, like grape-seed extract, ashwagandha, and alpha-lipoic acid.

It's hard to know whether a multivitamin is a winner, however. Many contain large amounts of vitamins and minerals most people don't need to supplement with, such as manganese, molybdenum, and the B vitamins (apart from niacin), as well as potentially harmful superdoses of others like retinol (vitamin A) and vitamin E. Cheap and less effective forms of ingredients are common too (to save money), and sometimes needlessly expensive ones are used only because they make for better marketing.

For example, it's often assumed that the natural forms of vitamins found in food are always better than their synthetic counterparts. Some supplement sellers and authorities even claim that synthetic vitamins are outright harmful. The truth, however, is that not all natural vitamins are better than artificial ones, and not all synthetics are bad. Certain natural forms have unique and desirable properties, such as vitamin E, and several synthetic vitamins outperform natural ones, such as folic acid, which is absorbed better than natural folate.

Another strike against multivitamins is the popularity of products that claim to provide 100 percent of everything you need in just one daily pill. The only way to get to one pill per day is by using too little of some key nutrients and none of others. Thus, most good multivitamins require taking at least a few pills per day because that allows for optimal dosing and absorption.

You should also be skeptical of multivitamins that are supposedly formulated for middle-aged people. Often these formulations aren't unique—and even when they are, they're usually flawed in the same ways described above (underdosing and overdosing; random, undesirable, or missing ingredients; and so on).

How do you find a good multivitamin, then? Here are a few tips:

1. Stay away from one-a-day products. A high-quality multivitamin will require taking at least two or three pills per day.

2. Stay away from tablets because they're not absorbed as well as pills.

3. Stay away from products that contain exactly 100 percent of RDI (*Reference Daily Intake*, or the amount of a nutrient required daily to maintain health in most people) of many vitamins and minerals. This is a sign the formulators didn't understand or consider actual dietary patterns and nutritional needs because proper dosing often ranges from a fraction of RDI in some cases to a multiple of it in others.

4. Stay away from products that contain retinol. This form of vitamin A should never be used orally because of the potential for liver damage at higher doses. Instead, *carotenoids* (pigments found in plants) should be used, which the body converts into retinol as needed and otherwise uses as antioxidants or eliminates.

5. The inclusion of *5-MTHF* is a good sign. This is short for *5-methyltetrahydrofolate*, and it's the active (usable by the body) form of the B vitamin folic acid (B9). When we eat foods with folate, our body converts it into 5-MTHF, which is then used for various physiological processes. Research shows that many people have a genetic mutation that hinders the production of 5-MTHF, however, and this can lead to a deficiency despite substantial folate or folic acid intake through healthy eating and supplementation. By supplementing with 5-MTHF directly, those with and without the genetic mutation can maintain sufficiency without any downsides, making it clearly the superior option for meeting this nutritional need. Many multivitamin formulators don't know this, however, and opt for folate or folic acid instead, and many that do understand the significance of 5-MTHF don't or can't use it because it's expensive. Thus, when a multivitamin contains 5-MTHF, it suggests the formulators may have known more about the subtleties of human nutrition than many of their peers and may have had a larger budget to work with.

How to Take a Multivitamin

Multivitamins should be taken with meals, ideally ones containing a bit of dietary fat, as this helps with nutrient absorption.

VITAMIN D

Not too long ago, vitamin D was simply known as a "bone vitamin," and even today many physicians still believe it's essential only for bone health. Recent research shows otherwise, however. Nearly every type of tissue and cell in the body has vitamin D receptors, including your heart, brain, and even fat cells, and it plays a vital role in many physiological processes, such as immune function, metabolism, and cell growth.

Furthermore, insufficient vitamin D intake is associated with an increased risk of many types of disease, including osteoporosis, heart disease, stroke, some cancers, type 1 diabetes, multiple sclerosis, tuberculosis, and even the flu. The importance of vitamin D is even more pronounced in people in their forties and beyond—studies show that many age-related diseases like osteoporosis, type 2 diabetes, cancer, and immune dysfunction are associated with low levels of vitamin D.

Getting vitamin D is tricky, too, because the human body is designed to make it when exposed to the sun, and most people aren't in the sun enough to maintain vitamin D sufficiency. Depending on your diet, latitude, and lifestyle, you'd need to sunbathe anywhere from fifteen to sixty minutes per day to maintain sufficient levels of vitamin D—and even if that's workable for you, unless you live in California or Hawaii, you'll be out of luck in the winter.

Food isn't a great option either, considering how much vitamin D we need to maintain optimal health. There are small amounts in foods like beef liver, cheese, and egg yolks, which have anywhere from 10 to 60 IU per ounce, and slightly larger amounts in fatty fish like salmon, tuna, and mackerel, which contain between 50 and 150 IU per ounce. Vitamin D is also added to various "fortified" foods like milk, breakfast cereals, orange juice, and margarine, but a wholesome meal plan never contains much of them.

Most multivitamins contain vitamin D, which is why I ranked a multivitamin above a standalone vitamin D supplement, but dosing can vary considerably, and sometimes a separate vitamin D supplement is needed as well.

How to Take Vitamin D

According to a committee of the Endocrine Society convened in 2011, 1,500 to 2,000 IU of vitamin D per day is adequate for ages 19 and up. Assuming you're in that age range, I recommend you start at 2,000 IU per day, and then, if you're experiencing any symptoms of low vitamin D levels (fatigue, bone pain, muscle weakness, and mood changes are several), get blood-tested for your levels of *25-hydroxyvitamin D* (the usable form of vitamin D your body creates) to determine your status and adjust your intake according to your doctor's recommendations.

Like a multivitamin, vitamin D should be taken with meals, and ideally ones containing a bit of dietary fat.

FISH OIL

Fish oil is, well, oil from fish, such as salmon, herring, mackerel, sardines, and anchovies, and an excellent source of two valuable omega-3 essential fatty acids: *eicosapentaenoic acid* (EPA) and *docosahexaenoic acid* (DHA).

Studies show that the average person's diet provides just one-tenth of the EPA and DHA needed to preserve health and prevent disease, and this can increase the risk of heart disease, Alzheimer's, dementia, depression, cancer, and other health conditions. What's more, maintaining sufficient EPA and DHA intake offers many other benefits, including:

+ Faster fat loss
+ Less fat gain
+ More muscle growth
+ Improved mood (lower levels of depression, anxiety, and stress)
+ Better cognitive performance (memory, attention, and reaction time)

- ✦ Enhanced immunity
- ✦ Reduced muscle and joint soreness

You have several options for increasing your intake of EPA and DHA through diet alone, but fatty fish is best. Grass-fed meat, free-range eggs, and vegetable oils can help, but omega-3 levels are much lower in meat and eggs than in fish, and vegetable oils contain not EPA and DHA but the fatty acid *alpha-linolenic acid* (ALA). The body converts ALA into EPA, which is then converted into DHA, but this conversion process is inefficient, so you have to eat large amounts of ALA to supply your body with enough EPA and DHA. This is one reason vegans often have omega-3 fatty acid deficiencies.

For those of us who don't want to eat a couple of servings of fatty fish per week (while also ensuring we avoid those highest in pollutants), a fish oil supplement is ideal. Hence its inclusion in my list of supplements worth taking.

There are three forms of fish oil supplements on the market today:

1. Triglyceride. Triglyceride fish oil is created by processing raw fish oil to remove impurities without changing its chemical form. This type of fish oil is as close to what you'd get from real fish as you can get.
2. Ethyl ester. Ethyl ester fish oil is created by processing natural triglycerides to replace the glycerol molecules they contain with ethanol (alcohol). This removes impurities and increases EPA and DHA levels.
3. Re-esterified triglyceride. Re-esterified triglyceride fish oil is created by using enzymes to convert ethyl ester oil back into a triglyceride form.

All three are viable choices, but you'd probably assume that a natural triglyceride fish oil supplement is your best choice. Not necessarily. Natural triglyceride oils have two significant drawbacks:

1. Because of the low level of processing, they can have higher levels of contaminants.
2. They're often lower in EPA and DHA per serving than the other two forms, which means you have to take more, and this can be expensive in dollars and calories.

As for ethyl ester fish oil, it gets the job done, but research shows that re-esterified triglyceride fish oil is better absorbed by the body, resulting in larger increases in plasma (blood) EPA and DHA levels. Another downside is that ethyl ester oil oxidizes (goes bad) more easily at all temperatures.

That leaves re-esterified triglyceride oil, which is the gold standard of fish oil supplements for four reasons:

+ High bioavailability (well-absorbed)
+ High concentrations of EPA and DHA
+ Low levels of toxins and pollutants
+ Resistance to oxidation (stays fresh longer)

How to Take Fish Oil

Research shows that a combined intake of 500 milligrams to 1.8 grams of EPA and DHA per day is adequate for general health, and for physically active people, 2 to 3 grams of combined EPA and DHA per day is reasonable. I don't recommend you take more than this, however, because higher doses can have immunosuppressive effects, which is more of a concern among the middle-aged and elderly than the young.

Take your fish oil with meals to maximize absorption and effectiveness, and to prevent nasty fish-oil burps (unlikely but possible with a high-quality supplement), store the pills in the freezer.

CREATINE

Creatine is a natural compound made up of the amino acids *L-arginine*, *glycine*, and *methionine* and is present in almost all cells, where it acts as an energy reserve. Our body can produce creatine, but also gets it from foods like meat, eggs, and fish.

Of all the sports supplements on the market today, creatine stands out as one of the absolute best. It's the most-researched molecule in all of sports nutrition—the subject of hundreds of scientific studies—and the benefits are clear:

+ More muscle growth
+ Faster strength gain
+ Greater anaerobic endurance
+ Better post-workout recovery

Creatine does all these things safely as well. Despite what you may have heard, if you have healthy kidneys, research shows that you have nothing to fear from creatine, and even if you have impaired kidney function, you're unlikely to experience any problems. Just to be safe, however, if you have any kidney issues, check with your doctor before you start supplementing with creatine.

And speaking of doctor visits, one reason that people (including many physicians) still think creatine stresses the kidneys is related to a substance known as *creatinine*, which is produced when your body metabolizes creatine. In sedentary people not supplementing with creatine, elevated creatinine levels can indicate kidney problems; but in people exercising regularly and supplementing with creatine, high creatinine levels are normal. Many active people taking creatine (and sometimes their doctors) don't know this, though, and are alarmed by high creatinine numbers popping up on a blood test.

Creatine supplements come in many forms, including creatine monohydrate, creatine ethyl ester, buffered creatine, and others. We could discuss them one by one, but here's all you need to know: go with powdered creatine monohydrate. It's the best-researched form by which all others are judged.

How to Take Creatine

Five grams of creatine monohydrate per day is optimal for enhancing muscle growth and recovery. When you start taking creatine, you can "load" it by taking 20 grams per day for the first five to seven days and see benefits sooner, but this can also upset your stomach, so I generally don't recommend it.

You can take creatine whenever to good effect, but taking it post-workout may be optimal. That said, it's unclear how important creatine timing is, so first and foremost, just make sure you take it every day.

JOINT SUPPORT

People often say you're as old as you feel, but I think it's more accurate to say you're as old as your *joints* feel. This is especially true for people with an active lifestyle—nothing can put the kibosh on our lifestyle like joint problems.

Temperamental shoulders can shut down upper-body workouts. Achy knees give a whole new reason to dread cardio and leg days. And a bitter lower back can impede just about everything we like to do in and out of the gym.

On the other hand, healthy, functional, pain-free joints make our training (and day-to-day life) more enjoyable and productive, which is one of the many reasons to be a stickler about eating right, training properly, and ensuring we get adequate rest and recovery.

Supplementation can help as well, with three natural ingredients standing out in particular: undenatured type-II collagen, boswellia, and curcumin.

Undenatured Type-II Collagen

We recall that collagen is the main protein in connective tissues in animals, and type-II collagen makes up your joint cartilage.

"Undenatured" is often a meaningless marketing buzzword, but in this case, it's a pivotal part of the supplement. *Denaturation* is the alteration of the natural structure of a substance, and research shows that denatured collagen has no beneficial effects on joint inflammation. Undenatured collagen, however, is a more natural form of the substance, and studies show that it's effective for regulating the immune response that inflames joints and destroys cartilage and bone.

It accomplishes this by "teaching" the body's immune system to stop attacking its collagen as a foreign substance, working almost like a natural vaccine against an inflammatory response in the body to collagen. These effects have been found both in people with arthritic conditions and in those with healthy joints, so whether you have joint problems or not, you can benefit from supplementing with undenatured type-II collagen.

How to Take Undenatured Type-II Collagen

Ten to 40 milligrams of undenatured type-II collagen per day is effective for improving joint health. This is a large range, but studies have found benefits at various doses, and more isn't always better. For instance, we know that 10 milligrams works, but two, three, or four times that amount doesn't appear to double, triple, or quadruple efficacy. Therefore, it's safe to say that 20 milligrams per day is sufficient, and 40 milligrams per day is at least slightly better but also significantly more expensive.

You can take undenatured type-II collagen with or without meals, but it may be most effective by itself or with a small meal (but not a large one).

Boswellia

Boswellia serrata is a plant native to much of India and Pakistan. It produces an aromatic substance known as *frankincense*, which has been used in Ayurvedic medicine for thousands of years to treat various disorders related to inflammation.

Thanks to modern science, we now know why. Frankincense contains molecules called *boswellic acids*—including the VIP *acetyl-11-keto-ß-boswellic acid* (or AKBA)—that inhibit the production of proteins that cause inflammation in the body. This effect extends to the joints. Studies show that boswellia reduces joint inflammation and pain, and inhibits the autoimmune response that eats away at joint cartilage, causing arthritis.

How to Take Boswellia

Boswellia is effective between 100 and 200 milligrams per day, depending on its boswellic acid content. High-quality boswellia supplements are usually around 20 percent AKBA by weight.

You can take boswellia with or without meals, but with food may be better for absorption.

Curcumin

Curcumin is the orange pigment found in the turmeric plant, which is the main spice in most curry blends. It has been used therapeutically in Ayurvedic medicine for thousands of years, and the roster of health benefits associated with curcumin is impressive and growing as scientists continue investigating its effects on a variety of diseases, including cancer, cardiovascular disease, osteoporosis, diabetes, Alzheimer's, and more.

Curcumin also produces healthier, less painful joints by inhibiting an inflammatory enzyme known as *cyclooxygenase* (COX).

Unfortunately, however, it's poorly absorbed in the intestines—so much so, studies show that to reap most of its benefits, you must take a patented form of curcumin (Meriva) that's combined with a natural substance known as *phosphatidylcholine* or combine generic curcumin with another ingredient to enhance absorption, such as black pepper extract.

How to Take Curcumin

Most studies proving curcumin's effectiveness have used 200 to 500 milligrams per day of an absorption-enhanced form like the Meriva phosphatidylcholine-curcumin complex or generic curcumin with black pepper extract (which is often included at 20 milligrams).

You can take curcumin with or without meals, but with food may be better for absorption.

VITALITY SUPPORT

Above all, I wrote this book to help people who might think they're over the hill regain much of the confidence, beauty, and energy of their younger years. Proper nutrition, exercise, rest, and stress management do most of the heavy lifting (ha ha), but there are natural supplements that can further bolster your resilience, stamina, and spirit. My favorites are DHEA, rhodiola, ashwagandha, and maca.

DHEA

DHEA, short for *dehydroepiandrosterone*, is a hormone produced by our adrenal glands and artificially created from substances in wild yam and soy. Our body converts DHEA into male and female sex hormones, including testosterone and estrogen, and natural production peaks in our early thirties and gradually declines as we get older.

Research shows that supplementing with DHEA increases testosterone production in older men and estrogen production in older women, making it an ideal supplement for supporting healthy hormone levels as we age. Therefore, I recommend DHEA to anyone over 40 with any steroid hormonal issues (such as low testosterone, estrogen, or progesterone levels), and to anyone over 60 regardless of hormone health.

How to Take DHEA

DHEA dosing is simple: 50 to 100 milligrams of DHEA per day gets the job done. You need to ensure you're taking DHEA, however, and not *7-Keto DHEA*, which is produced by your body when it metabolizes DHEA and works differently when supplemented.

You can take DHEA with or without meals, but with food may be better for absorption.

Rhodiola

Rhodiola rosea (also known as golden root) is a plant that grows in cold parts of the world, including the Arctic regions of Europe, Asia, and North America. It's known as an *adaptogen*, which is a substance that causes an imperceptible level of stress in the body and trains it to better handle future stresses.

The major benefit of rhodiola is a reduction in fatigue from prolonged stressors, meaning it helps protect against burnout caused by too much physical or mental effort and stress. Research also shows that it can enhance, or at least preserve, cognition and mood during strenuous periods.

How to Take Rhodiola

Studies on rhodiola have used doses ranging from 50 to 700 milligrams, with higher amounts used for acute benefits and lower ones for long-term supplementation. Additionally, most of the research on rhodiola used an extract known as *SHR-5*, which is standardized to contain a certain number of molecules known as *rosavins* and *salidrosides* that are responsible for most of rhodiola's benefits.

Thus, as we're interested in rhodiola's chronic effects, I recommend 100 to 200 milligrams of the SHR-5 extract per day or the same amount of another extract that's at least 3 percent rosavins by weight and 1 percent salidrosides. If you'd prefer to use the raw root of the plant, 5 to 6 grams per day is the recommended dose.

You can take rhodiola with or without meals, but with food may be better for absorption.

Ashwagandha

Ashwagandha is derived from a plant important in Ayurvedic medicine, and—fun fact—it means "smell of horse" in Sanskrit because it smells like horse sweat and was once thought to give you horselike strength.

Ashwagandha is also an adaptogen that helps your body grow stronger by exposing it to minor stress, and research shows that it can benefit us in many ways, including . . .

+ Increasing power and strength
+ Reducing chronic and acute cortisol increases from stress
+ Lowering feelings of stress and anxiety
+ Restoring fertility in men
+ Improving immune function
+ Increasing cardiovascular endurance
+ Protecting against pigments that accumulate during Alzheimer's disease and possibly producing a therapeutic effect in those with the disease

How to Take Ashwagandha

Most research on ashwagandha used doses between 500 and 600 milligrams per day. Studies of athletes and anxious people used an extract known as *KSM-66*, which is standardized to contain 5 percent of molecules called *withanolides* by weight.

Therefore, to ensure you get the most from your ashwagandha supplementation, take 500 to 600 milligrams of KSM-66 per day or the same amount of another extract providing a similar amount of withanolides (20 to 30 milligrams per serving).

You can take ashwagandha with or without meals, but with food may be better for absorption.

Maca

Maca is a plant related to cruciferous vegetables that has been grown in mountainous regions of Peru for nearly two thousand years. It too is an adaptogen, and its primary benefits are improved libido and sexual function in men and women and enhanced mood in postmenopausal women.

How to Take Maca

Studies on maca that have demonstrated notable benefits used a dose of 3 grams of the root per day (or a concentrated extract providing the equivalent of this), so that's my recommendation.

You can buy maca in pill and powder form, and if you want pills, pick an extract that's between 4:1 and 6:1, allowing you to take just 500 to 800 milligrams per day.

You can take maca with or without meals, but with food may be better for absorption.

Let's now see how these guidelines translate into structured plans you can easily reference and follow.

THE BASIC SUPPLEMENTATION PLAN

If you want to enhance your results on the *Muscle for Life* program but don't have the budget or desire to take many supplements, this plan is for you.

What	Why	When	How
Protein powder	Helps you eat enough high-quality protein to improve your body composition and health	Whenever (pre- and/or post-workout and midafternoon is common)	20 to 40 grams per serving, no more than 50 percent of daily protein from powder
Multivitamin	Boosts intake of vital nutrients that enhance health and well-being	With meal	Follow instructions
Vitamin D	Enhances health and well-being and reduces the risk of many diseases	With meal	2,000 IU per day
Fish oil	Provides essential omega-3 fatty acids that improve health and reduce the risk of disease	With meal	2 to 3 grams of combined EPA and DHA per day
Creatine monohydrate	Increases post-workout recovery and muscle and strength gain	Whenever, although post-workout may be ideal	5 grams per day

THE ALL-IN SUPPLEMENTATION PLAN

If you want all the possible benefits supplementation has to offer, follow this plan.

What	Why	When	How
Protein powder	Helps you eat enough high-quality protein to improve your body composition and health	Whenever (pre- and/or post-workout and midafternoon is common)	20 to 40 grams per serving, no more than 30 percent of daily calories from powders
Multivitamin	Boosts intake of vital nutrients that enhance health and well-being	With meal	Follow instructions
Vitamin D	Enhances health and well-being and reduces the risk of many diseases	With meal	2,000 IU per day
Fish oil	Provides essential omega-3 fatty acids that improve halth and reduce the risk of disease and dysfunction	With meal	2 to 3 grams of combined EPA and DHA per day
Creatine monohydrate	Increases post-workout recovery and muscle and strength gain	Whenever, although post-workout may be ideal	5 grams per day
Undenatured type-II collagen	Reduces joint inflammation and helps preserve cartilage	Whenever, by itself or with small meal	20 milligrams per day

What	Why	When	How
Boswellia	Reduces joint swelling and pain	Whenever, ideally with meal	100 to 200 milligrams per day
Curcumin	Reduces joint inflammation and pain and improves joint mobility	Whenever, ideally with meal	200 to 500 milligrams per day of an absorption-enhanced form like Meriva or generic curcumin with black pepper extract (which is often included at 20 milligrams)
DHEA (*not* 7-Keto DHEA)	Improves hormone profile	Whenever, ideally with meal	50 to 100 milligrams of DHEA per day
Rhodiola (SHR-5 extract)	Reduces mental and physical fatigue	Whenever, ideally with meal	100 to 200 milligrams per day
Ashwagandha (KSM-66 extract)	Increases physical performance and immunity and reduces stress and anxiety	Whenever, ideally with meal	500 to 600 milligrams of KSM-66 per day
Maca	Enhances libido and sexual function	Whenever, ideally with meal	3 grams of root equivalent per day

Supplementation is a complex and overwhelming subject, and if you take many of the marketing claims at face value, your cabinets can quickly fill with expensive bottles and bags that deliver minimal benefits, if any at all. Remember, then, that you don't need to use any supplements to reach your health and fitness goals, including the products highlighted in this chapter. If you're willing to eat enough of the right foods (and spend some time in the sun), you can give your body everything it needs to thrive.

Many people struggle to do that, however, and even if they can make it work, they'll still miss out on the additional benefits that smart supplementation can offer. Therefore, it's prudent to at least consider following the basic supplementation plan, and if it makes sense to you given your circumstances and goals, choose the full regimen.

Once you've made up your mind, go ahead and order any supplements you want to take. If you'd like specific product recommendations from me, you'll find them in the free bonus material that comes with this book (www .muscleforlifebook.com/bonus).

Then, keep reading, because in the next section of this book, I'll share with you more insights and tactics that'll help you troubleshoot and get the most from this program.

KEY TAKEAWAYS

- ✦ A great protein powder has several hallmarks: it tastes good, it mixes well, it's high in protein and low in carbohydrate and fat, it's rich in essential amino acids, it's absorbed well by the body, and it's affordable.
- ✦ Artificial sweeteners and food dyes may not be as dangerous as alarmists would have you believe, but studies do show that they can cause adverse reactions in some people.
- ✦ Whey isolate and hydrolysate have advantages—more protein by weight, no lactose, better mixability and digestibility, and some

would say better taste—but as far as bottom-line results go, a high-quality whey concentrate works just fine.

✦ Casein protein comes from milk and is highly effective for muscle building, but unlike whey, casein digests slowly, resulting in a steadier, more gradual release of amino acids into the blood—a property that makes it no better or worse for our purposes.

✦ If you're a man, avoid soy protein powder because it may negatively affect male hormones. If you're a woman, however, soy protein is a wonderful plant-based source of protein with no known risks or downsides.

✦ Rice protein has a high biological value of about 80 percent (similar to beef's), a robust amino acid profile (similar to soy's), a mild taste, and a pleasant texture and mouthfeel, making it an all-around winner for plant-based protein supplementation.

✦ Pea protein has a high biological value (about the same as that of rice) and a large amount of leucine, making it effective in promoting muscle gain.

✦ Getting too much of your daily protein from powders can cause gastrointestinal distress, so don't get more than 50 percent of your daily protein from protein powders, and don't eat more than 40 to 50 grams of protein from powder in one sitting.

✦ Here are a few tips to help you find a good multivitamin:

    ✦ Stay away from one-a-day products—high-quality multivitamin supplements will require taking at least two or three pills per day.

    ✦ Stay away from tablets because they're not absorbed as well as pills.

- Stay away from products that contain exactly 100 percent of RDI of many vitamins and minerals.
- Stay away from products that contain retinol.
- The inclusion of 5-MTHF is a good sign.

+ Creatine helps you build muscle and get stronger faster, and improves both anaerobic endurance and muscle recovery.

+ Supplementing with undenatured type-II collagen, boswellia, and curcumin can help keep your joints healthy, functional, and pain-free.

+ Proper nutrition, exercise, rest, and stress management will help you regain much of the confidence, beauty, and energy of your younger years, but natural supplements like DHEA, rhodiola, ashwagandha, and maca can further bolster your resilience, stamina, and spirit.

PART 5

THE BEGINNING

16

Frequently Asked Questions

Don't sacrifice who you could be for who you are.
—DR. JORDAN B. PETERSON

At this point, we've covered all of the most important aspects of the *Muscle for Life* program, but you may have lingering doubts or uncertainties. That's perfectly normal, so let's see if we can't tackle some of them here.

Q: Can I do strength training with arthritis?

A: Yes, but you should consult your doctor first. Research shows that moderate- and high-intensity strength training like you do in *Muscle for Life* rarely aggravates arthritis symptoms and is actually *better* for improving arthritic joints than the low-intensity training often prescribed for people with osteo- or rheumatoid arthritis.

Some exercises may be uncomfortable or even mildly (operative word here) painful for the first few weeks of training, but stick with it because most people with joint issues experience significant relief within their first month.

Q: Can I do strength training with high blood pressure?

A: Yes, but you should consult with your doctor first. Although strength training temporarily increases blood pressure during workouts, studies show that it can substantially decrease blood pressure on the whole, sometimes almost as much as cardio.

That said, as you learned in chapter 2, a combination of strength training and cardio is best for lowering blood pressure. There's a notable exception to this observation, however: if you have very high blood pressure (usually defined as >140/90 mm Hg, also known as *stage 2 hypertension*), your cardiovascular system may not be up to intense exercise yet. Again, discuss this with your doctor before beginning the *Muscle for Life* program (or any other exercise routine).

Q: I only have dumbbells. Can I do this program?

A: For the most part, yes. You can follow the beginner and intermediate routines fairly easily—all you have to do is make a few substitutions for the machines you don't have access to and the trap-bar deadlift (in the case of the intermediate program). The advanced routines will require more substitutions since they introduce more barbell exercises, but it's still feasible.

Here's a chart that'll help you make the right choices:

Instead of the . . .	Do the . . .
Machine Chest Press	Push-up, Dumbbell Bench Press, or Chest Dip
Trap-Bar Deadlift	Dumbbell Deadlift
Leg Curl	Dumbbell Romanian Deadlift
Lat Pulldown	One-Arm Dumbbell Row
Cable Triceps Pushdown	Dumbbell Triceps Overhead Press
Leg Press	Dumbbell Goblet Squat
Seated Cable Row	One-Arm Dumbbell Row
Cable Biceps Curl	Alternating Dumbbell Curl
Machine Shoulder Press	Seated Dumbbell Overhead Press

Q: I travel regularly. Can I do this program?

A: Yes, but it'll require some forethought. Booking hotels close to a gym helps greatly if you're following an intermediate or advanced strength training routine (hotel gyms are usually inadequate), and determining beforehand when you'll work out helps with scheduling. If you can't do either of those things, however, any training when traveling is better than none, so do whatever you can, even if it's just bodyweight exercises and cardio (applying everything you've learned in this book to make those workouts as productive as possible).

As for your diet when traveling, you have three options:

1. Make a meal plan with simple foods you can pick up at a local grocery store and prepare and store in your hotel room. Good choices include salad, rotisserie chicken, high-protein dairy, protein bars and powders, fruit, nuts, precut vegetables/crudités, hummus, and the like. A grocery delivery service like Instacart (www.instacart .com) or Amazon Prime Now (primenow.amazon.com) can be helpful here too.

2. Track your calories/macros with an app like MyFitnessPal if you have to do most of your eating on the go. Try to keep your calories and protein in the right range.

3. Eat according to your appetite and use what you know about the foods you like to eat enough protein and keep your calories in check.

If you travel a lot and still want to make good progress, options one and two are best. Option three works fine for the occasional trip, but not for frequent travel.

Q: I can't do a specific exercise in a workout. What should I do?

A: It depends on why you can't do the exercise.

If it's because you're not strong enough yet, substitute an easier exercise you can do. For instance, if you're following the women's intermediate strength training routine and struggling with the trap-bar deadlift, you can continue doing the dumbbell deadlift instead until you're strong enough to progress.

If you can't do an exercise because you don't have the right equipment, substitute a comparable exercise you *do* have the equipment for. Keep in mind, however, that some exercises don't have great substitutes. For instance, the dumbbell deadlift and goblet squat can't hold a candle to the barbell versions of the exercises, and even though the lat pulldown is similar to the pull-up and chin-up, the latter are much more difficult and thus not viable alternatives for people new to strength training.

To avoid substitution problems, try not to let a lack of proper equipment get in the way of your results. A simple home gym setup or a gym membership may seem expensive, but remember—that money is an investment in your health and wellness, not a frivolous expense.

If you can't do an exercise because of pain or physical limitation, swap it for a similar exercise you can do comfortably. Suppose you're following the men's advanced strength training routine, and you can't do the incline barbell bench press because of an old shoulder injury. In this case, you'd pick a comparable push exercise from either the advanced or intermediate routines (the beginner exercises will be too easy for you), such as the incline dumbbell bench press, which is easier on the shoulders.

Here are some commonly workable substitutions for when pain is the problem:

If You Can't Do the . . .	Do the . . .
Dumbbell Bench Press	Machine Chest Press
Incline Barbell Bench Press	Incline Dumbbell Bench Press
Barbell Bench Press	Dumbbell Bench Press
Barbell Deadlift	Trap-Bar Deadlift
Trap-Bar Deadlift	Dumbbell Deadlift
Seated Dumbbell Overhead Press	Machine Shoulder Press
Barbell Romanian Deadlift	Leg Curl
One-Arm Dumbbell Row	Seated Cable Row
Dumbbell Split Squat	Leg Press

Q: What should I do if I miss or have to skip a workout?

A: If you miss a workout or two in a week, you can either do them on other days of the week or skip them and carry on as if you'd done them, depending on your circumstances and preferences. For example, let's say your normal schedule looks like this:

Mon	Tue	Wed	Thu	Fri	Sat	Sun
Upper Body A	Lower Body A	Rest	Upper Body B	Cardio	Rest	Cardio

You miss your Lower Body A workout for one reason or another, and so you could do it the following day (Wednesday); or if you don't like doing three workouts in a row, you could do it Wednesday, rest on Thursday, and do your Upper Body B workout on Friday or Saturday.

If you can't make up for a missed workout or two by shuffling around your schedule, don't sweat it. The occasional skipped session won't make any measurable difference in your overall results, so just let it slide and carry on as you normally would.

What if you miss a week or two of training, though, or even a month or more because of vacation, work, the birth of a child, etc.? If you've only missed a week or two, you should be able to resume where you left off without issue because it takes at least three to four weeks of no training for most people to lose a noticeable amount of muscle or strength. If you've missed several weeks or more, however, you'll need to reduce your training weights when you get back in the gym, but I have good news: no matter how long it has been and how much progress you feel you've lost, you'll gain it all back quickly—much faster than it took to get there in the first place.

This is mostly because of a phenomenon known as *muscle memory*, which refers to how muscle fibers can regain their former size and strength quicker than the first time around. Scientists are still investigating how this works, but strength training appears to permanently alter the physiology of muscle cells in a way that primes them for rapid regrowth.

So, to restart your strength training after an extended break, reduce your previous training weights by . . .

- ✦ 20 percent if it has been one to two months since you last worked out
- ✦ 30 percent if it has been three to four months since you last worked out
- ✦ 50 percent if it has been five to six months since you last worked out

And before long, you'll have returned to form.

Q: What if I have to cut a workout short?

A: This isn't an issue if it happens occasionally, but try not to make a habit of it. If you're interrupting one or more workouts per week for a couple of weeks in a row (or a couple of weeks per month), you need to adjust your schedule or priorities or both. Also, if you do shorten a workout, don't try to make it up in your next one—just carry on like it never happened.

Q: What can I do to be less hungry while cutting?

A: My three favorite ways to feel fuller and cut hunger and cravings are:

1. Drink plenty of water.

   Research shows that increasing water intake (especially when added to meals) can be an effective way to increase fullness, fight off hunger, and stick to your diet. And remember: the National Academy of Medicine recommends a baseline intake of about ¾ of a gallon of water per day for adult men and women, with an additional 1 to 1.5 liters of water per hour of sweaty physical activity.

2. Get plenty of sleep.

   Undersleeping is a powerful way to sabotage your self-control, spike your hunger, and blunt the satisfaction you get from eating. A study conducted by scientists at the European Center for Taste Sciences found that people who slept four hours per night ate almost 600 calories more the next day *and* experienced more hunger before meals than people who slept eight hours per night. Other research shows that just a single night of sleep deprivation increases brain activity associated with hunger when people look at images of food.

Recall that sleep needs vary from individual to individual, but according to the National Sleep Foundation, adults need seven to nine hours of sleep per night to maintain sleep sufficiency.

3. Eat slowly and mindfully.

   Slow eating is exactly what it sounds like—eating your food gradually by taking smaller bites and deliberately chewing and savoring each. Mindful eating involves paying attention to your meal while you're eating (as opposed to your TV, computer, smartphone, etc.).

   Here are a few easy ways to eat slower and more mindfully:

   + Take at least fifteen to twenty minutes to finish your larger meals.
   + Chew each bite thoroughly and swallow before taking your next one.
   + Use smaller utensils to help you take smaller bites.
   + Put your utensils down between bites.
   + Focus on your food and conversation with others when eating, not on an electronic device.

Q: Why aren't there any core exercises in the program?

A: There are!

They're called: the squat, deadlift, seated dumbbell overhead press, bench press, chin-up, pull-up, one-arm dumbbell row, and others.

My point is, while there are no direct ab exercises in the program, like crunches, planks, and sit-ups, many of the exercises in it heavily train your abdominals, obliques, and other core muscles.

Q: I'm not getting very sore. Is that a problem?

A: I used to think perpetual muscle soreness was a price you had to pay to get bigger, something like a badge of honor. "Damn straight I have to walk down stairs backward! My legs will be *huge*!"

I assumed that a major reason we trained our muscles was to damage them, which resulted in soreness, and therefore considerable soreness meant considerable damage that would lead to considerable muscle growth, right? Not quite.

Research shows that muscle damage may contribute to growth, but it isn't a requirement. Workouts that produce large amounts of muscle soreness can generate little growth (downhill running and heavy eccentric training, for instance), and ones that produce very little soreness can cause significant growth. Further complicating matters is the fact that the amount of soreness you experience after a workout isn't a reliable indicator of the degree of muscle damage—a high or low amount of soreness doesn't always reflect a high or low amount of damage.

These phenomena aren't fully understood yet, but one study conducted by scientists at Concordia University found that at least some of the pain we're feeling in post-workout soreness stems from the connective tissue holding muscle fibers together, not from the actual fibers themselves. Therefore, what we think is muscle soreness is at least partially (if not mostly) connective tissue soreness.

So, the key takeaway is if you aren't too sore after your workouts, it doesn't mean you're doing anything wrong.

Q: Can I train muscles that are still sore from a previous workout?

A: Yes. Training sore muscles doesn't necessarily hinder recovery and prevent muscle growth. However, if you generally train too hard, you can experience chronic soreness and fatigue that compromises your performance and eventually your health. If you follow the *Muscle for Life* program as it's laid out, though, this shouldn't happen.

Q: I'm having trouble eating enough to gain weight. What should I do?

A: Here are three easy ways to get in enough calories to grow that don't involve double-fisting cheeseburgers and pizza every day:

1. Eat more calorie-dense foods.

   This is by far the easiest way to kick-start weight gain. When you're struggling to eat enough calories, eat plenty of foods higher in calories and lower in fiber and water (less filling) to help hit your daily calorie target. Some good options include:

   + White rice
   + Bread
   + Pasta
   + Dried fruit
   + Eggs
   + Fatty cuts of meat and seafood (steak, duck, salmon, etc.)
   + Oats
   + Breakfast cereal
   + Cheese, yogurt, milk, and other high-fat dairy products
   + Nuts and nut butters
   + Sauces like pesto, mole, aioli, chimichurri, teriyaki, and good ol'-fashioned gravy

2. Don't do too much cardio.

   Past a certain point, the more cardio you do, the harder it'll be to gain muscle and strength. Thus, try to do no more than a couple of hours of cardio per week when lean gaining, and stick with walking or cycling if you want to minimize the negative impact cardio can have on strength training.

3. Drink calories if necessary.

   Some people (skinny guys and gals, usually) need to eat an uncomfortably large number of calories every day to gain weight—so much that they struggle to do this with whole foods alone. Drinking calories can help tremendously. Milk, protein and meal replacement shakes, and no-sugar-added fruit juices are popular choices.

Q: How often should I change my workouts?

A: If you follow the routines that I provide in the back of the book, you don't need to make any changes to your workouts because the routines switch up exercises and rep ranges as you progress from one phase and difficulty level to the next.

That said, if you'd like to create your own workouts or routines to follow based on the information you've learned, I have three tips for you:

1. Try not to change your workout routine more than once every six to eight weeks. Remember that your primary goal in strength training is improving your whole-body strength, and if you change your workouts—and especially the exercises you're doing—too often, you'll progress slower, not faster.

2. Do your hardest exercises first in your workouts, followed by your

easier exercises. For example, if you want to do an upper-body workout that includes the barbell bench press and the one-arm dumbbell row, do the bench press first.

3. When swapping exercises in a workout, choose ones that target the same muscle groups and aren't significantly easier or harder to do. For instance, if you've just wrapped up eight weeks of training and want to replace the leg press in a lower-body workout, the dumbbell lunge would work well (because it's similar in difficulty) but the hamstring curl (much easier) or an upper-body exercise (different muscle group) wouldn't.

You may also plan on following the workouts I've created for you but wonder what to do if you've completed all three phases of a routine but don't yet qualify for the harder routine. Should you just upgrade anyway? No. Just restart with the first phase, and eventually you'll be eligible for the next routine.

Q: Should I exercise when I'm sick?

A: No. At least not intensely.

I understand the desire to train when sick, however. Once you've established a good workout habit, skipping days can be harder than going to the gym even when you're not feeling well. Force yourself to rest, though, because your normal workouts will only make things worse by depressing immune function.

That said, animal research has found that light exercise (twenty to thirty minutes of light running) while infected with the influenza virus can boost immunity and recovery. Similar effects have been seen in human studies as well. If you do any exercise while under the weather, then, make it twenty minutes or less of light cardio per day, like walking.

Q: Should I eat a meal before and after working out?

A: You can if you want to, but it won't make a big difference either way. Here's my general recommendation:

+ If you haven't eaten at least one portion of protein or carbs in the three to five hours preceding your workout, eat 20 to 40 grams of protein and carbs thirty to sixty minutes before your workout. If you have eaten at least a portion of protein and carbs in the couple of hours preceding a workout, you don't need to eat again before you train.

+ If you ate a meal one to two hours before a workout, you don't need to eat again immediately after you train (just wait until your next planned meal). If you didn't eat before, eat 20 to 40 grams of protein within thirty to sixty minutes of finishing your workout (and have carbs and fat as desired).

Q: What do people who achieve their fitness goals all have in common?

A: The men and women who lose the most fat and gain the most muscle and strength and then continue getting fitter over time usually aren't exceptionally disciplined, driven, or diehard. Out of all the positive habits and traits these people develop and embody, the factor most responsible for their success is *consistency*.

Invariably, they're just the ones who miss the fewest workouts and make the fewest dietary mistakes. They're far from perfect, too—just good enough most of the time—and that's why I'm so confident you'll succeed on the *Muscle for Life* program. The fact that you've made it to the end of this book tells me you have the will and wherewithal to win, and now you also have the way. Follow it, and I'll see you on the other side.

17

Epilogue

*To be yourself in a world that is constantly trying to make you
something else is the greatest accomplishment.*
—RALPH WALDO EMERSON

My goal is to help you reach *your* goals, and I know that if we work together as a team, we can and will succeed. And by "work together," I mean it—I want to connect with you, keep tabs on your progress, answer any questions or address any concerns you may have, and one day feature you as a success story on my website!

The best way to reach me is e-mail: mikem@legionsupplements.com. I get a lot of e-mails every day, so it may take a week or two for me to get back to you, but you *will* get a reply.

I also want to invite you to join my Facebook group, which is a community of thousands of positive, supportive, like-minded people who can answer your questions, cheer your victories, and soothe your setbacks. You can find it at www.muscleforlife.group, and all you have to do is visit that URL and click the "+ Join Group" button, and one of my team members will approve your application.

And speaking of social media, here's where you can find me on the major networks:

- ✦ Instagram: www.instagram.com/muscleforlifefitness
- ✦ Facebook: www.facebook.com/muscleforlifefitness
- ✦ YouTube: www.youtube.com/muscleforlifefitness
- ✦ Twitter: www.twitter.com/muscleforlife

If you plan on publicly announcing that you're starting *Muscle for Life*, definitely tag me and add the #MuscleForLife hashtag so other people on the program can find you and follow your journey.

Also, if you've enjoyed this book and are better off after reading it, please pass it on to someone you care about. Let them borrow your copy, or, better yet, get them their own as a gift and say, "I love and appreciate you and want to help you live your best life, so I got you this. Read it." My personal mission is to get this information into as many hands as possible, and I can't do that without your help. So please spread the word.

Thank you so much, and I hope to hear from you soon.

18

Free Bonus Material (Videos, Tools, and More!)

Giving up on our long-term goals for immediate gratification,
my friends, is procrastination.

—DAN ARIELY

Thank you for reading *Muscle for Life*. I hope you've found it insightful, inspiring, and practical, and I hope it helps you forever change your body and your life.

I want to make sure you receive as much value from this book as possible, so I've put together free resources to help you, including:

+ A savable, shareable, printable reference guide with all of this book's key takeaways, checklists, and action items.

+ Links to form demonstration videos for all *Muscle for Life* exercises.

+ An entire year's worth of *Muscle for Life* workouts neatly laid out and provided in several formats, including PDF, Excel, and Google Sheets. And if you'd prefer to use an app, check out my free workout app Stacked (www.getstackedapp.com), which comes with the *Muscle for Life* workouts.

- 20 *Muscle for Life* meal plans for losing fat and gaining muscle.
- A list of my favorite tools for getting and staying motivated and on track inside and outside of the gym.
- And more.

To get instant access to all of those free bonuses (plus a few additional surprise gifts), go here now:

→ www.muscleforlifebook.com/bonus

I also have a small favor to ask: Would you mind taking a minute to write a blurb online about this book? I check all my reviews and love getting honest feedback.

To leave me a quick review, you can go here:

→ www.muscleforlifebook.com/review

APPENDIX

MEAL PLANS FOR CUTTING

Meal	Food	Portion	Calories	Protein	Carbs	Fat
Cutting Meal Plan for a 140-Pound Woman (Moderate-Carb)						
Breakfast	Egg, whole	1	70	6	0	5
	2% cottage cheese	1	150	20	10	3
	Avocado	1	120	1	6	10
	Spinach	1	0	0	0	0
	Mushroom, chopped	1	30	2	6	0
	Sweet pepper, chopped	1	30	2	6	0
Total			400	31	28	18
Workout						
Post-workout Shake	Plain 2% yogurt	1	150	20	10	3
	Mango, frozen	1	60	1	15	0
	Blueberry, frozen	1	60	1	15	0
Total			270	22	40	3
Lunch	Skinless, boneless chicken breast	1	130	25	0	3
	Lettuce	1	0	0	0	0
	Carrot, chopped	½	15	1	3	0
	Tomato, chopped	½	15	1	3	0
	Balsamic vinaigrette	1	100	0	2	10
Total			260	27	8	13
Dinner	Tilapia, pan-seared	2	260	50	0	6
	Broccoli	1	30	2	6	0
	Zucchini	1	30	2	6	0
	Cauliflower	1	30	2	6	0
	Olive oil	1	120	0	0	14
Total			470	56	18	20
Daily Total			1,400	136	94	54
Daily Target			1,400	140	90	55

Cutting Meal Plan for a 160-Pound Woman (Moderate-Carb)						
Meal	**Food**	**Portion**	**Calories**	**Protein**	**Carbs**	**Fat**
Breakfast	Plain 2% Greek yogurt	2	300	40	20	6
	Peach	1	60	1	15	0
	Egg, whole	2	140	12	0	10
Total			500	53	35	16
Lunch	Shrimp	2	260	50	0	6
	Broccoli	3	90	6	18	0
	Olive oil	1	120	0	0	14
Total			470	56	18	20
Snack	Almond	2	160	6	6	14
Total			160	6	6	14
Workout						
Dinner	Tilapia, cooked	1	130	25	0	3
	Green bean	3	90	6	18	0
	Light ice cream (such as Halo Top)	1⅓ cup	180	12	42	4
Total			400	43	60	7
Daily Total			1,530	158	119	57
Daily Target			1,600	160	120	55

\multicolumn{7}{l}{Cutting Meal Plan for a 200-Pound Woman (Low-Carb)}
Meal	**Food**	**Portion**	**Calories**	**Protein**	**Carbs**	**Fat**
Breakfast	Egg, whole	3	210	18	0	15
	Ham	1	130	25	0	3
	Tomato, chopped	1	30	2	6	0
	Spinach	1	0	0	0	0
	Mushroom, chopped	1	30	2	6	0
	Sweet pepper, chopped	1	30	2	6	0
	Total		430	49	18	18
Lunch	Skinless, boneless chicken breast	2	260	50	0	6
	Lettuce	2	0	0	0	0
	Arugula	1	0	0	0	0
	Carrot, chopped	½	15	1	3	0
	Cucumber, chopped	½	15	1	3	0
	Onion, chopped	½	15	1	3	0
	Sweet pepper, chopped	1	30	2	6	0
	Ranch dressing	2	200	0	4	20
	Total		535	55	19	26
\multicolumn{7}{c}{**Workout**}
Snack	2% cottage cheese	2	300	40	20	6
	Blueberry	1	60	1	15	0
	Total		360	41	35	6
Dinner	Salmon	2	400	40	0	24
	Brussels sprout	2	60	4	12	0
	Yellow squash	1	30	2	6	0
	Asparagus	1	30	2	6	0
	Eggplant	1	30	2	6	0
	Olive oil	1	120	0	0	14
	Total		670	50	30	38
\multicolumn{3}{c}{**Daily Total**}	1,995	195	102	88
\multicolumn{3}{c}{**Daily Target**}	2,000	200	100	90

Cutting Meal Plan for a 160-Pound Man (Moderate-Carb)						
Meal	**Food**	**Portion**	**Calories**	**Protein**	**Carbs**	**Fat**
Breakfast	Egg, whole	2	140	12	0	10
	Egg white	1	130	27	2	0
	Banana	2	120	2	30	0
	Butternut squash	3	90	6	18	0
	Apple	1	120	0	0	14
Total			600	47	50	24
Workout						
Lunch	Tilapia, pan-seared	2	260	50	0	6
	Zucchini	2	60	4	12	0
	Carrot	2	60	4	12	0
	Olive oil	1	120	0	0	14
Total			500	58	24	20
Dinner	Skinless, boneless chicken breast	2	260	50	0	6
	Broccoli	3	90	6	18	0
	Butter	1	120	0	0	14
	Light ice cream (such as Halo Top)	$2/3$ cup	90	60	21	2
Total			560	62	39	22
Daily Total			1,630	165	107	66
Daily Target			1,600	160	100	60

Cutting Meal Plan for a 200-Pound Man (Moderate-Carb)						
Meal	Food	Portion	Calories	Protein	Carbs	Fat
Breakfast	Ham	1	130	25	0	3
	2% cottage cheese	1	150	20	10	3
	Cooked oats	1	120	3	25	1
	Apple	1	60	1	15	0
Total			460	49	50	7
Lunch	Skinless, boneless chicken breast	2	260	50	0	6
	Asparagus	2	60	4	12	0
	Cauliflower	2	60	4	12	0
	Olive oil	1	120	0	0	14
Total			500	58	24	20
Snack	Plain 2% Greek yogurt	2	300	40	20	6
Total			300	40	20	6
Workout						
Dinner	Ribeye steak, trimmed of visible fat	2	400	40	0	24
	Green bean	3	90	6	18	0
	Yellow squash	2	60	4	12	0
	Snickers bar	1.5 ounces	215	3	28	11
Total			765	53	58	35
Daily Total			2,025	200	152	68
Daily Target			2,000	200	150	65

Cutting Meal Plan for a 240-Pound Man (Moderate-Carb)						
Meal	**Food**	**Portion**	**Calories**	**Protein**	**Carbs**	**Fat**
Breakfast	Plain full-fat Greek yogurt	2	440	40	20	20
	Banana	2	120	2	30	0
	Almond	2	160	6	6	14
	Total		720	48	56	34
Lunch	Turkey breast	2	260	50	0	6
	Cheddar cheese	2	240	12	2	20
	Lettuce	½	0	0	0	0
	Tomato	½	15	1	3	0
	Sauerkraut	½	15	1	3	0
	Broccoli	2	60	4	12	0
	Kraft light mayonnaise (or similar)	2	70	0	4	6
	Dijon mustard	3 tsp	15	1	2	0
	Whole-grain bread (such as Dave's Killer Bread)	1 slice	110	5	22	2
	Total		785	74	48	34
Snack	Whey protein powder	2	200	40	4	4
	Apple	2	120	2	30	0
	Total		320	42	34	4
Workout						
Dinner	Pork chop, trimmed of visible fat	3	390	75	0	9
	Collard greens	2	60	4	12	0
	Butter	1	120	0	0	14
	Total		570	79	12	23
	Daily Total		2,395	243	150	95
	Daily Target		2,400	240	150	95

MEAL PLANS FOR LEAN GAINING

Lean Gaining Meal Plan for a 100-Pound Woman (Moderate-Carb)						
Meal	Food	Portion	Calories	Protein	Carbs	Fat
Breakfast	Egg, whole	1	70	6	0	5
	Spinach	1	0	0	0	0
	Mushroom, chopped	1	30	2	6	0
	Sweet pepper, chopped	1	30	2	6	0
	Cooked oats	1	120	3	25	1
	Avocado	1	120	1	6	10
Total			370	14	43	16
Workout						
Post-workout Shake	Plain 2% yogurt	1	150	20	10	3
	Whey protein powder	1	100	20	2	2
	Mango, frozen	1	60	1	15	0
	Blueberry, frozen	2	120	2	30	0
Total			430	43	57	5
Lunch	Skinless, boneless chicken breast	1	130	25	0	3
	Lettuce	1	0	0	0	0
	Carrot, chopped	½	15	1	3	0
	Tomato, chopped	½	15	1	3	0
	Sweet pepper, chopped	1	30	2	6	0
	Balsamic vinaigrette	2	200	0	4	20
Total			390	29	16	23
Dinner	Tilapia, pan-seared	1	130	25	0	3
	Broccoli	2	60	4	12	0
	Zucchini	2	60	4	12	0
	Cauliflower	2	60	4	12	0
	Brown rice	1	120	3	25	1
	Olive oil	1	120	0	0	14
Total			550	40	61	18
Daily Total			1,740	126	177	62
Daily Target			1,700	130	170	55

Lean Gaining Meal Plan for a 120-Pound Woman (Moderate-Carb)						
Meal	Food	Portion	Calories	Protein	Carbs	Fat
Breakfast	Plain 2% Greek yogurt	2	300	40	20	6
	Banana	2	120	2	30	0
	Kiwi	1	60	1	15	0
	Peach	1	60	1	15	0
	Almond	1	80	3	3	7
Total			620	47	83	13
Lunch	Shrimp	2	260	50	0	6
	Broccoli	3	90	6	18	0
	Brown rice	2	240	6	50	2
	Olive oil	1	120	0	0	14
Total			710	62	68	22
Workout						
Dinner	Adobo Sirloin (page 138)	1	237	39	2	7
	Green bean	2	60	4	12	0
	Sweet potato	1	120	3	25	1
	Butter	1	120	0	0	14
	Dark chocolate, 85% cocoa	1 ounce	170	4	11	14
Total			707	50	50	36
Daily Total			2,037	159	201	71
Daily Target			2,040	155	205	70

Lean Gaining Meal Plan for a 140-Pound Woman (Moderate-Carb)						
Meal	**Food**	**Portion**	**Calories**	**Protein**	**Carbs**	**Fat**
Breakfast	Egg, whole	3	210	18	0	15
	Ham	1	130	25	0	3
	Tomato, chopped	1	30	2	6	0
	Spinach	1	0	0	0	0
	Mushroom, chopped	1	30	2	6	0
	Sweet pepper, chopped	1	30	2	6	0
	Whole-grain bread	2 slices	220	10	44	4
	Total		650	59	62	22
Lunch	Skinless, boneless chicken breast	1	130	25	0	3
	Lettuce	2	0	0	0	0
	Arugula	1	0	0	0	0
	Carrot, chopped	1	30	2	6	0
	Cucumber, chopped	½	15	1	3	0
	Onion, chopped	½	15	1	3	0
	Sweet pepper, chopped	1	30	2	6	0
	Chickpea	1	120	3	25	1
	Ranch dressing	2	200	0	4	20
	Total		540	34	47	24
Snack	Plain 2% Greek yogurt	2	300	40	20	6
	Banana	4	240	4	60	0
	Total		540	44	80	6
Workout						
Dinner	Salmon, farm-raised	2	400	40	0	24
	Brussels sprout	1	30	2	6	0
	Yellow squash	1	30	2	6	0
	Asparagus	1	30	2	6	0
	Eggplant	1	30	2	6	0
	White potato	1	120	3	25	1
	Total		640	51	49	25
	Daily Total		2,370	188	238	77
	Daily Target		2,380	180	240	80

Appendix

Lean Gaining Meal Plan for a 140-Pound Man (Moderate-Carb)						
Meal	Food	Portion	Calories	Protein	Carbs	Fat
Breakfast	Egg, whole	3	210	18	0	15
	Egg white	1	130	27	2	0
	Banana	2	120	2	30	0
	Butternut squash	3	90	6	18	0
	Butter	1	120	0	0	14
Total			670	53	50	29
Workout						
Snack	Whey protein powder	1	100	20	2	2
	Apple	2	120	2	30	0
Total			220	22	32	2
Lunch	Raspberry Walnut Chicken Salad Sandwich (page 136)	1	374	29	33	14
	Brown rice	1	120	3	25	0
Total			494	32	58	14
Dinner	Skinless, boneless chicken breast	2	260	50	0	6
	Broccoli	3	90	6	18	0
	Sweet potato	2	240	6	50	2
	Butter	1	120	0	0	14
	Ice cream	²/₃ cup	300	6	26	20
Total			1,010	68	94	42
Daily Total			2,394	175	234	87
Daily Target			2,380	180	240	80

Lean Gaining Meal Plan for a 160-Pound Man (Moderate-Carb)						
Meal	Food	Portion	Calories	Protein	Carbs	Fat
Breakfast	2% cottage cheese	2	300	40	20	6
	Cooked oats	2	240	6	50	2
	Apple	2	120	2	30	0
	Blueberry	1	60	1	15	0
	Almond	1	80	3	3	7
Total			800	52	118	15
Lunch	Skinless, boneless chicken breast	2	260	50	0	6
	Asparagus	2	60	4	12	0
	Cauliflower	2	60	4	12	0
	Olive oil	1	120	0	0	14
Total			500	58	24	20
Snack	Plain full-fat Greek yogurt	2	440	40	20	20
	Banana	2	120	2	30	0
Total			560	42	50	20
Workout						
Dinner	Rib eye steak, trimmed of visible fat	2	400	40	0	24
	Green bean	3	90	6	18	0
	Yellow squash	2	60	4	12	0
	White rice	1	120	3	25	1
	Snickers bar	1.5 ounces	215	3	28	11
Total			885	56	83	36
Daily Total			2,745	208	275	91
Daily Target			2,720	205	270	90

| \multicolumn{7}{c}{**Lean Gaining Meal Plan for a 180-Pound Man (Moderate-Carb)**} |
Meal	Food	Portion	Calories	Protein	Carbs	Fat
Breakfast	Creamy Blueberry-Banana Smoothie (page 134)	2	446	42	48	20
	Almond	2	160	6	6	14
	Cooked oats	2	240	6	50	2
Total			846	54	104	36
Lunch	Turkey breast	2	260	50	0	6
	Cheddar cheese	2	240	12	2	20
	Lettuce	½	0	0	0	0
	Tomato, sliced	½	15	1	3	0
	Sauerkraut	½	15	1	3	0
	Broccoli	2	60	4	12	0
	Kraft light mayonnaise (or similar)	2	70	0	4	6
	Dijon mustard	3 tsp	15	1	2	0
	Whole-grain bread (such as Dave's Killer Bread)	2 slices	220	10	44	4
Total			895	79	70	36
Snack	Plain 2% Greek yogurt	2	300	40	20	6
	Apple	2	120	2	30	0
	Hummus	½ cup	200	10	17	11
Total			620	52	67	17
\multicolumn{7}{c}{**Workout**}
Dinner	Lasagna with Cottage Cheese and Butternut Squash (page 139)	1	419	38	48	8
	Zucchini	2	60	4	12	0
	Dark chocolate, 85% cocoa	1 ounce	170	4	11	14
Total			649	46	71	22
Daily Total			3,010	231	312	111
Daily Target			3,060	230	305	100

WOMEN'S STRENGTH TRAINING WORKOUTS

Beginner Routine
Phase One

Workout 1 Lower Body A	Workout 2 Upper Body A	Workout 3 Lower Body B
Bodyweight Squat 3 hard sets of 12–15 reps	Push-up 3 hard sets of 12–15 reps	Dumbbell Deadlift 3 hard sets of 10–15 reps
Dumbbell Deadlift 3 hard sets of 12–15 reps	Lat Pulldown 3 hard sets of 12–15 reps	Bodyweight Lunge 3 hard sets of 12–15 reps
Bodyweight Split Squat 3 hard sets of 12–15 reps	Machine Chest Press 3 hard sets of 12–15 reps	Leg Press 3 hard sets of 12–15 reps
Triceps Dip 3 hard sets of 12–15 reps	Bodyweight Row 3 hard sets of 12–15 reps	Leg Curl 3 hard sets of 12–15 reps

Phase Two

Workout 1 Lower Body A	Workout 2 Upper Body A	Workout 3 Lower Body B
Bodyweight Lunge 3 hard sets of 12–15 reps	Push-up 3 hard sets of 12–15 reps	Dumbbell Deadlift 3 hard sets of 12–15 reps
Dumbbell Deadlift 3 hard sets of 12–15 reps	One-Arm Dumbbell Row 3 hard sets of 12–15 reps	Bodyweight Step-up 3 hard sets of 12–15 reps
Bodyweight Squat 3 hard sets of 12–15 reps	Machine Shoulder Press 3 hard sets of 12–15 reps	Leg Extension 3 hard sets of 12–15 reps
Triceps Dip 3 hard sets of 12–15 reps	Bodyweight Row 3 hard sets of 12–15 reps	Glute Bridge 3 hard sets of 12–15 reps

Phase Three

Workout 1 Lower Body A	Workout 2 Upper Body A	Workout 3 Lower Body B
Bodyweight Squat 3 hard sets of 12–15 reps	Push-up 3 hard sets of 12–15 reps	Dumbbell Deadlift 3 hard sets of 12–15 reps
Dumbbell Deadlift 3 hard sets of 12–15 reps	Lat Pulldown 3 hard sets of 12–15 reps	Bodyweight Lunge 3 hard sets of 12–15 reps
Bodyweight Split Squat 3 hard sets of 12–15 reps	Machine Chest Press 3 hard sets of 12–15 reps	Leg Press 3 hard sets of 12–15 reps
Triceps Dip 3 hard sets of 12–15 reps	Bodyweight Row 3 hard sets of 12–15 reps	Leg Curl 3 hard sets of 12–15 reps

Intermediate Routine
Phase One

Workout 1 Lower Body A	Workout 2 Upper Body A	Workout 3 Lower Body B
Trap-Bar Deadlift 3 hard sets of 10–12 reps	Dumbbell Bench Press 3 hard sets of 10–12 reps	Dumbbell Lunge 3 hard sets of 10–12 reps
Dumbbell Split Squat 3 hard sets of 10–12 reps	Lat Pulldown 3 hard sets of 10–12 reps	Dumbbell Romanian Deadlift 3 hard sets of 10–12 reps
Leg Curl 3 hard sets of 10–12 reps	Seated Dumbbell Overhead Press 3 hard sets of 10–12 reps	Leg Press 3 hard sets of 10–12 reps
Dumbbell Goblet Squat 3 hard sets of 10–12 reps	Seated Cable Row 3 hard sets of 10–12 reps	Leg Curl 3 hard sets of 10–12 reps

Phase Two

Workout 1 Lower Body A	Workout 2 Upper Body A	Workout 3 Lower Body B
Trap-Bar Deadlift 3 hard sets of 10–12 reps	Incline Dumbbell Bench Press 3 hard sets of 10–12 reps	Dumbbell Goblet Squat 3 hard sets of 10–12 reps
Dumbbell Lunge 3 hard sets of 10–12 reps	One-Arm Dumbbell Row 3 hard sets of 10–12 reps	Dumbbell Deadlift 3 hard sets of 10–12 reps
Dumbbell Romanian Deadlift 3 hard sets of 10–12 reps	Dumbbell Bench Press 3 hard sets of 10–12 reps	Leg Extension 3 hard sets of 10–12 reps
Dumbbell Goblet Squat 3 hard sets of 10–12 reps	Seated Cable Row 3 hard sets of 10–12 reps	Leg Curl 3 hard sets of 10–12 reps

Phase Three

Workout 1 Lower Body A	Workout 2 Upper Body A	Workout 3 Lower Body B
Trap-Bar Deadlift 3 hard sets of 10–12 reps	Seated Dumbbell Overhead Press 3 hard sets of 10–12 reps	Dumbbell Lunge 3 hard sets of 10–12 reps
Dumbbell Goblet Squat 3 hard sets of 10–12 reps	Seated Cable Row 3 hard sets of 10–12 reps	Dumbbell Romanian Deadlift 3 hard sets of 10–12 reps
Glute Bridge 3 hard sets of 10–12 reps	Incline Dumbbell Bench Press 3 hard sets of 10–12 reps	Leg Press 3 hard sets of 10–12 reps
Dumbbell Split Squat 3 hard sets of 10–12 reps	Lat Pulldown 3 hard sets of 10–12 reps	Leg Curl 3 hard sets of 10–12 reps

Advanced Routine
Phase One

Workout 1 Lower Body A	Workout 2 Upper Body A	Workout 3 Lower Body B
Barbell Back Squat 3 hard sets of 8–10 reps	Barbell Bench Press 3 hard sets of 8–10 reps	Dumbbell Lunge 3 hard sets of 8–10 reps
Barbell Deadlift 3 hard sets of 8–10 reps	Lat Pulldown 3 hard sets of 8–10 reps	Barbell Romanian Deadlift 3 hard sets of 8–10 reps
Leg Curl 3 hard sets of 8–10 reps	Incline Barbell Bench Press 3 hard sets of 8–10 reps	Leg Press 3 hard sets of 8–10 reps
Dumbbell Lunge 3 hard sets of 8–10 reps	One-Arm Dumbbell Row 3 hard sets of 8–10 reps	Chest Dip 3 hard sets of 8–10 reps

Phase Two

Workout 1 Lower Body A	Workout 2 Upper Body A	Workout 3 Lower Body B
Barbell Back Squat 3 hard sets of 8–10 reps	Barbell Bench Press 3 hard sets of 8–10 reps	Barbell Deadlift 3 hard sets of 8–10 reps
Barbell Romanian Deadlift 3 hard sets of 8–10 reps	Chin-up 3 hard sets of 8–10 reps	Dumbbell Lunge 3 hard sets of 8–10 reps
Leg Extension 3 hard sets of 8–10 reps	Chest Dip 3 hard sets of 8–10 reps	Incline Barbell Bench Press 3 hard sets of 8–10 reps
Leg Curl 3 hard sets of 8–10 reps	Seated Cable Row 3 hard sets of 8–10 reps	Leg Press 3 hard sets of 8–10 reps

Phase Three

Workout 1 Lower Body A	Workout 2 Upper Body A	Workout 3 Lower Body B
Barbell Back Squat 3 hard sets of 8–10 reps	Barbell Bench Press 3 hard sets of 8–10 reps	Dumbbell Lunge 3 hard sets of 8–10 reps
Barbell Deadlift 3 hard sets of 8–10 reps	Pull-up 3 hard sets of 8–10 reps	Barbell Romanian Deadlift 3 hard sets of 8–10 reps
Leg Curl 3 hard sets of 8–10 reps	Incline Barbell Bench Press 3 hard sets of 8–10 reps	Leg Press 3 hard sets of 8–10 reps
Dumbbell Lunge 3 hard sets of 8–10 reps	One-Arm Dumbbell Row 3 hard sets of 8–10 reps	Chest Dip 3 hard sets of 8–10 reps

MEN'S STRENGTH TRAINING WORKOUTS

Beginner Routine
Phase One

Workout 1 Upper Body A	Workout 2 Lower Body A	Workout 3 Upper Body B
Push-up 3 hard sets of 12–15 reps	Bodyweight Squat 3 hard sets of 12–15 reps	Machine Shoulder Press 3 hard sets of 12–15 reps
Lat Pulldown 3 hard sets of 12–15 reps	Dumbbell Deadlift 3 hard sets of 12–15 reps	Bodyweight Row 3 hard sets of 12–15 reps
Machine Chest Press 3 hard sets of 12–15 reps	Leg Press 3 hard sets of 12–15 reps	Machine Chest Press 3 hard sets of 12–15 reps
Bodyweight Row 3 hard sets of 12–15 reps	Leg Curl 3 hard sets of 12–15 reps	Cable Biceps Curl 3 hard sets of 12–15 reps

Phase Two

Workout 1 Upper Body A	Workout 2 Lower Body A	Workout 3 Upper Body B
Push-up 3 hard sets of 12–15 reps	Bodyweight Split Squat 3 hard sets of 12–15 reps	Machine Chest Press 3 hard sets of 12–15 reps
Lat Pulldown 3 hard sets of 12–15 reps	Dumbbell Deadlift 3 hard sets of 12–15 reps	Machine Row 3 hard sets of 12–15 reps
Machine Shoulder Press 3 hard sets of 12–15 reps	Leg Extension 3 hard sets of 12–15 reps	Push-up 3 hard sets of 12–15 reps
One-Arm Dumbbell Row 3 hard sets of 12–15 reps	Glute Bridge 3 hard sets of 12–15 reps	Alternating Dumbbell Curl 3 hard sets of 12–15 reps

Phase Three

Workout 1 Upper Body A	Workout 2 Lower Body A	Workout 3 Upper Body B
Push-up 3 hard sets of 12–15 reps	Bodyweight Squat 3 hard sets of 12–15 reps	Machine Shoulder Press 3 hard sets of 12–15 reps
Lat Pulldown 3 hard sets of 12–15 reps	Dumbbell Deadlift 3 hard sets of 12–15 reps	Bodyweight Row 3 hard sets of 12–15 reps
Machine Chest Press 3 hard sets of 12–15 reps	Bodyweight Lunge 3 hard sets of 12–15 reps	Machine Chest Press 3 hard sets of 12–15 reps
Bodyweight Row 3 hard sets of 12–15 reps	Leg Curl 3 hard sets of 12–15 reps	Triceps Dip 3 hard sets of 12–15 reps

Intermediate Routine
Phase One

Workout 1 Upper Body A	Workout 2 Lower Body A	Workout 3 Upper Body B
Dumbbell Bench Press 3 hard sets of 10–12 reps	Trap-Bar Deadlift 3 hard sets of 10–12 reps	Seated Dumbbell Overhead Press 3 hard sets of 10–12 reps
Lat Pulldown 3 hard sets of 10–12 reps	Dumbbell Goblet Squat 3 hard sets of 10–12 reps	Seated Cable Row 3 hard sets of 10–12 reps
Machine Chest Press 3 hard sets of 10–12 reps	Leg Curl 3 hard sets of 10–12 reps	Machine Chest Press 3 hard sets of 10–12 reps
Seated Cable Row 3 hard sets of 10–12 reps	Dumbbell Split Squat 3 hard sets of 10–12 reps	Alternating Dumbbell Curl 3 hard sets of 10–12 reps

Phase Two

Workout 1 Upper Body A	Workout 2 Lower Body A	Workout 3 Upper Body B
Incline Dumbbell Bench Press 3 hard sets of 10–12 reps	Trap-Bar Deadlift 3 hard sets of 10–12 reps	Seated Dumbbell Overhead Press 3 hard sets of 10–12 reps
Lat Pulldown 3 hard sets of 10–12 reps	Dumbbell Lunge 3 hard sets of 10–12 reps	One-Arm Dumbbell Row 3 hard sets of 10–12 reps
Machine Chest Press 3 hard sets of 10–12 reps	Leg Curl 3 hard sets of 10–12 reps	Dumbbell Bench Press 3 hard sets of 10–12 reps
Machine Row 3 hard sets of 10–12 reps	Leg Press 3 hard sets of 10–12 reps	Cable Biceps Curl 3 hard sets of 10–12 reps

Phase Three

Workout 1 Upper Body A	Workout 2 Lower Body A	Workout 3 Upper Body B
Dumbbell Bench Press 3 hard sets of 10–12 reps	Trap-Bar Deadlift 3 hard sets of 10–12 reps	Seated Dumbbell Overhead Press 3 hard sets of 10–12 reps
Lat Pulldown 3 hard sets of 10–12 reps	Dumbbell Split Squat 3 hard sets of 10–12 reps	Seated Cable Row 3 hard sets of 10–12 reps
Machine Chest Press 3 hard sets of 10–12 reps	Leg Curl 3 hard sets of 10–12 reps	Machine Chest Press 3 hard sets of 10–12 reps
Seated Cable Row 3 hard sets of 10–12 reps	Dumbbell Lunge 3 hard sets of 10–12 reps	Alternating Dumbbell Curl 3 hard sets of 10–12 reps

Advanced Routine
Phase One

Workout 1 Upper Body A	Workout 2 Lower Body A	Workout 3 Upper Body B
Barbell Bench Press 3 hard sets of 8–10 reps	Barbell Back Squat 3 hard sets of 8–10 reps	Seated Dumbbell Overhead Press 3 hard sets of 8–10 reps
Lat Pulldown 3 hard sets of 8–10 reps	Barbell Deadlift 3 hard sets of 8–10 reps	One-Arm Dumbbell Row 3 hard sets of 8–10 reps
Dumbbell Bench Press 3 hard sets of 8–10 reps	Dumbbell Split Squat 3 hard sets of 8–10 reps	Dumbbell Bench Press 3 hard sets of 8–10 reps
One-Arm Dumbbell Row 3 hard sets of 8–10 reps	Leg Curl 3 hard sets of 8–10 reps	Alternating Dumbbell Curl 3 hard sets of 8–10 reps

Phase Two

Workout 1 Upper Body A	Workout 2 Lower Body A	Workout 3 Upper Body B
Incline Barbell Bench Press 3 hard sets of 8–10 reps	Barbell Back Squat 3 hard sets of 8–10 reps	Seated Dumbbell Overhead Press 3 hard sets of 8–10 reps
Chin-up 3 hard sets of 8–10 reps	Barbell Deadlift 3 hard sets of 8–10 reps	Seated Cable Row 3 hard sets of 8–10 reps
Chest Dip 3 hard sets of 8–10 reps	Dumbbell Lunge 3 hard sets of 8–10 reps	Dumbbell Bench Press 3 hard sets of 8–10 reps
Seated Cable Row 3 hard sets of 8–10 reps	Dumbbell Romanian Deadlift 3 hard sets of 8–10 reps	Dumbbell Triceps Overhead Press 3 hard sets of 8–10 reps

Phase Three

Workout 1 Upper Body A	Workout 2 Lower Body A	Workout 3 Upper Body B
Barbell Bench Press 3 hard sets of 8–10 reps	Barbell Back Squat 3 hard sets of 8–10 reps	Seated Dumbbell Overhead Press 3 hard sets of 8–10 reps
Pull-up 3 hard sets of 8–10 reps	Barbell Deadlift 3 hard sets of 8–10 reps	One-Arm Dumbbell Row 3 hard sets of 8–10 reps
Incline Dumbbell Bench Press 3 hard sets of 8–10 reps	Leg Press 3 hard sets of 8–10 reps	Dumbbell Bench Press 3 hard sets of 8–10 reps
One-Arm Dumbbell Row 3 hard sets of 8–10 reps	Barbell Romanian Deadlift 3 hard sets of 8–10 reps	Cable Biceps Curl 3 hard sets of 8–10 reps

References

Chapter 2: The Promise

17 *More and more scientific research is showing:* Giuseppe Passarino, Francesco De Rango, and Alberto Montesanto, "Human Longevity: Genetics or Lifestyle? It Takes Two to Tango," *Immunity and Ageing* 13, no. 12 (April 2016), doi: 10.1186/s12979-016-0066-z.

18 *you lose about 1 percent of your muscle mass per year after age 30:* Walter R. Frontera et al., "Aging of Skeletal Muscle: A 12-Yr Longitudinal Study," *Journal of Applied Physiology (1985)* 88, no. 4 (2000): 1321–6, doi: 10.1152/jappl.2000.88.4.1321; Bret H. Goodpaster et al., "The Loss of Skeletal Muscle Strength, Mass, and Quality in Older Adults: The Health, Aging, and Body Composition Study," *Journals of Gerontology: Series A, Biological Sciences and Medical Sciences* 61, no. 10 (2006): 1059–64, doi: 10.1093/gerona/61.10.1059.

18 *you can not only prevent muscle loss in your forties:* Maren S. Fragala et al., "Resistance Training for Older Adults: Position Statement from the National Strength and Conditioning Association," *Journal of Strength and Conditioning Research* 33, no. 8 (Aug 2019): 2019–52, doi: 10.1519/JSC.0000000000003230.

18 *In a study conducted by scientists at the University of Oklahoma:* Chad M. Kerksick et al., "Early-Phase Adaptations to a Split-Body, Linear Periodization Resistance Training Program in College-Aged and Middle-Aged Men," *Journal of Strength and Conditioning Research* 23, no. 3 (2009): 962–71, doi: 10.1519/JSC.0b013e3181a00baf.

18 *seen in a study conducted by scientists at the University of Maryland:* F. Marty Ivey et al., "Effects of Age, Gender, and Myostatin Genotype on the Hypertrophic Response to Heavy Resistance Strength Training," *Journals of Gerontology: Series A, Biological Sciences and Medical Sciences* 55, no. 11 (2000): 641–48, doi: 10.1093/gerona/55.11.m641.

19 *In a study conducted at Brigham Young University:* Larry A. Tucker, "Physical Activity and Telomere Length in U.S. Men and Women: An NHANES Investigation," *Preventive Medicine* 100 (2017): 145–51, doi: 10.1016/j.ypmed.2017.04.027.

19 *A study conducted by scientists at the University of Giessen:* Petra Lührmann et al., "Longitudinal Changes in Energy Expenditure in an Elderly German Population: A 12-Year Follow-Up," *European Journal of Clinical Nutrition* 63, no. 8 (2009): 986–92, doi: 10.1038/ejcn.2009.1.

20 *As scientists at Hiroshima University observed in another study:* H. Shimokata and F. Kuzuya, "[Aging, basal metabolic rate, and nutrition]," *Nihon Ronen Igakkai Zasshi / Japanese Journal of Geriatrics* 30, no. 7 (1993): 572–6, doi: 10.3143/geriatrics.30.572.

21 *In a study conducted by scientists at Brigham and Women's Hospital:* Robert H. Demling and Leslie DeSanti, "Effect of a Hypocaloric Diet, Increased Protein Intake and Resistance Training on Lean Mass Gains and Fat Mass Loss in Overweight Police Officers," *Annals of Nutrition and Metabolism* 44, no. 1 (2000): 21–9, doi: 10.1159/000012817.

21 *In an extensive five-year study:* Patricia A. Brill et al., "Muscular Strength and Physical Function," *Medicine and Science in Sports and Exercise* 32, no. 2 (2000): 412–16, doi: 10.1097/00005768-200002000-00023.

22 *this greatly reduces the risk of fracture:* A. Menkes et al., "Strength Training Increases Regional Bone Mineral Density and Bone Remodeling in Middle-Aged and Older Men," *Journal of Applied Physiology (1985)* 74, no. 5 (1993): 2478–84, doi: 10.1152/jappl.1993.74.5.2478.

22 *Heart health is an essential aspect of longevity:* George A. Kelley and Kristi Sharpe Kelley, "Progressive Resistance Exercise and Resting Blood Pressure: A Meta-analysis of Randomized Controlled Trials," *Hypertension* 35, no. 3 (2000): 838–43, doi: 10.1161/01.hyp.35.3.838; Steven Mann, Christopher Beedie, and Alfonso Jimenez, "Differential Effects of Aerobic Exercise, Resistance Training and Combined Exercise Modalities on Cholesterol and the Lipid Profile: Review, Synthesis, and Recommendations," *Sports Medicine* 44, no. 2 (2014): 211–21, doi: 10.1007/s40279-013-0110-5; Salameh Bweir et al., "Resistance Exercise Training Lowers HbA1c More than Aerobic Training in Adults with Type 2 Diabetes," *Diabetology and Metabolic Syndrome* 1, no. 27 (December 2009), doi: 10.1186/1758-5996-1-27.

22 *strength training combats it by reducing blood sugar levels:* Bweir et al., "Resistance Exercise Training Lowers HbA1c."

22 *strength training is as effective:* Barbara Strasser, Uwe Siebert, and Wolfgang Schobersberger, "Resistance Training in the Treatment of the Metabolic Syndrome: A Systematic Review and Meta-analysis of the Effect of Resistance Training on Metabolic Clustering in Patients with Abnormal Glucose Metabolism," *Sports Medicine* 40, no. 5 (2010): 397–415, doi: 10.2165/11531380-000000000-00000; Casey Irvine and Nicholas F. Taylor, "Progressive Resistance Exercise Improves Glycaemic Control in People with Type 2 Diabetes Mellitus: A Systematic Review," *Australian Journal of Physiotherapy* 55, no. 4 (2009): 237–46, doi: 10.1016/s0004-9514(09)70003-0; Neil J. Snowling and Will G. Hopkins, "Effects of Different Modes of Exercise Training on Glucose Control and Risk Factors for Complications in Type 2 Diabetic Patients: A Meta-analysis," *Diabetes Care* 29, no. 11 (2006): 2518–27, doi: 10.2337/dc06-1317.

22 *In a study conducted at the University of British Columbia:* Teresa Liu-Ambrose et al., "Resistance Training and Executive Functions: A 12-Month Randomized

Controlled Trial," *Archives of Internal Medicine* 170, no. 2 (2010): 170–8, doi: 10.1001/archinternmed.2009.494.

22 *researchers analyzed these scans:* John R. Best et al., "Long-Term Effects of Resistance Exercise Training on Cognition and Brain Volume in Older Women: Results from a Randomized Controlled Trial," *Journal of the International Neuropsychological Society* 21, no. 10 (2015): 745–56, doi: 10.1017/S1355617715000673.

24 *doing both reduces blood pressure the most:* Linda S. Pescatello and Jonna M. Kulikowich, "The After Effects of Dynamic Exercise on Ambulatory Blood Pressure," *Medicine and Science in Sports and Exercise* 33, no. 11 (2001): 1855–61, doi: 10.1097/00005768-200111000-00009; Véronique A. Cornelissen and Robert H. Fagard, "Effects of Endurance Training on Blood Pressure, Blood Pressure–Regulating Mechanisms, and Cardiovascular Risk Factors," *Hypertension* 46, no. 4 (2005): 667–75, doi: 10.1161/01.HYP.0000184225.05629.51; Vitor O. Carvalho et al., "Effect of Exercise Training on 24-Hour Ambulatory Blood Pressure Monitoring in Heart Failure Patients," *Congestive Heart Failure* 15, no. 4 (2009): 176–80, doi: 10.1111/j.1751-7133.2009.00093.x; Mireille Marceau et al., "Effects of Different Training Intensities on 24-Hour Blood Pressure in Hypertensive Subjects," *Circulation* 88, no. 6 (1993): 2803–11, doi: 10.1161/01.cir.88.6.2803.

24 *helps keep your arteries flexible and responsive to changes in blood flow:* Ammar W. Ashor et al., "Effects of Exercise Modalities on Arterial Stiffness and Wave Reflection: A Systematic Review and Meta-analysis of Randomized Controlled Trials," *PLoS One* 9, no. 10 e110034 (October 2014), doi: 10.1371/journal.pone.0110034.

24 *people who do the most cardio have the supplest arteries:* Giacomo Pucci, Francesca Battista, and Giuseppe Schillaci, "Aerobic Physical Exercise and Arterial

De-stiffening: A Recipe for Vascular Rejuvenation," *Hypertension Research* 35, no. 10 (2012): 964–6, doi: 10.1038/hr.2012.107; Hirofumi Tanaka, "Anti-aging Effects of Aerobic Exercise on Systemic Arteries," *Hypertension* 74, no. 2 (2019): 237–243, doi: 10.1161/hypertensionaha.119.13179.

24 *cardio can significantly increase capillary density:* Matthew Cocks et al., "Effect of Resistance Training on Microvascular Density and eNOS Content in Skeletal Muscle of Sedentary Men," *Microcirculation* 21, no. 8 (2014): 738–46, doi: 10.1111/micc.12155; Matthew Cocks et al., "Sprint Interval and Endurance Training Are Equally Effective in Increasing Muscle Microvascular Density and eNOS Content in Sedentary Males," *Journal of Physiology* 591, no. 3 (2013): 641–56, doi: 10.1113/jphysiol.2012.239566.

24 *Cardio also burns substantially more calories:* Joseph E. Donnelly et al., "Aerobic Exercise Alone Results in Clinically Significant Weight Loss for Men and Women: Midwest Exercise Trial 2," *Obesity* 21, no. 3 (2013): E219–28, doi: 10.1002/oby.20145; Dale A. Schoeller, Kathyjo Shay, and Robert F. Kushner, "How Much Physical Activity Is Needed to Minimize Weight Gain in Previously Obese Women?," *American Journal of Clinical Nutrition* 66, no. 3 (1997): 551–6, doi: 10.1093/ajcn/66.3.551.

25 *those who ate the most protein lost 40 percent less muscle:* Denise K. Houston et al., "Dietary Protein Intake Is Associated with Lean Mass Change in Older, Community-Dwelling Adults: The Health, Aging, and Body Composition (Health ABC) Study," *American Journal of Clinical Nutrition* 87, no. 1 (2008): 150–5, doi: 10.1093/ajcn/87.1.150.

25 *notably less likely to become physically impaired:* Nuno Mendonça et al., "Protein Intake and Disability Trajectories in Very Old Adults: The Newcastle 85+ Study," *Journal of the American Geriatrics Society* 67, no. 1 (2019): 50–56, doi: 10.1111/jgs.15592; Adela Hruby et al., "Protein Intake and Functional Integ-

rity in Aging: The Framingham Heart Study Offspring," *Journals of Gerontology: Series A, Biological Sciences and Medical Sciences* 75, no. 1 (2020): 123–130, doi: 10.1093/gerona/gly201.

25 *An extraordinary amount of evidence:* Simin Liu et al., "Fruit and Vegetable Intake and Risk of Cardiovascular Disease: The Women's Health Study," *American Journal of Clinical Nutrition* 72, no. 4 (2000): 922–8, doi: 10.1093/ajcn/72.4.922; Gladys Block, Blossom Patterson, and Amy Subar, "Fruit, Vegetables, and Cancer Prevention: A Review of the Epidemiological Evidence," *Nutrition and Cancer* 18, no. 1 (1992): 1–29, doi: 10.1080/01635589209514201; Jian Zhan et al., "Fruit and Vegetable Consumption and Risk of Cardiovascular Disease: A Meta-analysis of Prospective Cohort Studies," *Critical Reviews in Food Science and Nutrition* 57, no. 8 (2017): 1650–1663, doi: 10.1080/10408398.2015.1008980.

25 *A team of scientists from around the world conducted a study:* Ashkan Afshin et al., "Health Effects of Dietary Risks in 195 Countries, 1990–2017: A Systematic Analysis for the Global Burden of Disease Study 2017," *Lancet* 393, no. 10184 (2019): 1958–1972, doi: 10.1016/S0140-6736(19)30041-8.

25 *a third of adults over the age of 65 meet the bare minimum requirements:* Adam Drewnowski and J. M. Shultz, "Impact of Aging on Eating Behaviors, Food Choices, Nutrition, and Health Status," *Journal of Nutrition, Health and Aging* 5, no. 2 (2001): 75–9, https://pmid.us/11426286; M. K. Serdula et al., "Fruit and Vegetable Intake among Adults in 16 States: Results of a Brief Telephone Survey," *American Journal of Public Health* 85, no. 2 (1995): 236–9, doi: 10.2105/ajph.85.2.236; Susan M. Krebs-Smith et al., "US Adults' Fruit and Vegetable Intakes, 1989 to 1991: A Revised Baseline for the Healthy People 2000 Objective," *American Journal of Public Health* 85, no. 12 (1995): 1623–9, doi: 10.2105/ajph.85.12.1623.

26 *which aren't necessary for life but are still healthful:* Hongwei Si and Dongmin

Liu, "Dietary Antiaging Phytochemicals and Mechanisms Associated with Prolonged Survival," *Journal of Nutritional Biochemistry* 25, no. 6 (2014): 581–91, doi: 10.1016/j.jnutbio.2014.02.001.

26 *fantastic for controlling calorie intake and avoiding chronic hunger or cravings:* Monica Nour et al., "The Relationship between Vegetable Intake and Weight Outcomes: A Systematic Review of Cohort Studies," *Nutrients* 10, no. 11 (November 2018): 1626, doi: 10.3390/nu10111626.

26 *Studies have shown repeatedly:* Nour et al., "The Relationship between Vegetable Intake and Weight Outcomes"; Stephan J. Guyenet, "Impact of Whole, Fresh Fruit Consumption on Energy Intake and Adiposity: A Systematic Review," *Frontiers in Nutrition* 6, no. 66 (May 2019), doi: 10.3389/fnut.2019.00066.

26 *how full we feel after a meal is affected more by volume:* Barbara J. Rolls, Adam Drewnowski, and Jenny H. Ledikwe, "Changing the Energy Density of the Diet as a Strategy for Weight Management," *Journal of the American Dietetic Association* 105, no. 5 Suppl 1 (2005): S98–103, doi: 10.1016/j.jada.2005.02.033.

27 *It improves fat loss, muscle growth, immunity, telomere length, and cognition:* Arlet V. Nedeltcheva et al., "Insufficient Sleep Undermines Dietary Efforts to Reduce Adiposity," *Annals of Internal Medicine* 153, no. 7 (2010): 435–41, doi: 10.7326/0003-4819-153-7-201010050-00006; Murilo Dattilo et al., "Sleep and Muscle Recovery: Endocrinological and Molecular Basis for a New and Promising Hypothesis," *Medical Hypotheses* 77, no. 2 (2011): 220–2, doi: 10.1016/j.mehy.2011.04.017; Sheldon Cohen et al., "Sleep Habits and Susceptibility to the Common Cold," *Archives of Internal Medicine* 169, no. 1 (2009): 62–7, doi: 10.1001/archinternmed.2008.505; Marta Jackowska et al., "Short Sleep Duration Is Associated with Shorter Telomere Length in Healthy Men: Findings from the Whitehall II Cohort Study," *PloS One* 7, no. 10 (2012): e47292, doi: 10.1371/journal.pone.0047292; Paula Alhola and Päivi Polo-Kantola, "Sleep Deprivation: Impact on Cognitive Performance,"

Neuropsychiatric Disease and Treatment 3, no. 5 (2007): 553–67, https://pmid
.us/19300585; Tina Sundelin et al., "Negative Effects of Restricted Sleep on
Facial Appearance and Social Appeal," *Royal Society Open Science* 4, no. 5 (May
2017): 160918, doi: 10.1098/rsos.160918.

27 *increases your risk of just about every disease:* Guglielmo Beccuti and Silvana Pan-
nain, "Sleep and Obesity," *Current Opinion in Clinical Nutrition and Metabolic
Care* 14, no. 4 (2011): 402–12, doi: 10.1097/MCO.0b013e3283479109;
Christopher B. Cooper et al., "Sleep Deprivation and Obesity in Adults:
A Brief Narrative Review," *BMJ Open Sport and Exercise Medicine* 4, no. 1
(October 2018): e000392, doi: 10.1136/bmjsem-2018-000392; Kristen
L. Knutson and Eve Van Cauter, "Associations between Sleep Loss and In-
creased Risk of Obesity and Diabetes," *Annals of the New York Academy of
Sciences* 1129 (2008): 287–304, doi: 10.1196/annals.1417.033; Adam P.
Spira et al., "Impact of Sleep on the Risk of Cognitive Decline and Demen-
tia," *Current Opinion in Psychiatry* 27, no. 6 (2014): 478–83, doi: 10.1097
/YCO.0000000000000106; Janet M. Mullington et al., "Cardiovascular, Inflam-
matory, and Metabolic Consequences of Sleep Deprivation," *Progress in Cardiovascular Diseases* 51, no. 4 (2009): 294–302, doi: 10.1016/j.pcad.2008.10.003;
Yuheng Chen et al., "Sleep Duration and the Risk of Cancer: A Systematic Review and Meta-analysis Including Dose-Response Relationship," *BMC Cancer*
18, no. 1 (November 2018): 1149, doi: 10.1186/s12885-018-5025-y; Aric A.
Prather et al., "Behaviorally Assessed Sleep and Susceptibility to the Common
Cold," *Sleep* 38, no. 9 (September 2015): 1353–9, doi: 10.5665/sleep.4968.

27 *most of us need 7 to 9 hours of sleep:* Michael A. Grandner, "Sleep Duration across
the Lifespan: Implications for Health," *Sleep Medicine Reviews* 16, no. 3 (2012):
199–201, doi: 10.1016/j.smrv.2012.02.001.

27 *While there is a tiny fraction of the population:* Amita Sehgal and Emmanuel

Mignot, "Genetics of Sleep and Sleep Disorders," *Cell* 146, no. 2 (2011): 194–207, doi: 10.1016/j.cell.2011.07.004.

28 *proven to enhance muscle and strength gain:* Robert Cooper et al., "Creatine Supplementation with Specific View to Exercise/Sports Performance: An Update," *Journal of the International Society of Sports Nutrition* 9, no. 1 (July 2012): 33, doi: 10.1186/1550-2783-9-33.

28 *may also improve cognition in older people:* Terry McMorris et al., "Creatine Supplementation and Cognitive Performance in Elderly Individuals," *Neuropsychology, Development, and Cognition: Section B, Aging, Neuropsychology, and Cognition* 14, no. 5 (2007): 517–28, doi: 10.1080/13825580600788100.

28 *most people don't get enough of these nutrients:* P. M. Kris-Etherton et al., "Polyunsaturated Fatty Acids in the Food Chain in the United States," *American Journal of Clinical Nutrition* 71, no. 1 Suppl (2000): 179S–88S, doi: 10.1093/ajcn/71.1.179S; Alessio Molfino et al., "The Role for Dietary Omega-3 Fatty Acids Supplementation in Older Adults," *Nutrients* 6, no. 10 (October 2014): 4058–73, doi: 10.3390/nu6104058; Charles Couet et al., "Effect of Dietary Fish Oil on Body Fat Mass and Basal Fat Oxidation in Healthy Adults," *International Journal of Obesity and Related Metabolic Disorders* 21, no. 8 (1997): 637–43, doi: 10.1038/sj.ijo.0800451; Gordon I. Smith et al., "Omega-3 Polyunsaturated Fatty Acids Augment the Muscle Protein Anabolic Response to Hyperinsulinaemia-Hyperaminoacidaemia in Healthy Young and Middle-Aged Men and Women," *Clinical Science* 121, no. 6 (2011): 267–78, doi: 10.1042/CS20100597.

Chapter 5: How to Master the "Inner Game" of Fitness

42 *A study conducted by scientists at the University of Pennsylvania:* Christopher N. Cascio et al., "Self-affirmation Activates Brain Systems Associated with Self-Related Processing and Reward and Is Reinforced by Future Orientation," *So-*

cial Cognitive and Affective Neuroscience 11, no. 4 (2016): 621–29, doi: 10.1093 /scan/nsv136; Philine S. Harris et al., "Self-Affirmation Improves Performance on Tasks Related to Executive Functioning," *Journal of Experimental Social Psychology* 70 (2017): 281–85, doi: 10.1016/j.jesp.2016.11.011.

53 *According to research conducted by scientists at Stanford University:* Christopher D. Gardner et al., "Effect of Low-Fat vs Low-Carbohydrate Diet on 12-Month Weight Loss in Overweight Adults and the Association with Genotype Pattern or Insulin Secretion: The DIETFITS Randomized Clinical Trial," *JAMA* 319, no. 7 (2018): 667–79, doi: 10.1001/jama.2018.0245.

54 *this type of response in times of frustration and failure:* Michael Wohl et al., "I Forgive Myself, Now I Can Study: How Self-Forgiveness for Procrastinating Can Reduce Future Procrastination," *Personality and Individual Differences* 48, no. 7 (2010): 803–8, doi: 10.1016/j.paid.2010.01.029; Mark R. Leary et al., "Self-Compassion and Reactions to Unpleasant Self-Relevant Events: The Implications of Treating Oneself Kindly," *Journal of Personality and Social Psychology* 92, no. 5 (2007): 887–904, doi: 10.1037/0022-3514.92.5.887; Ashley Batts Allen and Mark R. Leary, "Self-Compassion, Stress, and Coping," *Social and Personality Psychology Compass* 4, no. 2 (2010): 107–18, doi: 10.1111/j.1751-9004.2009.00246.x; Sarah Milne, Sheina Orbell, and Paschal Sheeran, "Combining Motivational and Volitional Interventions to Promote Exercise Participation: Protection Motivation Theory and Implementation Intentions," *British Journal of Health Psychology* 7, pt. 2 (2002): 163–84, doi: 10.1348/135910702169420.

59 *it can increase your motivation to overcome obstacles:* Andreas Kappes, Henrik Singmann, and Gabriele Oettingen, "Mental Contrasting Instigates Goal Pursuit by Linking Obstacles of Reality with Instrumental Behavior," *Journal of Experimental Social Psychology* 48, no. 4 (2012), 811–18, doi: 10.1016/j.jesp.2012.02.002.

Chapter 6: It's All in Your Body Composition

66 *the math behind the* body mass index *(BMI):* Eugenia Cheng, "Weight Loss Is Harder than Rocket Science," *Wall Street Journal* website, January 30, 2020, https://www.wsj.com/articles/weight-loss-is-harder-than-rocket-science-11580 396067.

67 *there are many people who have a "normal weight" BMI:* A. Janet Tomiyama et al., "Misclassification of Cardiometabolic Health When Using Body Mass Index Categories in NHANES 2005–2012," *International Journal of Obesity* 40, no. 5 (2016): 883–86, doi: 10.1038/ijo.2016.17.

68 *Mark Haub . . . who lost 27 pounds in ten weeks eating Hostess cupcakes:* Madison Park, "Twinkie Diet Helps Nutrition Professor Lose 27 Pounds," *CNN* online, November 8, 2010, http://www.cnn.com/2010/HEALTH/11/08/twinkie.diet .professor/index.html.

68 *John Cisna, who lost 56 pounds in six months eating nothing but McDonald's*: Hayley Peterson, "A teacher Who Lost 56 Pounds Eating Only McDonald's Is Starring in a Documentary to Show Kids about 'Healthy' Eating," *Business Insider* website, October 13, 2015, https://www.businessinsider.com/how-to -lose-weight-eating-only-mcdonalds-2015-10.

69 *Kai Sedgwick, who got into the best shape of his life:* Emma Innes, "Fitness fa-natic Claims to Be in the Best Shape of His Life Despite Only Eating MCDONALD'S for a Month," *Daily Mail* website, May 30, 2014, https:// www.dailymail.co.uk/health/article-2643936/Fitness-fanatic-claims-best -shape-life-despite-ONLY-eating-McDonalds.html.

69 *dozens of studies that have found no difference in weight or fat loss between low- and high-carb and low- and high-sugar diets:* Carol S. Johnston et al., "Ketogenic Low-Carbohydrate Diets Have No Metabolic Advantage over Nonketogenic Low-Carbohydrate Diets," *American Journal of Clinical Nutrition* 83, no. 5 (2006): 1055–61, doi: 10.1093/ajcn/83.5.1055; Shane A. Phillips et al., "Bene-

fit of Low-Fat over Low-Carbohydrate Diet on Endothelial Health in Obesity," *Hypertension* 51, no. 2 (2008): 376–82, doi: 10.1161/hypertensionaha.107 .101824; Frank M. Sacks et al., "Comparison of Weight-Loss Diets with Different Compositions of Fat, Protein, and Carbohydrates," *New England Journal of Medicine* 360, no. 9 (2009): 859–73, doi: 10.1056/NEJMoa0804748; Christopher D. Gardner et al., "Effect of Low-Fat vs Low-Carbohydrate Diet on 12-Month Weight Loss in Overweight Adults and the Association with Genotype Pattern or Insulin Secretion: The DIETFITS Randomized Clinical Trial," *JAMA* 319, no. 7 (2018): 667–79, doi: 10.1001/jama.2018.0245; Richard S. Surwit et al., "Metabolic and Behavioral Effects of a High-Sucrose Diet during Weight Loss," *American Journal of Clinical Nutrition* 65, no. 4 (1997): 908–15, doi: 10.1093 /ajcn/65.4.908; J. A. West and Anne de Looy, "Weight Loss in Overweight Subjects Following Low-Sucrose or Sucrose-Containing Diets," *International Journal of Obesity and Related Metabolic Disorders* 25, no. 8 (2001): 1122–28, doi: 10.1038/sj.ijo.0801652.

71 *meaningful weight loss requires energy expenditure to exceed energy intake:* Isabelle Romieu et al., "Energy Balance and Obesity: What Are the Main Drivers?," *Cancer Causes and Control* 28, no. 3 (2017): 247–58, doi: 10.1007 /s10552-017-0869-z; Kevin D. Hall et al., "Energy Balance and Its Components: Implications for Body Weight Regulation," *American Journal of Clinical Nutrition* 95, no. 4 (2012): 989–94, doi: 10.3945/ajcn.112.036350; Michael E. J. Lean, Arne Astrup, and Susan B. Roberts, "Making Progress on the Global Crisis of Obesity and Weight Management," *BMJ* 361 (June 2018): k2538, doi: 10.1136/bmj.k2538; James O. Hill, Holly R. Wyatt, and John C. Peters, "Energy Balance and Obesity," *Circulation* 126, no. 1 (2012): 126–32, doi: 10.1161/circulationaha.111.087213.

71 *these outcomes have been demonstrated with many diets:* Carol S. Johnston et al., "Ketogenic Low-Carbohydrate Diets Have No Metabolic Advantage

over Nonketogenic Low-Carbohydrate Diets," *American Journal of Clinical Nutrition* 83, no. 5 (2006): 1055–61, doi: 10.1093/ajcn/83.5.1055; Iris Shai et al., "Weight Loss with a Low-Carbohydrate, Mediterranean, or Low-Fat Diet," *New England Journal of Medicine* 359, no. 3 (2008): 229–41, doi: 10.1056/NEJMoa0708681; Kate Jolly et al., "Comparison of Range of Commercial or Primary Care Led Weight Reduction Programmes with Minimal Intervention Control for Weight Loss in Obesity: Lighten Up Randomised Controlled Trial," *BMJ* 343 (November 2011): d6500, doi: 10.1136/bmj.d6500; Deirdre K. Tobias et al., "Effect of Low-Fat Diet Interventions versus Other Diet Interventions on Long-Term Weight Change in Adults: A Systematic Review and Meta-analysis," *Lancet Diabetes and Endocrinology* 3, no. 12 (2015): 968–79, doi: 10.1016/S2213-8587(15)00367-8; Arne Astrup et al., "The Role of Low-Fat Diets in Body Weight Control: A Meta-analysis of Ad Libitum Dietary Intervention Studies," *International Journal of Obesity and Related Metabolic Disorders* 24, no. 12 (2000): 1545–52, doi: 10.1038/sj.ijo.0801453; Jayson B. Calton, "Prevalence of Micronutrient Deficiency in Popular Diet Plans," *Journal of the International Society of Sports Nutrition* 7, no. 24 (June 2010), doi: 10.1186/1550-2783-7-24; Staffan Lindeberg et al., "A Palaeolithic Diet Improves Glucose Tolerance More Than a Mediterranean-Like Diet in Individuals with Ischaemic Heart Disease," *Diabetologia* 50, no. 9 (2007): 1795–1807, doi: 10.1007/s00125-007-0716-y; Suruchi Mishra et al., "A Multicenter Randomized Controlled Trial of a Plant-Based Nutrition Program to Reduce Body Weight and Cardiovascular Risk in the Corporate Setting: The GEICO Study," *European Journal of Clinical Nutrition* 67, no. 7 (2013): 718–24, doi: 10.1038/ejcn.2013.92.

72 *it could easily be 1,200, 1,500, or more:* Steven W Lichtman et al., "Discrepancy between Self-Reported and Actual Caloric Intake and Exercise in Obese Subjects," *New England Journal of Medicine* 327, no. 27 (1992): 1893–98, doi:

10.1056/NEJM199212313272701; Danit R. Shahar et al., "Misreporting of Energy Intake in the Elderly Using Doubly Labeled Water to Measure Total Energy Expenditure and Weight Change," *Journal of the American College of Nutrition* 29, no. 1 (2010): 14–24, doi: 10.1080/07315724.2010.10719812.

72   *In a study conducted by scientists at York University:* Ruth E. Brown et al., "Calorie Estimation in Adults Differing in Body Weight Class and Weight Loss Status," *Medicine and Science in Sports and Exercise* 48, no. 3 (2016): 521–26, doi: 10.1249/MSS.0000000000000796.

73   *energy balance works the same in the lean and the obese:* Eric R. Helms, Alan A. Aragon, and Peter J. Fitschen, "Evidence-Based Recommendations for Natural Bodybuilding Contest Preparation: Nutrition and Supplementation," *Journal of the International Society of Sports Nutrition* 11, no. 20 (May 2014), doi: 10.1186/1550-2783-11-20; Gilbert B. Forbes, "Body Fat Content Influences the Body Composition Response to Nutrition and Exercise," *Annals of the New York Academy of Sciences* 904, no. 1 (2000): 359–65. doi: 10.1111/j.1749 -6632.2000.tb06482.x; Karen E. Foster-Schubert et al., "Effect of Diet and Exercise, Alone or Combined, on Weight and Body Composition in Overweight-to-Obese Postmenopausal Women," *Obesity* 20, no. 8 (2012): 1628–38, doi: 10.1038/oby.2011.76; Sarah Steven et al., "Very Low-Calorie Diet and 6 Months of Weight Stability in Type 2 Diabetes: Pathophysiological Changes in Responders and Nonresponders," *Diabetes Care* 39, no. 5 (2016): 808–15, doi: 10.2337/dc15-1942; Monica C. Serra et al., "Effects of a Hypocaloric, Nutritionally Complete, Higher Protein Meal Plan on Regional Body Fat and Cardiometabolic Biomarkers in Older Adults with Obesity," *Annals of Nutrition and Metabolism* 74, no. 2 (2019): 149–55, doi: 10.1159/000497066.

75   *you also impair your body's ability to build muscle:* Christina I. Zito et al., "SHP-2 Regulates Cell Growth by Controlling the mTOR/S6 Kinase 1 Pathway," *Jour-*

nal of Biological Chemistry 282, no. 10 (2007): 6946–53, doi: 10.1074/jbc
.M608338200; Roberto Cangemi et al., "Long-Term Effects of Calorie Restriction on Serum Sex-Hormone Concentrations in Men," *Aging Cell* 9, no. 2
(2010): 236–42, doi: 10.1111/j.1474-9726.2010.00553.x; A. Janet Tomiyama
et al., "Low Calorie Dieting Increases Cortisol," *Psychosomatic Medicine* 72,
no. 4 (2010): 357–64, doi: 10.1097/PSY.0b013e3181d9523c.

76 *people who eat more protein:* N. Santesso et al., "Effects of Higher- versus Lower-
Protein Diets on Health Outcomes: A Systematic Review and Meta-analysis,"
European Journal of Clinical Nutrition 66, no. 7 (2012): 780–88, doi: 10.1038
/ejcn.2012.37.

76 *Lose fat faster:* Ellen M. Evans et al., "Effects of Protein Intake and Gender
on Body Composition Changes: A Randomized Clinical Weight Loss Trial,"
Nutrition and Metabolism 9, no. 1 (June 2012): 55, doi: 10.1186/1743-7075
-9-55.

76 *Gain more muscle:* Eric R. Helms, Alan A. Aragon, and Peter J. Fitschen,
"Evidence-Based Recommendations for Natural Bodybuilding Contest Prepa-
ration: Nutrition and Supplementation," *Journal of the International Society of
Sports Nutrition* 11, no. 20 (May 2014), doi: 10.1186/1550-2783-11-20.

76 *Burn more calories:* Klaas R. Westerterp, "Diet Induced Thermogenesis," *Nutrition and Metabolism* 1, no. 1 (August 2004): 5, doi: 10.1186/1743-7075-1-5.

76 *Experience less hunger:* Douglas Paddon-Jones et al., "Protein, Weight Management, and Satiety," *American Journal of Clinical Nutrition* 87, no. 5 (2008):
1558S–1561S, doi: 10.1093/ajcn/87.5.1558S.

76 *Have stronger bones:* Wayne W. Campbell and Minghua Tang, "Protein Intake,
Weight Loss, and Bone Mineral Density in Postmenopausal Women," *Journals of Gerontology: Series A, Biological Sciences and Medical Sciences* 65, no. 10
(2010): 1115–22, doi: 10.1093/gerona/glq083.

76 *Enjoy better moods:* Eric R. Helms, Alan A. Aragon, and Peter J. Fitschen, "Evidence-Based Recommendations for Natural Bodybuilding Contest Preparation: Nutrition and Supplementation," *Journal of the International Society of Sports Nutrition* 11, no. 20 (May 2014), doi: 10.1186/1550-2783-11-20.

77 *working out increases your body's need for amino acids:* Stuart M. Phillips and Luc J. C. Van Loon, "Dietary Protein for Athletes: From Requirements to Optimum Adaptation," *Journal of Sports Sciences* 29, Suppl 1 (2011): S29–S38, doi: 10.1080/02640414.2011.619204.

77 *it helps preserve lean mass while dieting:* James W. Krieger et al., "Effects of Variation in Protein and Carbohydrate Intake on Body Mass and Composition during Energy Restriction: A Meta-Regression," *American Journal of Clinical Nutrition* 83, no. 2 (2006): 260–74, doi: 10.1093/ajcn/83.2.260.

77 *mice burn about seven times more calories per pound of body weight than humans:* A. H. Terpstra, "Differences between Humans and Mice in Efficacy of the Body Fat Lowering Effect of Conjugated Linoleic Acid: Role of Metabolic Rate," *Journal of Nutrition* 131, no. 7 (2001): 2067–68, doi: 10.1093/jn/131.7.2067.

77 *statistical models developed by scientists at Texas A&M:* Carlos A. Silva and Kalyan Annamalai, "Entropy Generation and Human Aging: Lifespan Entropy and Effect of Diet Composition and Caloric Restriction Diets," *Journal of Thermodynamics* (2009): 1–10, doi: 10.1155/2009/186723.

77 *low-protein dieting is associated with a higher incidence of muscle loss:* Jane E. Kerstetter, Anne M. Kenny, and Karl L. Insogna, "Dietary Protein and Skeletal Health: A Review of Recent Human Research," *Current Opinion in Lipidology* 22, no. 1 (2011): 16–20, doi: 10.1097/MOL.0b013e3283419441; Rachel R. Deer and Elena Volpi, "Protein Intake and Muscle Function in Older Adults," *Current Opinion in Clinical Nutrition and Metabolic Care* 18, no. 3 (2015): 248–53, doi: 10.1097/MCO.0000000000000162; Bernhard Franzke et al.,

"Dietary Protein, Muscle and Physical Function in the Very Old," *Nutrients* 10, no. 7 (July 2018): 935, doi: 10.3390/nu10070935; Hélio J. Coelho-Júnior et al., "Protein-Related Dietary Parameters and Frailty Status in Older Community-Dwellers across Different Frailty Instruments," *Nutrients* 12, no. 2 (February 2020): 508, doi: 10.3390/nu12020508.

78   *the mineral zinc, which is abundant in foods like beef, seeds, and legumes:* Eric R. Helms, Alan A. Aragon, and Peter J. Fitschen, "Evidence-Based Recommendations for Natural Bodybuilding Contest Preparation: Nutrition and Supplementation," *Journal of the International Society of Sports Nutrition* 11, no. 20 (May 2014), doi: 10.1186/1550-2783-11-20.

78   *In a case study conducted by scientists at the University of Massachusetts:* Christy Maxwell and Stella Lucia Volpe, "Effect of Zinc Supplementation on Thyroid Hormone Function: A Case Study of Two College Females," *Annals of Nutrition and Metabolism* 51, no. 2 (2007): 188–94, doi: 10.1159/000103324.

79   *Whole-grain bread with less-processed (cheddar) cheese has a TEF:* Sadie B. Barr and Jonathan C. Wright, "Postprandial Energy Expenditure in Whole-Food and Processed-Food Meals: Implications for Daily Energy Expenditure," *Food and Nutrition Research* 54 (July 2010), doi: 10.3402/fnr.v54i0.5144.

79   *a slice of white bread with highly processed (American) cheese has a TEF:* Barr and Wright, "Postprandial Energy Expenditure."

80   *Eating enough fiber reduces the risk of many types of disease:* Yikyung Park et al., "Dietary Fiber Intake and Mortality in the NIH-AARP Diet and Health Study," *Archives of Internal Medicine* 171, no. 12 (2011): 1061–68, doi: 10.1001/archinternmed.2011.18; Marc P. McRae, "Dietary Fiber Intake and Type 2 Diabetes Mellitus: An Umbrella Review of Meta-Analyses," *Journal of Chiropractic Medicine* 17, no. 1 (2018): 44–53, doi: 10.1016/j.jcm.2017.11.002.

80   *children and adults consume 14 grams of fiber for every 1,000 calories:* Wendy J.

Dahl and Maria L. Stewart, "Position of the Academy of Nutrition and Dietetics: Health Implications of Dietary Fiber," *Journal of the Academy of Nutrition and Dietetics* 115, no. 11 (2015): 1861–70, doi: 10.1016/j.jand.2015.09.003.

81   *This helps explain why there's an association:* Rachel K. Johnson et al., "Dietary Sugars Intake and Cardiovascular Health: A Scientific Statement from the American Heart Association," *Circulation* 120, no. 11 (2009): 1011–20, doi: 10.1161/circulationaha.109.192627; Kelly D. Brownell et al., "The Public Health and Economic Benefits of Taxing Sugar-Sweetened Beverages," *New England Journal of Medicine* 361, no. 16 (2009): 1599–1605, doi: 10.1056/NEJMhpr0905723.

82   *those associated with health benefits like whole grains, fruit, vegetables, and legumes:* Sonia S. Anand et al., "Food Consumption and Its Impact on Cardiovascular Disease: Importance of Solutions Focused on the Globalized Food System: A Report from the Workshop Convened by the World Heart Federation," *Journal of the American College of Cardiology* 66, no. 14 (2015): 1590–1614, doi: 10.1016/j.jacc.2015.07.050.

82   *this inhibits workout performance:* Pim Knuiman, Maria T. E. Hopman, and Marco Mensink, "Glycogen Availability and Skeletal Muscle Adaptations with Endurance and Resistance Exercise," *Nutrition and Metabolism* 12, no. 59 (December 2015), doi: 10.1186/s12986-015-0055-9; Louise M. Burke et al., "Carbohydrates for Training and Competition," *Journal of Sports Sciences* 29, Suppl 1 (2011): S17–S27, doi: 10.1080/02640414.2011.585473; Andrew Creer et al., "Influence of Muscle Glycogen Availability on ERK1/2 and Akt Signaling after Resistance Exercise in Human Skeletal Muscle," *Journal of Applied Physiology (1985)* 99, no. 3 (2005): 950–56, doi: 10.1152/japplphysiol.00110.2005.

82   *restricting your carbs also raises your cortisol and lowers your testosterone:* Amy R. Lane, Joseph W. Duke, and Anthony C. Hackney, "Influence of Dietary Car-

bohydrate Intake on the Free Testosterone: Cortisol Ratio Responses to Short-Term Intensive Exercise Training," *European Journal of Applied Physiology* 108, no. 6 (2010): 1125–31, doi: 10.1007/s00421-009-1220-5.

82   *athletes who eat low-carb diets recover more slowly:* Lyonel Benjamin, Peter Blan-pied, and Linda Lamont, "Dietary Carbohydrate and Protein Manipulation and Exercise Recovery in Novice Weight-Lifters," *Journal of Exercise Physiology* 12, no. 6 (2009): 33–39, https://www.researchgate.net/publication/258242414 _Dietary_carbohydrate_and_protein_manipulation_and_exercise_recovery_in _novice_weight-Lifters; Krista R. Howarth et al., "Effect of Glycogen Avail-ability on Human Skeletal Muscle Protein Turnover during Exercise and Re-covery," *Journal of Applied Physiology* 109, no. 2 (2010): 431–38, doi: 10.1152 /japplphysiol.00108.2009.

84   *a weak albeit consistent correlation between high saturated fat intake and heart dis-ease:* Joyce Nettleton et al., "Saturated Fat Consumption and Risk of Coronary Heart Disease and Ischemic Stroke: A Science Update," *Annals of Nutrition and Metabolism* 70, no. 1 (2017): 26–33, doi: 10.1159/000455681; Mark Hous-ton, "The Relationship of Saturated Fats and Coronary Heart Disease: Fa(c)t or Fiction? A Commentary," *Therapeutic Advances in Cardiovascular Disease* 12, no. 2 (2018): 33–37, doi: 10.1177/1753944717742549; Jan I. Pedersen et al., "The Importance of Reducing SFA to Limit CHD," *British Journal of Nutrition* 106, no. 7 (2011): 961–63 doi: 10.1017/S000711451100506X; Daan Krom-hout et al., "The Confusion about Dietary Fatty Acids Recommendations for CHD Prevention," *British Journal of Nutrition* 106, no. 5 (2011): 627–32, doi: 10.1017/S0007114511002236.

84   *we should follow the generally accepted dietary guidelines:* Houston, "The Rela-tionship of Saturated Fats."

85   *it can reduce the risk of heart disease:* Lukas Schwingshackl and Georg Hoffmann, "Monounsaturated Fatty Acids, Olive Oil and Health Status: A Systematic Re-

view and Meta-analysis of Cohort Studies," *Lipids in Health and Disease* 13, no. 1 (2014): 154, doi: 10.1186/1476-511X-13-154; Francesco Sofi et al., "Accruing Evidence on Benefits of Adherence to the Mediterranean Diet on Health: An Updated Systematic Review and Meta-analysis," *American Journal of Clinical Nutrition* 92, no. 5 (2010): 1189–96, doi: 10.3945/ajcn.2010.29673.

85 *the absolute amount of omega-3 fatty acids in the diet may be more important:* Penny M. Kris-Etherton et al., "Polyunsaturated Fatty Acids in the Food Chain in the United States," *American Journal of Clinical Nutrition* 71, no. 1 (2000): 179S–188S, doi: 10.1093/ajcn/71.1.179S.

86 *high levels of LDL in your blood can lead to an accumulation of fat in your arteries:* Brian A. Ference et al., "Low-density Lipoproteins Cause Atherosclerotic Cardiovascular Disease. 1. Evidence from Genetic, Epidemiologic, and Clinical Studies. A Consensus Statement from the European Atherosclerosis Society Consensus Panel," *European Heart Journal* 38, no. 31 (2017): 2459–72, doi: 10.1093/eurheartj/ehx144.

86 *food that can raise LDL levels . . . is considered bad for your heart:* Sonia S. Anand et al., "Food Consumption and Its Impact on Cardiovascular Disease: Importance of Solutions Focused on the Globalized Food System: A Report from the Workshop Convened by the World Heart Federation," *Journal of the American College of Cardiology* 66, no. 14 (2015): 1590–1614, doi: 10.1016/j.jacc.2015.07.050; Taraka Vijay Gadiraju et al., "Fried Food Consumption and Cardiovascular Health: A Review of Current Evidence," *Nutrients* 7, no. 10 (2015): 8424–30, doi: 10.3390/nu7105404.

87 *you want to ensure that your LDL levels aren't too high:* "HDL: The Good, but Complex, Cholesterol," *Harvard Health* website, last modified August 6, 2019, https://www.health.harvard.edu/newsletter_article/hdl-the-good-but-complex-cholesterol.

87 *eating low-cholesterol foods and avoiding saturated fat won't cut it:* Bradley C.

Johnston et al., "Unprocessed Red Meat and Processed Meat Consumption: Dietary Guideline Recommendations from the Nutritional Recommendations (NutriRECS) Consortium," *Annals of Internal Medicine* 171, no. 10 (2019): 756, doi: 10.7326/M19-1621; Julie Hjerpsted et al., "Cheese Intake in Large Amounts Lowers LDL-Cholesterol Concentrations Compared with Butter Intake of Equal Fat Content," *American Journal of Clinical Nutrition* 94, no. 6 (2011): 1479–84, doi: 10.3945/ajcn.111.022426.

87 *Exercising regularly (especially intense exercise, including strength training):* Carl J. Lavie et al., "Exercise and the Cardiovascular System: Clinical Science and Cardiovascular Outcomes," *Circulation Research* 117, no. 2 (2015): 207–19, doi: 10.1161/circresaha.117.305205; Steven Mann et al., "Differential Effects of Aerobic Exercise, Resistance Training, and Combined Exercise Modalities on Cholesterol and the Lipid Profile: Review, Synthesis, and Recommendations," *Sports Medicine* 44, no. 2 (2014): 211–21, doi: 10.1007/s40279-013-0110-5.

87 *Maintaining healthy body fat levels:* Michael L. Dansinger et al., "Comparison of the Atkins, Ornish, Weight Watchers, and Zone Diets for Weight Loss and Heart Disease Risk Reduction: A Randomized Trial," *JAMA* 293, no. 1 (2005): 43–53, doi: 10.1016/j.accreview.2005.02.079; Paul T. Williams et al., "The Effects of Weight Loss by Exercise or by Dieting on Plasma High-Density Lipoprotein (HDL) Levels in Men with Low, Intermediate, and Normal-to-High HDL at Baseline," *Metabolism* 43, no. 7 (1994): 917–24, https://pmid.us/8028519.

87 *Getting enough sleep:* Yoshitaka Kaneita et al., "Associations of Usual Sleep Duration with Serum Lipid and Lipoprotein Levels," *Sleep* 31, no. 5 (2008): 645–52, doi: 10.1093/sleep/31.5.645; Matthew S. Mosca and Brooke Aggarwal, "Sleep Duration, Snoring Habits, and Cardiovascular Disease Risk Factors in an Ethnically Diverse Population," *Journal of Cardiovascular Nursing* 27, no. 4 (2012): 263–69, doi: 10.1097/JCN.0b013e31821e7ad1.

87 *Not smoking:* Sara C. Campbell et al., "Smoking and Smoking Cessation—the Relationship between Cardiovascular Disease and Lipoprotein Metabolism: A Review," *Atherosclerosis* 201, no. 2 (2008): 225–35, doi: 10.1016/j.atherosclerosis.2008.04.046; *How Tobacco Smoke Causes Disease: The Biology and Behavioral Basis for Smoking-Attributable Disease: A Report of the Surgeon General* (Rockville, MD: US Department of Health and Human Services, Public Health Service, Office of the Surgeon General, 2010), 351–409, https://www.ncbi.nlm.nih.gov/books/NBK53017/pdf/Bookshelf_NBK53017.pdf.

87 *exercise alone can neutralize at least some of the downsides:* Luigi Fontana et al., "Long-Term Low-Calorie Low-Protein Vegan Diet and Endurance Exercise Are Associated with Low Cardiometabolic Risk," *Rejuvenation Research* 10, no. 2 (2007): 225–34, doi: 10.1089/rej.2006.0529.

Chapter 7: Welcome to the Easiest Diet in the World

94 *you can maintain a calorie deficit large enough to produce rapid fat loss:* Ina Garthe et al., "Effect of Two Different Weight-Loss Rates on Body Composition and Strength and Power-Related Performance in Elite Athletes," *International Journal of Sport Nutrition and Exercise Metabolism* 21, no. 2 (2011): 97–104, doi: 10.1123/ijsnem.21.2.97.

95 *A study conducted by scientists at Finland's University of Jyväskylä:* Heikki T. Huovinen et al., "Body Composition and Power Performance Improved after Weight Reduction in Male Athletes without Hampering Hormonal Balance," *Journal of Strength and Conditioning Research* 29, no. 1 (2015): 29–36, doi: 10.1519/JSC.0000000000000619.

95 *the less body fat you have, the more susceptible you are to losing muscle:* Gilbert B. Forbes, "Body Fat Content Influences the Body Composition Response to

Nutrition and Exercise," *Annals of the New York Academy of Sciences* 904 (2000): 359–65, doi: 10.1111/j.1749-6632.2000.tb06482.x.

95 *Other studies on calorie restriction:* J. E. Donnelly et al., "Muscle Hypertrophy with Large-Scale Weight Loss and Resistance Training," *American Journal of Clinical Nutrition* 58, no. 4 (1993): 561–65, doi: 10.1093/ajcn/58.4.561.

97 *this point of diminishing returns is somewhere around 110 percent:* Juma Iraki et al., "Nutrition Recommendations for Bodybuilders in the Off-Season: A Narrative Review," *Sports (Basel)* 7, no. 7 (2019): 154, doi: 10.3390/sports7070154; Ina Garthe et al., "Effect of Nutritional Intervention on Body Composition and Performance in Elite Athletes," *European Journal of Sports Science* 13, no. 3 (2013): 295–303, doi: 10.1080/17461391.2011.643923.

99 *a fantastic summary of the literature was coauthored by my friend Dr. Eric Helms:* Eric R. Helms, Alan A. Aragon, and Peter J. Fitschen, "Evidence-Based Recommendations for Natural Bodybuilding Contest Preparation: Nutrition and Supplementation," *Journal of the International Society of Sports Nutrition* 11, no. 20 (May 2014), doi: 10.1186/1550-2783-11-20.

106 *they're usually less wholesome than and don't trigger satiety as effectively as food:* Richard D. Mattes, RD, and Wayne W. Campbell, "Effects of Food Form and Timing of Ingestion on Appetite and Energy Intake in Lean Young Adults and in Young Adults with Obesity," *Journal of the American Dietetic Association* 109, no. 3 (2009): 430–37, doi: 10.1016/j.jada.2008.11.031.

106 *people who drink calories are much more likely to overeat:* David B. Allison, "Liquid Calories, Energy Compensation, and Weight: What We Know and What We Still Need to Learn," *British Journal of Nutrition* 111, no. 3 (2014): 384–86, doi: 10.1017/S0007114513003309.

106 *a clear association between a greater intake of sugar-sweetened beverages and weight gain:* Allison, "Liquid Calories"; Vasanti S. Malik et al., "Intake of

Sugar-Sweetened Beverages and Weight Gain: A Systematic Review," *American Journal of Clinical Nutrition* 84, no. 2 (2006): 274–88, doi: 10.1093/ajcn/84.1.274.

106 *dehydration impairs cognition and endurance:* Ana Adan, "Cognitive Performance and Dehydration," *Journal of the American College of Nutrition* 31, no. 2 (2012): 71–78, doi: 10.1080/07315724.2012.10720011; Serge P. Von Duvillard et al., "Fluids and Hydration in Prolonged Endurance Performance," *Nutrition* 20, no. 7–8 (2004): 651–56, doi: 10.1016/j.nut.2004.04.011; Kentaro Murakami et al., "Association between Dietary Fiber, Water and Magnesium Intake and Functional Constipation among Young Japanese Women," *European Journal of Clinical Nutrition* 61, no. 5 (2007): 616–22, doi: 10.1038/sj.ejcn.1602573; Jacqueline Chan et al., "Water, Other Fluids, and Fatal Coronary Heart Disease: The Adventist Health Study," *American Journal of Epidemiology* 155, no. 9 (2002): 827–33, doi: 10.1093/aje/155.9.827.

107 *recommends a baseline intake of about ¾ of a gallon: Dietary Reference Intakes for Water, Potassium, Sodium, Chloride, and Sulfate* (Washington, DC: National Academies Press, 2005), https://www.nap.edu/read/10925/chapter/1; V. A. Convertino et al., "American College of Sports Medicine Position Stand: Exercise and Fluid Replacement," *Medicine and Science in Sports and Exercise* 28, no. 1 (1996): i–vii, doi: 10.1097/00005768-199610000-00045.

107 *it's minimal even at high doses (up to 500 milligrams per day):* Yang Zhang et al., "Caffeine and Diuresis during Rest and Exercise: A Meta-analysis," *Journal of Science and Medicine in Sport* 18, no. 5 (2015): 569–74, doi: 10.1016/j.jsams.2014.07.017.

113   *people new to strength training gain very little fat while in a calorie surplus:* Ralph Rozenek et al., "Effects of High-Calorie Supplements on Body Composition and Muscular Strength Following Resistance Training," *Journal of Sports Medicine and Physical Fitness* 42, no. 3 (2002): 340–47, https://pmid.us/12094125.

127   *no meaningful metabolic difference between eating many small and a few large meals:* France Bellisle et al., "Meal frequency and energy balance," *British Journal of Nutrition* 77, Suppl 1 (1997): S57-70, doi: 10.1079/bjn19970104.

127   *eating more frequently has no effect on hunger levels:* Heather J. Leidy et al., "The Effects of Consuming Frequent, Higher Protein Meals on Appetite and Satiety during Weight Loss in Overweight/Obese Men," *Obesity* 19, no. 4 (2011): 818–24, doi: 10.1038/oby.2010.203; Heather J. Leidy et al., "The Influence of Higher Protein Intake and Greater Eating Frequency on Appetite Control in Overweight and Obese Men," *Obesity* 18, no. 9 (2010): 1725–32, doi: 10.1038/oby.2010.45; Heather J. Leidy and Wayne W. Campbell, "The Effect of Eating Frequency on Appetite Control and Food Intake: Brief Synopsis of Controlled Feeding Studies," *Journal of Nutrition* 141, no. 1 (2011): 154–57, doi: 10.3945/jn.109.114389.

127   *eating just one meal per day can make it harder to gain and maintain muscle:* Brad J. Schoenfeld and Alan Albert Aragon, "How Much Protein Can the Body Use in a Single Meal for Muscle-Building? Implications for Daily Protein Distribution," *Journal of the International Society of Sports Nutrition* 15, no. 10 (2018), doi: 10.1186/s12970-018-0215-1.

144   *many underreport these numbers:* Lorien E. Urban et al., "Energy Contents of Frequently Ordered Restaurant Meals and Comparison with Human Energy Requirements and US Department of Agriculture Database Information: A Multisite Randomized Study," *Journal of the Academy of Nutrition and Dietetics* 116, no: 4 (2016): 590–8.e6, doi: 10.1016/j.jand.2015.11.009.

References

145 *moderate alcohol consumption is associated with lower, not higher, body weights*: Martin R. Yeomans, "Alcohol, Appetite and Energy Balance: Is Alcohol Intake a Risk Factor for Obesity?," *Physiology and Behavior* 100, no. 1 (2010): 82–89, doi: 10.1016/j.physbeh.2010.01.012; Marion Flechtner-Mors et al., "Effects of Moderate Consumption of White Wine on Weight Loss in Overweight and Obese Subjects," *International Journal of Obesity* 28 no. 11 (2004): 1420–26, doi: 10.1038/sj.ijo.0802786.

145 *an increase in calories from alcohol alone didn't result in the weight gain that would normally occur:* Harvey W. Gruchow et al., "Alcohol Consumption, Nutrient Intake and Relative Body Weight among US Adults," *American Journal of Clinical Nutrition* 42, no. 2 (1985): 289–95, doi: 10.1093/ajcn/42.2.289.

145 *alcohol can reduce your appetite:* Anna Kokavec, "Is Decreased Appetite for Food a Physiological Consequence of Alcohol Consumption?," *Appetite* 51, no. 2 (2008): 233–43, doi: 10.1016/j.appet.2008.03.011; Mark F. McCarty, "Does Regular Ethanol Consumption Promote Insulin Sensitivity and Leanness by Stimulating AMP-Activated Protein Kinase?," *Medical Hypotheses* 57, no.3 (2001): 405–7, doi: 10.1054/mehy.2001.1404; Barbara Ukropcova et al., "Dynamic Changes in Fat Oxidation in Human Primary Myocytes Mirror Metabolic Characteristics of the Donor," *Journal of Clinical Investigation* 115, no. 7 (2005): 1934–41, doi: 10.1172/JCI24332.

146 *the body has no way to directly convert alcohol into body fat:* Scott Q. Siler et al., "De novo Lipogenesis, Lipid Kinetics, and Whole-Body Lipid Balances in Humans after Acute Alcohol Consumption," *American Journal of Clinical Nutrition* 70, no. 5 (1999): 928–36, doi: 10.1093/ajcn/70.5.928.

146 *it suppresses physiological mechanisms related to fat burning and increases the conversion of carbs into body fat:* Yves Schutz, "Role of Substrate Utilization and Thermogenesis on Body-Weight Control with Particular Reference to Alcohol,"

Proceedings of the Nutrition Society 59, no. 4 (2000): 511–17, doi: 10.1017 /s0029665100000744.

151 *eating at least three servings of protein throughout the day is better:* José L. Areta et al., "Timing and Distribution of Protein Ingestion during Prolonged Recovery from Resistance Exercise Alters Myofibrillar Protein Synthesis," *Journal of Physiology* 591, no. 9 (2013): 2319–31, doi: 10.1113/jphysiol.2012.244897.

170 *The drawbacks of treating are obvious:* James J. DiNicolantonio et al., "Subclinical Magnesium Deficiency: A Principal Driver of Cardiovascular Disease and a Public Health Crisis," *Open Heart* 2018, no. 5 (2018): e000668, doi: 10.1136 /openhrt-2017-000668; Theresa Kulie et al., " Vitamin D: An Evidence-Based Review," *Journal of the American Board of Family Medicine* 22, no. 6 (November 2009): 698–706, doi: 10.3122/jabfm.2009.06.090037; Jeffrey L. Miller, "Iron Deficiency Anemia: A Common and Curable Disease," *Cold Spring Harbor Perspectives in Medicine* 3, no. 7 (July 2013): a011866, doi: 10.1101/cshperspect .a011866.

171 *the analysis of 360 dinner entrees at 123 nonchain restaurants:* Lorien E. Urban et al., "Energy Contents of Frequently Ordered Restaurant Meals and Comparison with Human Energy Requirements and U.S. Department of Agriculture Database Information: A Multisite Randomized Study," *Journal of the Academy of Nutrition and Dietetics* 116, no. 4 (April 2016): 590–598.e6, doi: 10.1016 /j.jand.2015.11.009.

171 *an analysis of restaurant foods conducted by scientists at the Center for Science in the Public Interest:* "Xtreme Eating 2014," Center for Science in the Public Interest Website, accessed August 22, 2018, https://cspinet.org/eating-healthy/foods -avoid/xtreme2014.

172 *research conducted by scientists at the University of Illinois at Urbana-Champaign:* Ruopeng An, "Fast-Food and Full-Service Restaurant Consumption and Daily

Energy and Nutrient Intakes in US Adults," *European Journal of Clinical Nutrition* 70, no. 1 (January 2016): 97–103, doi: 10.1038/ejcn.2015.104.

173 *a hormone called* leptin, *which is produced by body fat:* Eric Jéquier, "Leptin Signaling, Adiposity, and Energy Balance," *Annals of the New York Academy of Sciences* 967, no. 1 (June 2002): 379–388, doi: 10.1111/j.1749-6632.2002. tb04293.x.

174 *accomplishes this through several mechanisms:* Hyeong-Kyu Park and Rexford S. Ahima, "Physiology of Leptin: Energy Homeostasis, Neuroendocrine Function and Metabolism," *Metabolism* 64, no. 1 (January 2015): 24–34, doi: 10.1016 /j.metabol.2014.08.004.

174 *You can temporarily boost leptin production:* B. R. Olson et al., "Short-Term Fasting Affects Luteinizing Hormone Secretory Dynamics but Not Reproductive Function in Normal-Weight Sedentary Women," *Journal of Clinical Endocrinology & Metabolism* 80, no. 4 (April 1995): 1187–1193, doi:10.1210 /jcem.80.4.7714088.

174 *Research shows that eating a large amount of carbohydrate:* M. Dirlewanger et al., "Effects of Short-Term Carbohydrate or Fat Overfeeding on Energy Expenditure and Plasma Leptin Concentrations in Healthy Female Subjects," *International Journal of Obesity* 24 (2000): 1413–1418, doi: 10.1038 /sj.ijo.0801395.

Chapter 9: The Little Big Things about Building Lean Muscle (at Any Age)

180 *there are three primary "triggers" or "pathways" for muscle growth:* Brad J. Schoenfeld, "The Mechanisms of Muscle Hypertrophy and Their Application to Resistance Training," *Journal of Strength and Conditioning Research* 24, no. 10 (2010): 2857–72, doi: 10.1519/JSC.0b013e3181e840f3.

180 *It's unclear whether muscle damage directly stimulates muscle growth:* Felipe Damas

et al., "The Development of Skeletal Muscle Hypertrophy through Resistance Training: The Role of Muscle Damage and Muscle Protein Synthesis," *European Journal of Applied Physiology* 118, no. 3 (2018): 485–500, doi: 10.1007/s00421-017-3792-9.

180 *mechanical tension is the most important of these three:* Troy A. Hornberger and Shu Chien, "Mechanical Stimuli and Nutrients Regulate Rapamycin-Sensitive Signaling through Distinct Mechanisms in Skeletal Muscle," *Journal of Cellular Biochemistry* 97, no. 6 (2006): 1207–16, doi: 10.1002/jcb.20671; Herman H. Vandenburgh, "Motion into Mass: How Does Tension Stimulate Muscle Growth?," *Medicine and Science in Sports and Exercise* 19, 5 Suppl (1987): S142–S149, https://pmid.us/3316913; Brad J. Schoenfeld. "The Mechanisms of Muscle Hypertrophy and Their Application to Resistance Training"; Hans Hoppeler et al., "Gene Expression in Working Skeletal Muscle," *Advances in Experimental Medicine and Biology* 618 (2007): 245–54, doi: 10.1007/978-0-387-75434-5_19.

181 *also relate to what scientists call the* strength-endurance continuum*:* Gerson E. R. Campos et al., "Muscular Adaptations in Response to Three Different Resistance-Training Regimens: Specificity of Repetition Maximum Training Zones," *European Journal of Applied Physiology* 88, no. 1–2 (2002): 50–60, doi: 10.1007/s00421-002-0681-6.

182 *neither men nor women can "lengthen" and "tighten" their muscles:* Cynthia H. Weppler and Stig P. Magnusson, "Increasing Muscle Extensibility: A Matter of Increasing Length or Modifying Sensation?," *Physical Therapy* 90, no. 3 (2010): 438–49, doi: 10.2522/ptj.20090012; Anthony J. Blazevich et al., "Range of Motion, Neuromechanical, and Architectural Adaptations to Plantar Flexor Stretch Training in Humans," *Journal of Applied Physiology* 117, no. 5 (1985): 452–62, doi: 10.1152/japplphysiol.00204.2014.

Chapter 10: The 5 Commandments of Successful Strength Training

193 *around 20 percent of patients account for 80 percent of healthcare spending:* Bradley Sawyer and Gary Claxton, "Discussion of Health Spending often Focus on Averages, but a Small Share of the Population Incurs Most of the Cost," *Health System Tracker* website, January 16, 2019, https:/www .healthsystemtracker.org/chart-collection/health-expenditures-vary -across-population/#item-discussion-of-health-spending-often-focus-on -averages-but-a-small-share-of-the-population-incurs-most-of-the-cost_2016; Jeff Zimmerman, "Applying the Pareto Principle (80-20 Rule) to Baseball," *Beyond the Box Score* website, June 4, 2010, https://www.beyondtheboxscore .com/2010/6/4/1501048/applying-the-parento-principle-80; Avshalom Caspi et al., "Childhood Forecasting of a Small Segment of the Population with Large Economic Burden," *Nature Human Behaviour* 1 (2016): 0005, doi: 10.1038 /s41562-016-0005.

194 *it also accumulates fatigue that leads to reductions in speed:* Jeffrey B. Kreher and Jennifer Schwartz, "Overtraining Syndrome: A Practical Guide," *Sports Health: A Multidisciplinary Approach* 4, no. 2 (2012): 128–38, doi: 10.1177 /1941738111434406.

194 *this response to training may be more of a mental or emotional state:* Shona L. Halson and Asker E. Jeukendrup, "Does Overtraining Exist? An Analysis of Overreaching and Overtraining Research," *Sports Medicine* 34, no. 14 (2004): 967–81, doi: 10.2165/00007256-200434140-00003.

196 *the less frequently you can do them*: Daniel W. Robbins et al., "The Effect of Training Volume on Lower-Body Strength," *Journal of Strength and Conditioning Research* 26, no. 1 (2012): 34–39, doi: 10.1519/JSC.0b013e31821d5cc4.

197 *this threshold is likely between 8 and 10 hard sets:* Eric R. Helms et al., "Rec-

ommendations for Natural Bodybuilding Contest Preparation: Resistance and Cardiovascular Training," *Journal of Sports Medicine and Physical Fitness* 55, no. 3 (2015): 164–78, https://pmid.us/24998610.

197   *trainees need to do upward of 15 to 20 hard sets per week:* Theban Amirthalingam et al., "Effects of a Modified German Volume Training Program on Muscular Hypertrophy and Strength," *Journal of Strength and Conditioning Research* 31, no. 11 (2017): 3109–19, doi: 10.1519/JSC.0000000000001747.

197   *when sets are taken to or close to* muscle failure*:* Michael Matthews, "Research Review: What's the Best Rep Range for Building Muscle?," June 27, 2018, *Muscle for Life* podcast, https://legionathletics.com/rep-range-podcast/.

197   *training to muscle failure regularly isn't optimal:* Alex S. Ribeiro et al., "Acute Effects of Different Training Loads on Affective Responses in Resistance-Trained Men," *International Journal of Sports Medicine* 40, no. 13 (2019): 850–55, doi: 10.1055/a-0997-6680; Cody T. Haun et al., "Molecular, Neuromuscular, and Recovery Responses to Light versus Heavy Resistance Exercise in Young Men," *Physiological Reports* 5, no. 18 (2017): e13457, doi: 10.14814/phy2.13457.

198   *A study conducted by scientists at the State University of Rio de Janeiro:* Belmiro Freitas de Salles et al., "Rest Interval between Sets in Strength Training," *Sport Medicine* 39, no. 9 (2009): 765–77, doi: 10.2165/11315230-000000000-00000.

198   *in another study conducted at Eastern Illinois University:* Jeffrey M. Willardson and Lee N. Burkett, "The Effect of Different Rest Intervals between Sets on Volume Components and Strength Gains," *Journal of Strength Conditioning Research* 22, no. 1 (2008): 146–52, doi: 10.1519/JSC.0b013e31815f912d.

199   *envisioning the successful completion of a resistance training set beforehand can increase performance:* Florent Lebon et al., "Benefits of Motor Imagery Training on Muscle Strength," *Journal of Strength and Conditioning Research* 24, no. 6 (2010): 1680–87, doi: 10.1519/JSC.0b013e3181d8e936.

202   *it increases muscle and strength gain, and may also reduce the risk of injury:* Ronei S. Pinto et al., "Effect of Range of Motion on Muscle Strength and Thickness," *Journal of Strength and Conditioning Research* 26, no. 8 (2012): 2140–45, doi: 10.1519/JSC.0b013e31823a3b15.

202   *the burden shifts to other tendons and ligaments:* Tony Ciccone et al., "Deep Squats and Knee Health: A Scientific Review," Center for Sport Performance, accessed Jan 30, 2021, https://shruggedcollective.com/wp-content/uploads/2015/04/Deep Squat-Review-Barbell-Daily-3-27-15.pdf.

204   *Your instinctive answer will often be accurate:* Daniel A. Hackett et al., "Accuracy in Estimating Repetitions to Failure during Resistance Exercise," *Journal of Strength and Conditioning Research* 31, no. 8 (2017): 2162–68, doi: 10.1519 /JSC.0000000000001683.

204   *slow-rep training has been put to the test in quite a few studies:* Joanne Munn et al., "Resistance Training for Strength: Effect of Number of Sets and Contraction Speed," *Medicine and Science in Sports and Exercise* 37, no. 9 (2005): 1622–26, doi: 10.1249/01.mss.0000177583.41245.f8; Christopher M. Neils et al., "Influence of Contraction Velocity in Untrained Individuals over the Initial Early Phase of Resistance Training," *Journal of Strength and Conditioning Research* 19, no. 4 (2005): 883, doi: 10.1519/R-15794.1; Eonho Kim et al., "Effects of 4 Weeks of Traditional Resistance Training vs. Superslow Strength Training on Early Phase Adaptations in Strength, Flexibility, and Aerobic Capacity in College-Aged Women," *Journal of Strength and Conditioning Research* 25, no. 11 (2011): 3006–13, 10.1519/JSC.0b013e318212e3a2; Disa L. Hatfield et al., "The Impact of Velocity of Movement on Performance Factors in Resistance Exercise," *Journal of Strength and Conditioning Research* 20, no. 4 (2006): 760– 66, doi: 10.1519/R-155552.1.

204   *Time under tension isn't important enough to warrant special attention:* Sam-

uel Arlington Headley et al., "Effects of Lifting Tempo on One Repetition Maximum and Hormonal Responses to a Bench Press Protocol," *Journal of Strength and Conditioning Research* 25, no. 2 (2011): 406–13, doi: 10.1519 /JSC.0b013e3181bf053b.

204 *load and reps are major factors in how much muscle and strength you gain:* Thalita Leite et al., "Dose-Response of 1, 3, and 5 Sets of Resistance Exercise on Strength, Local Muscular Endurance, and Hypertrophy," *Journal of Strength and Conditioning Research* 29, no. 5 (2015): 1349–58, doi: 10.1519 /JSC.0000000000000758.

205 *Many strength training injuries aren't caused by training too hard:* U. M. Kujala et al., "Knee Injuries in Athletes: Review of Exertion Injuries and Retrospective Study of Outpatient Sports Clinic Material," *Sports Medicine* 3, no. 6 (1986): 447–60, doi: 10.2165/00007256-198603060-00006; Nicola Maffulli et al., "Sport Injuries: A Review of Outcomes," *British Medical Bulletin* 97, no. 1 (2011): 47–80, doi: 10.1093/bmb/ldq026.

Chapter 11: The Best Strength Exercises for Building Your Best Body Ever

210 *The more often you make a switch, the harder it is to become proficient:* Philip D. Chilibeck et al., "A Comparison of Strength and Muscle Mass Increases during Resistance Training in Young Women," *European Journal of Applied Physiology and Occupational Physiology* 77, no.1–2 (1998): 170–75, doi: 10.1007 /s004210050316.

Chapter 12: The *Muscle for Life* Workout Program

272 *it's not clear that heating up our muscles before loading them makes injury less likely:* Andrea J. Fradkin et al., "Does Warming Up Prevent Injury in Sport?,"

Journal of Science and Medicine in Sport 9, no. 3 (2006): 214–20, doi: 10.1016 /j.jsams.2006.03.026.

273 *the more times you perform an exercise correctly, the more that becomes your default way to move:* David A. Gabriel et al., "Neural Adaptations to Resistive Exercise: Mechanisms and Recommendations for Training Practices," *Sports Medicine* 36, no. 2 (2006): 133–49, doi: 10.2165/00007256-200636020 -00004.

273 *a short warm-up routine . . . can boost performance levels:* Andrea J. Fradkin et al., "Effects of Warming-Up on Physical Performance: A Systematic Review with Meta-analysis," *Journal of Strength and Conditioning Research* 24, no. 1 (2010): 140–48, doi: 10.1519/JSC.0b013e3181c643a0.

278 *cardio causes adaptations at a cellular level:* Vernon G. Coffey et al., "Early Signaling Responses to Divergent Exercise Stimuli in Skeletal Muscle from Well-Trained Humans," *FASEB Journal* 20, no. 1 (2006): 190–92, doi: 10.1096 /fj.05-4809fje.

279 *It can burn more than twice as many calories per unit of time:* Jenna B. Gillen et al., "Twelve Weeks of Sprint Interval Training Improves Indices of Cardiometabolic Health Similar to Traditional Endurance Training despite a Five-Fold Lower Exercise Volume and Time Commitment," Øyvind Sandbakk, ed., *PLoS One* 11, no. 4 (2016): e0154075, doi: 10.1371/journal.pone.0154075; Kyle J. Sevits et al., "Total Daily Energy Expenditure Is Increased Following a Single Bout of Sprint Interval Training," *Physiological Reports* 1, no. 5 (2013): e00131, doi: 10.1002/phy2.131.

279 *It also causes more fatigue, soreness, and muscle damage than lower-intensity cardio:* Eric R. Helms et al., "Recommendations for Natural Bodybuilding Contest Preparation: Resistance and Cardiovascular Training," *Journal of Sports Medicine and Physical Fitness* 55, no. 3: 164–78, https://pmid.us/24998610.

280 *these kinds of exercise cause little muscle damage or soreness:* David C. Nieman

et al., "Immune and Inflammation Responses to a 3-day Period of Intensified Running versus Cycling," *Brain, Behavior, and Immunity* 39 (July 2014): 180–85, doi: 10.1016/j.bbi.2013.09.004; Moritz Schumann and Bent R. Rønnestad, *Concurrent Aerobic and Strength Training* (Springer International Publishing, 2019), 19–34.

280 *it can enhance lower-body muscle growth:* Schumann and Rønnestad, *Concurrent Aerobic and Strength Training.*

Chapter 13: The Right (and Wrong) Ways to Track Your Progress

285 *these gadgets and software are notoriously inaccurate:* Anna Shcherbina et al., "Accuracy in Wrist-Worn, Sensor-Based Measurements of Heart Rate and Energy Expenditure in a Diverse Cohort," *Journal of Personalized Medicine* 7, no. 2 (2017): 3, doi: 10.3390/jpm7020003; Andrea C. Buchholz, "The Validity of Bioelectrical Impedance Models in Clinical Populations," *Nutrition in Clinical Practice* 19, no. 5 (2004): 433–46, doi: 10.1177/0115426504019005433; Kurusart Konharn et al., "Validity and Reliability of Smartphone Applications for the Assessment of Walking and Running in Normal-Weight and Overweight/Obese Young Adults," *Journal of Physical Activity and Health* 13, no.12 (2016): 1333–40, doi: 10.1123/jpah.2015-0544.

Chapter 14: The *Muscle for Life* Workout Quickstart Guide

312 *such feelings aren't a sign that something is wrong:* Alison Wood Brooks, "Get Excited: Reappraising Pre-performance Anxiety as Excitement," *Journal of Experimental Psychology General* 143, no. 3 (2014): 1144–58, doi: 10.1037/a0035325.

315 *a growing body of evidence shows they don't:* Robert R. Wolfe, "Branched-Chain Amino Acids and Muscle Protein Synthesis in Humans: Myth or Reality?," *Journal of the International Society of Sports Nutrition* 14, no. 1 (2017): 30, doi: 10.1186/s12970-017-0184-9.

315 *studies show that it's a flop:* Steven B. Heymsfield et al., "*Garcinia cambogia* (Hydroxycitric Acid) as a Potential Antiobesity Agent: A Randomized Controlled Trial," *JAMA* 280, no. 18 (1998): 1596–1600, doi: 10.1001/jama.280.18.1596; Ji-Eun Kim et al., "Does Glycine Max Leaves or *Garcinia cambogia* Promote Weight-Loss or Lower Plasma Cholesterol in Overweight Individuals: A Randomized Control Trial," *Nutrition Journal* 10, no. 1 (2011): 94, doi: 10.1186/1475-2891-10-94; Richard D. Mattes and Leslie Bormann, "Effects of (-)-Hydroxycitric Acid on Appetitive Variables," *Physiology and Behaviour* 71, no. 1–2 (2000): 87–94, doi: 10.1016/S0031-9384(00)00321-8.

315 *The same goes for the go-to supplement for boosting testosterone,* Tribulus terrestris*:* Shane Rogerson et al., "The Effect of Five Weeks of *Tribulus terrestris* Supplementation on Muscle Strength and Body Composition during Preseason Training in Elite Rugby League Players," *Journal of Strength and Conditioning Research* 21, no. 2 (2007): 348, doi: 10.1519/R-18395.1; Vladimir Neychev et al., "The Aphrodisiac Herb *Tribulus terrestris* Does Not Influence the Androgen Production in Young Men," *Journal of Ethnopharmacology* 101, no. 1–3 (2005): 319–23, doi: 10.1016/j.jep.2005.05.017; Christophe Saudan et al., "Short Term Impact of *Tribulus terrestris* Intake on Doping Control Analysis of Endogenous Steroids," *Forensic Science International* 178, no. 1 (2008): e7–e10, doi: 10.1016/j.forsciint.2008.01.003.

317 *they can cause adverse reactions in some people:* Jinhui Feng, Carl E. Cerniglia,

and Huizhong Chen, "Toxicological Significance of Azo Dye Metabolism by Human Intestinal Microbiota," *Frontiers in Bioscience* (Elite Edition) 4 (2012): 568–86, doi: 10.2741/400; Robin B. Kanarek, "Artificial Food Dyes and Attention Deficit Hyperactivity Disorder," *Nutrition Reviews* 69, no. 7 (2011): 385–91, doi: 10.1111/j.1753-4887.2011.00385.x; Joel T. Nigg et al., "Meta-Analysis of Attention-Deficit/Hyperactivity Disorder Symptoms, Restriction Diet, and Synthetic Food Color Additives," *Journal of the American Academy of Child and Adolescent Psychiatry* 51, no. 1 (2012): 86–97.e8, doi: 10.1016/j.jaac.2011.10.015; Donna McCann et al., "Food Additives and Hyperactive Behaviour in 3-Year-Old and 8/9-Year-Old Children in the Community: A Randomised, Double-Blinded, Placebo-Controlled Trial," *Lancet* 370, no. 9598 (2007): 1560–7, doi: 10.1016/S0140-6736(07)61306-3; Yonglin Gao et al., "Effect of Food Azo Dye Tartrazine on Learning and Memory Functions in Mice and Rats, and the Possible Mechanisms Involved," *Journal of Food Science* 76, no. 6 (2011): T125–9, doi: 10.1111/j.1750-3841.2011.02267.x.

318   *whey is digested and absorbed quickly and flush with the amino acid* leucine: Layne E. Norton et al., "Leucine Content of Dietary Proteins Is a Determinant of Postprandial Skeletal Muscle Protein Synthesis in Adult Rats," *Nutrition and Metabolism* 9, no. 1 (2012): 67, doi: 10.1186/1743-7075-9-67; Yves Boirie et al., "Slow and Fast Dietary Proteins Differently Modulate Postprandial Protein Accretion," *Proceedings of the National Academy of Sciences* 94, no. 26 (1997): 14930–35, doi: 10.1073/pnas.94.26.14930.

318   *it contains dietary fat and lactose:* Jay R. Hoffman and Michael J. Falvo, "Protein—Which Is Best?," *Journal of Sports Science and Medicine* 3, no. 3 (2004): 118–30, https://pmid.us/24482589.

318   *a high-quality whey concentrate works just fine:* Hoffman and Falvo, "Protein—Which Is Best?"; Paige E. Miller et al., "Effects of Whey Protein and Resistance

Exercise on Body Composition: A Meta-analysis of Randomized Controlled Trials," *Journal of the American College of Nutrition* 33, no. 2 (2014): 163–75, doi: 10.1080/07315724.2013.875365.

320 *casein digests slowly:* Yves Boirie et al., "Slow and Fast Dietary Proteins Differently Modulate Postprandial Protein Accretion," *Proceedings of the National Academy of Sciences* 94, no. 26 (1997): 14930–35, doi: 10.1073/pnas.94.26.14930.

321 *normal levels of soy and isoflavone intake don't alter male fertility or hormones:* Jorge E. Chavarro et al., "Soy Food and Isoflavone Intake in Relation to Semen Quality Parameters among Men from an Infertility Clinic," *Human Reproduction* 23, no. 11 (2008): 2584–90, doi: 10.1093/humrep/den243; Baohua Liu et al., "Equol-Producing Phenotype and in Relation to Serum Sex Hormones among Healthy Adults in Beijing," *Wei Sheng Yan Jiu* 40, no. 6 (2011): 727–31, https://pmid.us/22279666; Laura K. Beaton et al., "Soy Protein Isolates of Varying Isoflavone Content Do Not Adversely Affect Semen Quality in Healthy Young Men," *Fertility and Sterility* 94, no. 5 (2010): 1717–22, doi: 10.1016/j.fertnstert.2009.08.055.

321 *these effects can vary depending on the presence or absence of certain intestinal bacteria:* Cara L. Frankenfeld et al., "High Concordance of Daidzein-Metabolizing Phenotypes in Individuals Measured 1 to 3 Years Apart," *British Journal of Nutrition* 94, no. 6 (2005): 873–76, doi: 10.1079/bjn20051565.

321 *soy protein is a wonderful plant-based source of protein:* Johannes Huber et al., "Effects of Soy Protein and Isoflavones on Circulating Hormone Concentrations in Pre- and Post-menopausal Women: A Systematic Review and Meta-analysis," *Human Reproduction Update* 16, no. 1 (2010): 110–11, doi: 10.1093/humupd/dmp040; Meinan Chen et al., "Association between Soy Isoflavone Intake and Breast Cancer Risk For Pre- and Post-menopausal Women: A Meta-analysis of Epidemiological Studies," *PLoS One* 9, no. 2 (2014): e89288, doi: 10.1371/journal.pone.0089288.

321 *it's lacking in the essential amino acids most related to muscle growth:* J. E. Eastoe, "The Amino Acid Composition of Mammalian Collagen and Gelatin," *Biochemical Journal* 61, no. 4 (1955): 589–600, doi: 10.1042/bj0610589; Juha J. Hulmi et al., "Effect of Protein/Essential Amino Acids and Resistance Training on Skeletal Muscle Hypertrophy: A Case for Whey Protein," *Nutrition and Metabolism* 7, no. 51 (2010), doi: 10.1186/1743-7075-7-51.

321 *Collagen protein is low in sulfur:* Omer Kabil et al., "Sulfur as a Signaling Nutrient through Hydrogen Sulfide," *Annual Review of Nutrition* 34, (2014): 171–205, doi: 10.1146/annurev-nutr-071813-105654.

322 *protein in rice . . . has a high* biological value: Jordan M. Joy et al., "The Effects of 8 Weeks of Whey or Rice Protein Supplementation on Body Composition and Exercise Performance," *Nutrition Journal* 12, no. 1 (2013): 86, doi: 10.1186/1475-2891-12-86; V. W. Padhye and D. K. Salunkhe, "Extraction and Characterization of Rice Proteins," *Cereal Chemistry* 56, no. 5 (1979): 389–93; Douglas Kalman, "Amino Acid Composition of an Organic Brown Rice Protein Concentrate and Isolate Compared to Soy and Whey Concentrates and Isolates," *Foods* 3, no. 3 (2014): 394–402, doi: 10.3390/foods3030394.

322 *pea protein also has a high biological value:* François Mariotti et al., "The Influence of the Albumin Fraction on the Bioavailability and Postprandial Utilization of Pea Protein Given Selectively to Humans," *Journal of Nutrition* 131, no. 6 (2001): 1706–13, doi: 10.1093/jn/131.6.1706; Nicolas Babault et al., "Pea Proteins Oral Supplementation Promotes Muscle Thickness Gains during Resistance Training: A Double-Blind, Randomized, Placebo-Controlled Clinical Trial vs. Whey Protein," *Journal of the International Society of Sports Nutrition* 12, no. 1 (2015): 3, doi: 10.1186/s12970-014-0064-5.

323 *hemp protein isn't absorbed as well as soy, rice, or pea protein:* James D. House, "Evaluating the Quality of Protein from Hemp Seed (Cannabis sativa L.) Products through the Use of the Protein Digestibility-Corrected Amino Acid Score

Method," *Journal of Agricultural Food Chemistry* 58, no. 22 (2010): 11801–07, doi: 10.1021/jf102636b; Xian-Sheng Wang et al., "Characterization, Amino Acid Composition and *In Vitro* Digestibility of Hemp (*Cannabis sativa* L.) Proteins," *Food Chemistry* 107, no. 1 (2008): 11–18, doi: 10.1016/j.food chem.2007.06.064.

324   *According to research conducted by scientists at Colorado State University:* Loren Cordain et al., "Origins and Evolution of the Western Diet: Health Implications for the 21st Century," *American Journal of Clinical Nutrition* 81, no. 2 (2005): 341–54, doi: 10.1093/ajcn.81.2.341.

324   *A more recent study conducted by scientists at Tufts University:* Jeffrey B. Blumberg et al., "Impact of Frequency of Multi-Vitamin/Multi-Mineral Supplement Intake on Nutritional Adequacy and Nutrient Deficiencies in US Adults," *Nutrients* 9, no. 8 (2017): 849, doi: 10.3390/nu9080849.

324   *average vitamin K and D intake levels may be suboptimal:* Gerry Kurt Schwalfenberg, "Vitamins K1 and K2: The Emerging Group of Vitamins Required for Human Health," *Journal of Nutrition and Metabolism* 2017 (2017): 6254836, doi: 10.1155/2017/6254836; Matthias Wacker and Michael F. Holick, "Vitamin D—Effects on Skeletal and Extraskeletal Health and the Need for Supplementation," *Nutrients* 5, no. 1 (2013): 111–48, doi: 10.3390/nu5010111.

325   *Many contain large amounts of vitamins and minerals most people don't need to supplement:* Marie-Cécile Nollevaux et al., "Hypervitaminosis A-induced Liver Fibrosis: Stellate Cell Activation and Daily Dose Consumption," *Liver International* 26, no. 2 (2006): 182–86, doi: 10.1111/j.1478-3231.2005.01207.x; Edgar R. Miller 3rd et al., "Meta-analysis: High-Dosage Vitamin E Supplementation May Increase All-Cause Mortality," *Annals of International Medicine* 142, no. 1 (2005): 37–46, doi: 10.7326/0003-4819-142-1-200501040-00110.

325   *several synthetic vitamins outperform natural ones:* Maret G. Traber et al., "Syn-

thetic as Compared with Natural Vitamin E Is Preferentially Excreted as Alpha-CEHC in Human Urine: Studies Using Deuterated Alpha-Tocopheryl Acetates," *FEBS Letters* 437, no. 1–2 (1998): 145–48, doi: 10.1016/s0014-5793(98)01210-1; Francesco Scaglione and Giscardo Panzavolta, "Folate, Folic Acid and 5-methyltetrahydrofolate Are Not the Same Thing," *Xenobiotica* 44, no. 5 (2014): 480–88, doi: 10.3109/00498254.2013.845705.

327 *many people have a genetic mutation that hinders the production of 5-MTHF:* "MTHFR Gene Variant," *Genetic and Rare Diseases Information Center (GARD)* website, last updated January 25, 2018, https://rarediseases.info.nih.gov/diseases/10953/mthfr-gene-mutation.

328 *it plays a vital role in many physiological processes:* Michael Holick, "Vitamin D Is Essential to the Modern Indoor Lifestyle," *Science News* website, October 8, 2010, https://www.sciencenews.org/article/vitamin-d-essential-modern-indoor-lifestyle; Michael Holick, "Vitamin D: Evolutionary, Physiological and Health Perspectives," *Current Drug Targets* 12, no. 1 (2011): 4–18, doi: 10.2174/138945011793591635; Matthias Wacker and Michael F. Holick, "Vitamin D—Effects on Skeletal and Extraskeletal Health and the Need for Supplementation," *Nutrients* 5, no. 1 (2013): 111–48, doi: 10.3390/nu5010111.

328 *insufficient vitamin D intake is associated with an increased risk of many types of disease:* Bess Dawson-Hughes et al., "IOF Position Statement: Vitamin D Recommendations for Older Adults," *Osteoporosis International* 21, no. 7 (2010): 1151–54, doi: 10.1007/s00198-010-1285-3; Thomas J. Wang et al., "Vitamin D Deficiency and Risk of Cardiovascular Disease," *Circulation* 117, no. 4 (2008): 503–11, doi: 10.1161/circulationaha.107.706127; Stefan Pilz et al., "Low Vitamin D Levels Predict Stroke in Patients Referred to Coronary Angiography," *Stroke* 39, no. 9 (2008): 2611–13, doi: 10.1161/strokeaha.107.513655;

Edward Giovannucci, "Epidemiological Evidence for Vitamin D and Colorectal Cancer," *Journal of Bone and Mineral Research* 22, no. S2 (2007): V81–V85, doi: 10.1359/jbmr.07s206; Elina Hyppönen et al., "Intake of Vitamin D and Risk of Type 1 Diabetes: A Birth-Cohort Study," *Lancet* 358, no. 9292 (2001): 1500–03, doi: 10.1016/S0140-6736(01)06580-1; Kassandra L. Munger et al., "Serum 25-Hydroxyvitamin D Levels and Risk of Multiple Sclerosis," *JAMA* 296, no. 23 (2006): 2832 doi: 10.1001/jama.296.23.2832; Kelechi Ebere Nnoaham and Aileen Clarke, "Low Serum Vitamin D Levels and Tuberculosis: A Systematic Review and Meta-analysis," *International Journal of Epidemiology* 37, no. 1 (2008): 113–19, doi: 10.1093/ije/dym247; John J. Cannell et al., "Epidemic Influenza and Vitamin D," *Epidemiology and Infection* 134, no. 6 (2006): 1129, doi: 10.1017/S0950268806007175.

328   *many age-related diseases . . . are associated with low levels of vitamin D:* Lynette M. Smith and Christopher J. Gallagher, "Dietary Vitamin D Intake for the Elderly Population: Update on the Recommended Dietary Allowance for Vitamin D," *Endocrinology and Metabolism Clinics of North America* 46, no. 4 (2017): 871–84, doi: 10.1016/j.ecl.2017.07.003.

329   *According to a committee of the Endocrine Society:* Michael F. Holick et al., "Evaluation, Treatment, and Prevention of Vitamin D Deficiency: An Endocrine Society Clinical Practice Guideline," *Journal of Clinical Endocrinology and Metabolism* 96, no. 7 (2011): 1911–30, doi: 10.1210/jc.2011-0385.

329   *the average person's diet provides just one-tenth of the EPA and DHA needed:* Penny M. Kris-Etherton et al., "Polyunsaturated Fatty Acids in the Food Chain in the United States," *American Journal of Clinical Nutrition* 71, no. 1 (2000): 179S–188S, doi: 10.1093/ajcn/71.1.179S; Danielle Swanson et al., "Omega-3 Fatty Acids EPA and DHA: Health Benefits throughout Life," *Advances in Nutrition* 12, no. 3 (2012): 1–7, doi: 10.3945/an.111.000893; André Nkondjock and Parviz Ghadirian, "Intake of Specific Carotenoids and Essential Fatty Acids

and Breast Cancer Risk in Montreal, Canada," *American Journal of Clinical Nutrition* 79, no. 5 (2004): 857–64, doi: 10.1093/ajcn/79.5.857.

329 *Faster fat loss:* Charles Couet et al., "Effect of Dietary Fish Oil on Body Fat Mass and Basal Fat Oxidation in Healthy Adults," *International Journal of Obesity and Related Metabolic Disorders* 21, no. 8 (1997): 637–43, doi: 10.1038/sj.ijo.0800451.

329 *Less fat gain:* Jonathan D. Buckley and Peter R. C. Howe, "Anti-obesity Effects of Long-Chain Omega-3 Polyunsaturated Fatty Acids," *Obesity Reviews* 10, no. 6 (2009): 648–59, doi: 10.1111/j.1467-789X.2009.00584.x.

329 *More muscle growth:* Gordon I. Smith et al., "Omega-3 Polyunsaturated Fatty Acids Augment the Muscle Protein Anabolic Response to Hyperinsulinaemia–Hyperaminoacidaemia in Healthy Young and Middle-Aged Men and Women," *Clinical Science* 121, no. 6 (2011): 267–78, doi: 10.1042/CS20100597.

329 *Improved mood:* Gordon Parker et al., "Omega-3 Fatty Acids and Mood Disorders," *American Journal of Psychiatry* 163, no. 6 (2006): 969–78, doi: 10.1176/ajp.2006.163.6.969; Alan C. Logan, "Omega-3 Fatty Acids and Major Depression: A Primer for the Mental Health Professional," *Lipids in Health and Disease* 3, (2004): 25, doi: 10.1186/1476-511X-3-25; Janice Kiecolt-Glaser et al., "Omega-3 Supplementation Lowers Inflammation and Anxiety in Medical Students: A Randomized Controlled Trial," *Brain Behaviour and Immunity* 25, no. 8 (2011): 1725–34, doi: 10.1016/j.bbi.2011.07.229.

329 *Better cognitive performance:* S. Kalmijn et al., "Dietary Intake of Fatty Acids and Fish in Relation to Cognitive Performance at Middle Age," *Neurology* 62, no. 2 (2004): 275–80, doi: 10.1212/01.WNL.0000103860.75218.A5.

330 *Enhanced immunity:* Alessio Molfino et al., "The Role for Dietary Omega-3 Fatty Acids Supplementation in Older Adults," *Nutrients* 6, no. 10 (2014): 4058–73, doi: 10.3390/nu6104058.

330 *Reduced muscle and joint soreness:* Robert J. Goldberg and Joel Katz, "A Meta-

analysis of the Analgesic Effects of Omega-3 Polyunsaturated Fatty Acid Supplementation for Inflammatory Joint Pain," *Pain* 129, no. 1–2 (2007): 210–23, doi: 10.1016/j.pain.2007.01.020.

330   *omega-3 levels are much lower in meat and eggs than in fish:* Eric Ponnampalam et al., "Effect of Feeding Systems on Omega-3 Fatty Acids, Conjugated Linoleic Acid and Trans Fatty Acids in Australian Beef Cuts: Potential Impact on Human Health," *Asia Pacific Journal of Clinical Nutrition* 15, no. 1 (2006): 21–29, https://pmid.us/16500874.

330   *this conversion process is inefficient:* Hermant Poudyal et al., "Omega-3 Fatty Acids and Metabolic Syndrome: Effects and Emerging Mechanisms of Action," *Progress in Lipid Research* 50, no. 4 (2011): 372–87, doi: 10.1016/j.plipres.2011.06.003.

330   *vegans often have omega-3 fatty acid deficiencies:* Magdalena Rosell et al., "Long-Chain n–3 Polyunsaturated Fatty Acids in Plasma in British Meat-Eating, Vegetarian, and Vegan Men," *American Journal of Clinical Nutrition* 82, no. 2 (2005): 327–33, doi: 10.1093/ajcn.82.2.327.

331   *re-esterified triglyceride fish oil is better absorbed by the body:* Jørn Dyerberg et al., "Bioavailability of Marine n-3 Fatty Acid Formulations," *Prostaglandins Leukotrienes and Essential Fatty Acids* 83, no. 3 (2010): 137–41, doi: 10.1016/j.plefa.2010.06.007.

331   *ethyl ester oil oxidizes (goes bad) more easily:* H. Lee et al., "Analysis of Headspace Volatile and Oxidized Volatile Compounds in DHA-Enriched Fish Oil on Accelerated Oxidative Storage," *Journal of Food Science* 68, no. 7 (2003): 2169–77, doi: 10.1111/j.1365-2621.2003.tb05742.x.

331   *a combined intake of 500 milligrams to 1.8 grams of EPA and DHA per day is adequate:* Penny M. Kris-Etherton et al., "Fish Consumption, Fish Oil, Omega-3 Fatty Acids, and Cardiovascular Disease," *Circulation* 106, no. 21 (2002): 2747–57, doi: 10.1161/01.cir.0000038493.65177.94; Gordon Smith et al., "Omega-3

Polyunsaturated Fatty Acids Augment the Muscle Protein Anabolic Response to Hyperinsulinaemia–Hyperaminoacidaemia in Healthy Young and Middle-Aged Men and Women," *Clinical Science* 121, no. 6 (2011): 267–78, doi: 10.1042 /CS20100597.

332 *More muscle growth:* John David Branch, "Effect of Creatine Supplementation on Body Composition and Performance: A Meta-analysis," *International Journal of Sport Nutrition and Exercise Metabolism* 13, no. 2 (2003): 198–226, doi: 10.1123/ijsnem.13.2.198.

332 *Faster strength gain:* Jeff S. Volek et al., "The Effects of Creatine Supplementation on Muscular Performance and Body Composition Responses to Short-Term Resistance Training Overreaching," *European Journal of Applied Physiology* 91, no. 5–6 (2004): 628–37, doi: 10.1007/s00421-003-1031-z.

332 *Greater anaerobic endurance:* Joan Eckerson et al., "Effect of Creatine Phosphate Supplementation on Anaerobic Working Capacity and Body Weight after Two and Six Days of Loading in Men and Women," *Journal of Strength and Conditioning Research* 19, no. 4 (2005): 756, doi: 10.1519/R-16924.1.

332 *Better post-workout recovery:* Reinaldo Abunasser Bassit et al., "Effect of Short-Term Creatine Supplementation on Markers of Skeletal Muscle Damage after Strenuous Contractile Activity," *European Journal of Applied Physiology* 108, no. 5 (2010): 945–55, doi: 10.1007/s00421-009-1305-1.

332 *Creatine does all these things safely:* Geert Jan Groeneveld et al., "Few Adverse Effects of Long-Term Creatine Supplementation in a Placebo-Controlled Trial," *International Journal of Sports Medicine* 26, no. 4 (2005): 307–13, doi: 10.1055/s-2004-817917.

332 *you have nothing to fear from creatine:* Kurt A. Pline and Curtis L. Smith, "The Effect of Creatine Intake on Renal Function," *Annals of Pharmacotherapy* 39, no. 6 (2005): 1093–96, doi: 10.1345/aph.1E628.

333 *high creatinine levels are normal:* Giuseppe Banfi and Massimo Del Fabbro,

"Serum Creatinine Values in Elite Athletes Competing in 8 Different Sports: Comparison with Sedentary People," *Clinical Chemistry* 52, no. 2 (2006): 330–31, doi: 10.1373/clinchem.2005.061390.

333 *Five grams of creatine monohydrate once per day is optimal:* Michael G. Bemben and Hugh S. Lamont, "Creatine Supplementation and Exercise Performance: Recent Findings," *Sports Medicine* 35, no. 2 (2005): 107–25, doi: 10.2165/00007256-200535020-00002.

333 *you can "load" it by taking 20 grams per day:* Bemben and Lamont, "Creatine Supplementation."

333 *taking it post-workout may be optimal:* Scott C. Forbes and Darren G. Candow, "Timing of Creatine Supplementation and Resistance Training: A Brief Review," *Journal of Exercise and Nutrition* 1, no. 5 (2018): 1, https://www .researchgate.net/scientific-contributions/FM-Ivey-2036138657.

334 *denatured collagen has no beneficial effects on joint inflammation:* Cathryn Nagler-Anderson et al., "Suppression of Type II Collagen-Induced Arthritis by Intragastric Administration of Soluble Type II Collagen," *Proceedings of the National Academy of Sciences* 83, no. 19 (1986): 7443–46, doi: 10.1073 /pnas.83.19.7443.

334 *it's effective for regulating the immune response that inflames joints:* James P. Lugo et al., "Undenatured Type II Collagen (UC-II®) for Joint Support: A Randomized, Double-Blind, Placebo-Controlled Study in Healthy Volunteers," *Journal of the International Society of Sports Nutrition.* 10, no. 1 (2013): 48, doi: 10.1186/1550-2783-10-48.

334 *These effects have been found both in people with arthritic conditions and in those with healthy joints:* U. Gimsa et al., "Type II Collagen Serology: A Guide to Clinical Responsiveness to Oral Tolerance?," *Rheumatology International* 16, no. 6 (1997): 237–40, doi: 10.1007/BF01375655.

335 *Ten to 40 milligrams of undenatured type-II collagen per day is effective:* Martha L. Barnett et al., "Treatment of Rheumatoid Arthritis with Oral Type II Collagen: Results of a Multicenter, Double-Blind, Placebo-Controlled Trial," *Arthritis Rheumatology* 41, no. 2 (1998): 290–97, doi: 10.1002/1529-0131(199802)41:2<290::AID-ART13>3.0.CO;2-R; David C. Crowley et al., "Safety and Efficacy of Undenatured Type II Collagen in the Treatment of Osteoarthritis of the Knee: A Clinical Trial," *International Journal of Medical Sciences* 6, no. 6 (2009): 312–21, doi: 10.7150/ijms.6.312.

335 *Frankincense contains molecules called* boswellic acids*:* Eckart-Roderich Sailer et al., "Acetyl-11-Keto-Beta-Boswellic Acid (AKBA): Structure Requirements for Binding and 5-Lipoxygenase Inhibitory Activity," *British Journal of Pharmacology* 117, no. 4 (1996): 615–18, doi: 10.1111/j.1476-5381.1996.tb15235.x.

335 *boswellia reduces joint inflammation and pain:* Nitin Kimmatkar et al., "Efficacy and Tolerability of *Boswellia serrata* Extract in Treatment of Osteoarthritis of Knee: A Randomized Double Blind Placebo Controlled Trial," *Phytomedicine* 10, no. 1 (2003): 3–7, doi: 10.1078/094471103321648593; H. P. Ammon, "Boswellic Acids in Chronic Inflammatory Diseases," *Planta Medica* 72, no. 12 (2006): 1100–16, doi: 10.1055/s-2006-947227.

336 *the roster of health benefits associated with curcumin is impressive and growing:* Bharat B Aggarwal et al., "Curcumin: The Indian Solid Gold," *Advances in Experimental Medicine and Biology* 595 (2007): 1–75, doi: 10.1007/978-0-387-46401-5_1.

336 *Curcumin also produces healthier, less painful joints:* Sita Aggarwal et al., "Curcumin (Diferuloylmethane) Down-Regulates Expression of Cell Proliferation and Antiapoptotic and Metastatic Gene Products through Suppression of IkappaBalpha Kinase and Akt Activation," *Molecular Pharmacology* 69, no. 1 (2006): 195–206, doi: 10.1124/mol.105.017400.

336 *it's poorly absorbed in the intestines:* Preetha Anand et al., "Bioavailability of Curcumin: Problems and Promises," *Molecular Pharmaceutics* 4, no. 6 (2007): 807–18, doi: 10.1021/mp700113r.

336 *you must take a patented form of curcumin:* Giuseppe Garcea et al., "Consumption of the Putative Chemopreventive Agent Curcumin by Cancer Patients: Assessment of Curcumin Levels in the Colorectum and Their Pharmacodynamic Consequences," *Cancer Epidemiology Biomarkers and Prevention* 14, no. 1 (2005): 120–25, https://pmid.us/15668484.

337 *DHEA increases testosterone production in older men and estrogen production in older women:* Te-Chih Liu et al., "Effect of Acute DHEA Administration on Free Testosterone in Middle-Aged and Young Men Following High-Intensity Interval Training," *European Journal of Applied Physiology* 113, no. 7 (2013): 1783–92, doi: 10.1007/s00421-013-2607-x; Anne Kenny et al., "Dehydroepiandrosterone Combined with Exercise Improves Muscle Strength and Physical Function in Frail Older Women," *Journal of the American Geriatrics Society* 58, no. 9 (2010): 1707–14, doi: 10.1111/j.1532-5415.2010.03019.x.

338 *The major benefit of rhodiola is a reduction in fatigue:* Vahagn Darbinyan et al., "*Rhodiola rosea* in Stress Induced Fatigue: A Double Blind Cross-Over Study of a Standardized Extract SHR-5 with a Repeated Low-Dose Regimen on the Mental Performance of Healthy Physicians during Night Duty," *Phytomedicine* 7, no. 5 (2000): 365–71, doi: 10.1016/S0944-7113(00)80055-0.

338 *it can enhance, or at least preserve, cognition and mood:* Yevgeniya Lekomtseva et al., "*Rhodiola rosea* in Subjects with Prolonged or Chronic Fatigue Symptoms: Results of an Open-Label Clinical Trial," *Research in Complementary Medicine* 24, no. 1 (2017): 46–52, doi: 10.1159/000457918; Erik M. G. Olsson et al., "A Randomised, Double-Blind, Placebo-Controlled, Parallel-Group Study of the Standardised Extract SHR-5 of the Roots of *Rhodiola rosea* in the

Treatment of Subjects with Stress-Related Fatigue," *Planta Medica* 75, no. 2 (2009): 105–12, doi: 10.1055/s-0028-1088346; Mark Cropley, "The Effects of *Rhodiola rosea* L. Extract on Anxiety, Stress, Cognition, and Other Mood Symptoms," *Phytotherapy Research* 29, no. 12 (2015): 1934–39, doi: 10.1002/ptr.5486.

339 *Increasing power and strength*: Sachin Wankhede et al., "Examining the effect of *Withania somnifera* Supplementation on Muscle Strength and Recovery: A Randomized Controlled Trial," *Journal of the International Society of Sports Nutrition* 12, no. 1 (2015): 43, doi: 10.1186/s12970-015-0104-9.

339 *Reducing chronic and acute cortisol increases from stress*: Beenish Khan et al., "Augmentation and Proliferation of T Lymphocytes and Th-1 Cytokines by *Withania somnifera* in Stressed Mice," *International Immunopharmacology* 6, no. 9 (2006): 1394–1403, doi: 10.1016/j.intimp.2006.04.001; Biswajit Auddy et al., "A Standardized *Withania somnifera* Extract Significantly Reduces Stress-Related Parameters in Chronically Stressed Humans: A Double-Blind, Randomized, Placebo-Controlled Study," *Journal of the American Nutraceutical Association* 11 (2008): 50–6, https://www.researchgate.net/publication/242151370_A_Standardized_Withania_Somnifera_Extract_Significantly_Reduces_Stress-Related_Parameters_in_Chronically_Stressed_Humans_A_Double-Blind_Randomized_Placebo-Controlled_Study.

339 *Lowering feelings of stress and anxiety:* Chittaranjan Andrade et al., "A Double-Blind, Placebo-Controlled Evaluation of the Anxiolytic Efficacy of an Ethanolic Extract of *Withania somnifera*," *Indian Journal of Psychiatry* 42, no. 3 (2000): 295–301, https://pmid.us/21407960; Kieran Cooley et al., "Naturopathic Care for Anxiety: A Randomized Controlled Trial ISRCTN78958974," *PLoS One* 4, no. 8 (2009): e6628, doi: 10.1371/journal.pone.0006628; Auddy et al., "A Standardized *Withania somnifera* Extract."

339   *Restoring fertility in men:* Vijay Ambiye et al., "Clinical Evaluation of the Sper-matogenic Activity of the Root Extract of Ashwagandha (*Withania somnifera*) in Oligospermic Males: A Pilot Study," *Evidence-Based Complementary and Alternative Medicine* 2013, no. 4 (2013): 571420, doi: 10.1155/2013/571420.

339   *Improving immune function:* Jeremy Mikolai et al., "In vivo Effects of Ashwa-gandha (*Withania somnifera*) Extract on the Activation of Lymphocytes," *Journal of Alternative and Complementary Medicine* 15, no. 4 (2009): 423–30, doi: 10.1089/acm.2008.0215.

339   *Increasing cardiovascular endurance:* Shweta Shenoy et al., "Effects of Eight-Week Supplementation of Ashwagandha on Cardiorespiratory Endurance in Elite Indian Cyclists," *Journal of Ayurveda and Integrative Medicine* 3, no. 4 (2012): 209–14, doi: 10.4103/0975-9476.104444.

339   *Protecting against pigments that accumulate during Alzheimer's disease:* Neha Sehgal et al., "*Withania somnifera* Reverses Alzheimer's Disease Pathology by Enhancing Low-Density Lipoprotein Receptor-Related Protein in Liver," *Proceedings of the National Academy of Sciences* 109, no. 9 (2012): 3510–15, doi: 10.1073/pnas.1112209109; Kesavarao V. Kurapati et al., "Ashwagandha (*Withania somnifera*) Reverses ß-Amyloid$_{1-42}$ Induced Toxicity in Human Neuronal Cells: Implications in HIV-Associated Neurocognitive Disorders (HAND)," *PLoS One* 8, no. 10 (2013): e77624, doi: 10.1371/journal.pone.0077624.

340   *its primary benefits are improved libido and sexual function in men and women and enhanced mood:* Nicole A. Brooks et al., "Beneficial Effects of *Lepidium meyenii* (Maca) on Psychological Symptoms and Measures of Sexual Dys-function in Postmenopausal Women Are Not Related to Estrogen or An-drogen Content," *Menopause* 15, no. 6 (2008): 1157–62, doi: 10.1097/gme.0b013e3181732953; Teo Zenico et al., "Subjective Effects of *Lepidium meyenii* (Maca) Extract on Well-Being and Sexual Performances in Patients

with Mild Erectile Dysfunction: A Randomised, Double-Blind Clinical Trial," *Andrologia* 41, no. 2 (2009): 95–99, doi: 10.1111/j.1439-0272.2008.00892.x; Lily Stojanovska et al., "Maca Reduces Blood Pressure and Depression, in a Pilot Study in Postmenopausal Women," *Climacteric* 18, no. 1 (2015): 69–78, doi: 10.3109/13697137.2014.929649.

Chapter 16: Frequently Asked Questions

349 *moderate- and high-intensity strength training . . . rarely aggravates arthritis symptoms:* Nancy Latham and Chiung-Ju Liu, "Strength Training in Older Adults: The Benefits for Osteoarthritis," *Clinics in Geriatric Medicine* 26, no. 3 (2010): 445–59, doi: 10.1016/j.cger.2010.03.006; Arja Häkkinen, "Effectiveness and Safety of Strength Training in Rheumatoid Arthritis," *Current Opinion in Rheumatology* 16, no. 2 (2004): 132–37, doi: 10.1097/00002281 -200403000-00011; Zuzana de Jong et al., "Long Term High Intensity Exercise and Damage of Small Joints in Rheumatoid Arthritis," *Annals of the Rheumatic Diseases* 63, no. 11 (2004): 1399–1405, doi: 10.1136 /ard.2003.015826; Miriam E. Nelson et al., "Effects of High-Intensity Strength Training on Multiple Risk Factors for Osteoporotic Fractures: A Randomized Controlled Trial," *JAMA* 272, no. 24 (1994): 1909–14, doi: 10.1001 /jama.1994.03520240037038.

350 *it can substantially decrease blood pressure:* Véronique A. Cornelissen, "Effect of Resistance Training on Resting Blood Pressure: A Meta-analysis of Randomized Controlled Trials," *Journal of Hypertension* 23, no. 2 (2005): 251–59, doi: 10.1097/00004872-200502000-00003; George Kelley and Kristi S. Kelley, "Progressive Resistance Exercise and Resting Blood Pressure: A Meta-analysis of Randomized Controlled Trials," *Hypertension* 35, no. 3 (2000): 838–43, doi: 10.1161/01.HYP.35.3.838; Véronique A. Cornelissen and Neil A. Smart, "Exercise Training for Blood Pressure: A Systematic Review and Meta-analysis,"

Journal of the American Heart Association 2, no. 1 (2013): e004473, doi: 10.1161/JAHA.112.004473.

350 *your cardiovascular system may not be up to intense exercise yet:* Alexandra S. Ghadieh and Basem Saab, "Evidence for Exercise Training in the Management of Hypertension in Adults," *Canadian Family Physician* 61, no. 3 (2015): 233–39, https://pmid.us/25927108.

354 *it takes at least three to four weeks of no training:* Paul S. Hwang et al., "Resistance Training–Induced Elevations in Muscular Strength in Trained Men Are Maintained after 2 Weeks of Detraining and Not Differentially Affected by Whey Protein Supplementation," *Journal of Strength and Conditioning Research* 31, no. 4 (2017): 869–81, doi: 10.1519/JSC.0000000000001807.

354 *strength training appears to permanently alter the physiology of muscle cells:* Behzad Bazgir et al., "Satellite Cells Contribution to Exercise Mediated Muscle Hypertrophy and Repair," *Cell Journal* 18, no. 4 (2017): 473–84, doi: 10.22074/cellj.2016.4714.

355 *increasing water intake (especially when added to meals):* Elizabeth A. Dennis et al., "Water Consumption Increases Weight Loss During a Hypocaloric Diet Intervention in Middle-Aged and Older Adults," *Obesity* 18, no. 2 (2010): 300–7, doi: 10.1038/oby.2009.235; Raimo Lappalainen et al., "Drinking Water with a Meal: A Simple Method of Coping with Feelings of Hunger, Satiety and Desire to Eat," *European Journal of Clinical Nutrition* 47, no. 11 (1993): 815–19, https://pmid.us/8287852.

355 *the National Academy of Medicine recommends a baseline intake of about ¾ of a gallon of water per day:* American College of Sports Medicine et al., "American College of Sports Medicine Position Stand: Exercise and Fluid Replacement," *Medicine and Science in Sports and Exercise* 39, no. 2 (2007): 377–90, doi: 10.1249/mss.0b013e31802ca597.

355 *A study conducted by scientists at the European Center for Taste Sciences:* Lau-

rent Brondel, et al., "Acute Partial Sleep Deprivation Increases Food Intake in Healthy Men," *American Journal of Clinical Nutrition* 91, no. 6 (2010): 1550–59, doi: 10.3945/ajcn.2009.28523.

355 *just a single night of sleep deprivation increases brain activity associated with hunger:* Christian Benedict et al., "Acute Sleep Deprivation Enhances the Brain's Response to Hedonic Food Stimuli: An fMRI Study," *Journal of Clinical Endocrinology and Metabolism* 97, no. 3 (Mar 2012): E443–47, doi: 10.1210/jc.2011-2759.

356 *adults need seven to nine hours of sleep per night:* "How Much Sleep Do We Really Need?," National Sleep Foundation website, accessed August 26, 2018, https://sleepfoundation.org/how-sleep-works/how-much-sleep-do-we-really-need.

356 *Mindful eating involves paying attention to your meal while you're eating:* Gayle M. Timmerman and Adama Brown, "The Effect of a Mindful Restaurant Eating Intervention on Weight Management in Women," *Journal of Nutrition Education and Behavior* 44, no. 1 (2012): 22–28, doi: 10.1016/j.jneb.2011.03.143.

357 *muscle damage may contribute to growth, but it isn't a requirement:* Brad J. Schoenfeld, "The Mechanisms of Muscle Hypertrophy and Their Application to Resistance Training," *Journal of Strength and Conditioning Research* 24, no. 10 (2010): 2857–72, doi: 10.1519/JSC.0b013e3181e840f3.

357 *Workouts that produce large amounts of muscle soreness can generate little growth:* Kyle L. Flann, "Muscle Damage and Muscle Remodeling: No Pain, No Gain?," *Journal of Experimental Biology* 15, no. 214 (Feb 2011): 674–79, doi: 10.1242/jeb.050112; Kyung-Shin Park and Man-Gyoon Lee, "Effects of Unaccustomed Downhill Running on Muscle Damage, Oxidative Stress, and Leukocyte Apoptosis," *Journal of Exercise Nutrition and Biochemistry* 19, no. 2 (2015): 55–63, doi: 10.5717/jenb.2015.15050702; Jason P. Brandenburg and David Docherty, "The Effects of Accentuated Eccentric Loading on Strength, Mus-

cle Hypertrophy, and Neural Adaptations in Trained Individuals," *Journal of Strength and Conditioning Research* 16, no. 1 (2002): 25–32, https://pmid .us/11834103; Simon Walker et al., "Greater Strength Gains after Training with Accentuated Eccentric than Traditional Isoinertial Loads in Already Strength-Trained Men," *Frontiers in Physiology* 27, no. 7 (Apr 2016): 149, doi: 10.3389 /fphys.2016.00149.

357 *isn't a reliable indicator of the degree of muscle damage:* Kazunori Nosaka, Mike Newton, and Paul Sacco, "Delayed-Onset Muscle Soreness Does Not Reflect the Magnitude of Eccentric Exercise-Induced Muscle Damage," *Scandinavian Journal of Medicine and Science in Sports* 12, no. 6 (Dec 2002): 337–46, doi: 10.1034/j.1600-0838.2002.10178.x.

357 *stems from the connective tissue holding muscle fibers together:* R. M. Crameri et al., "Myofibre Damage in Human Skeletal Muscle: Effects of Electrical Stimulation versus Voluntary Contraction," *Journal of Physiology* 15, no. 583 (Aug 2007): 365–80, doi: 10.1113/jphysiol.2007.128827.

357 *Training sore muscles doesn't necessarily hinder recovery and prevent muscle growth:* Trevor C. Chen and Kazunori Nosaka, "Responses of Elbow Flexors to Two Strenuous Eccentric Exercise Bouts Separated by Three Days," *Journal of Strength and Conditioning Research* 20, no. 1 (2006):108, doi: 10.1519/R-16634.1.

360 *your normal workouts will only make things worse by depressing immune function:* Nicolette C. Bishop and Michael Gleeson, "Acute and Chronic Effects of Exercise on Markers of Mucosal Immunity," *Frontiers in Bioscience (Landmark Edition)* 14, (2009): 4444–56, doi: 10.2741/3540.

360 *light exercise . . . while infected with the influenza virus can boost immunity and recovery:* E. A. Murphy et al., "Exercise Stress Increases Susceptibility to Influenza Infection," *Brain, Behavior, and Immunity* 22, no. 8 (2008):1152–55, doi: 10.1016/j.bbi.2008.06.004.

360 *Similar effects have been seen in human studies:* Stephen A. Martin, Brandt D.

Pence, and Jeffrey A. Woods, "Exercise and Respiratory Tract Viral Infections," *Exercise and Sport Sciences Reviews* 37, no. 4 (Oct 2009): 157–64, doi: 10.1097/JES.0b013e3181b7b57b; T. G. Weidner et al., "The Effect of Exercise Training on the Severity and Duration of a Viral Upper Respiratory Illness," *Medicine and Science in Sports and Exercise* 30, no. 11 (November 1998): 1578–83, doi: 10.1097/00005768-199811000-00004.

Index

Whole foods, 78–80

Willpower, 54

Women

  advanced strength training routines, 269, 384–85

  beginner strength training routines, 267, 381–82

  intermediate strength training routines, 268, 382–83

  and musclehead myth, 182–83

  strength standards, 266

  strength training routines, 265

Workout gloves, 298

Wristwatch, 298

Z

Zinc, 78–79

About the Author

Mike Matthews is a certified personal trainer; the #1 bestselling fitness author in the world, with over 1.5 million books sold; and the founder of the #1 brand of all-natural sports supplements, Legion.

His simple and science-based approach to building muscle, losing fat, and getting healthy has helped tens of thousands of people build their best body ever, and his work has been featured in many popular outlets, including *Esquire*, *Men's Health*, *Elle*, *Women's Health*, *Muscle & Strength*, and more, as well as on Fox and ABC.